Medical Radiology

Diagnostic Imaging

For further volumes:
http://www.springer.com/series/4354

Emanuele Neri • Lorenzo Faggioni • Carlo Bartolozzi
Editors

CT Colonography Atlas

For the Practicing Radiologist

Foreword by
Maximilian F. Reiser

Springer

Editors
Emanuele Neri
Department of Diagnostic and Interventional Radiology
University of Pisa
Pisa
Italy

Carlo Bartolozzi
Department of Diagnostic and Interventional Radiology
University of Pisa
Pisa
Italy

Lorenzo Faggioni
Department of Diagnostic and Interventional Radiology
University of Pisa
Pisa
Italy

ISBN 978-3-642-11148-8 ISBN 978-3-642-11149-5 (eBook)
DOI 10.1007/978-3-642-11149-5
Springer Heidelberg New York Dordrecht London

Library of Congress Control Number: 2013941367

Printed on acid-free paper

Springer is part of Springer Science+Business Media (www.springer.com)

Foreword

Since the first introduction of CT Colonography, the technique and the clinical applications have matured in a very impressive manner. A large number of studies have shown that both sensitivity and specificity of the method are comparable with optical colonoscopy. Radiation exposure is definitely a major issue when using computed tomography for screening; however, by means of sophisticated CT technology including online dose modulation and iterative reconstruction of image data, CT Colonograpy has become a true "ultra low dose" application.

Patients' and screenies' compliance and acceptance were also investigated and CT Colonography proved to be well accepted. Since health care systems worldwide are under major financial pressure, cost-effectiveness studies have been performed, which demonstrate that CT Colonography is a cost-effective technique for the early detection of polyps prone to undergo malignant degeneration. Despite this success story, however, reimbursement for CT Colonography is problematic in various countries.

The editors and authors of the *CT Colonography Atlas* have great merits in compiling a beautiful collection of CT Colonography cases which are highly educational. In order to differentiate normal from abnormal findings, chapters tackling the normal colon, anatomical variants and pitfalls are included. In a logical manner, chapters about the large variety of pathological conditions involving the colon and rectum (diverticular disease, lipoma, inflammatory bowel diseases, polyps, flat lesions, colon cancer, rectal cancer, cancer of the ileo-cecal valve and post-surgical colon) with a large number of beautifully illustrated cases are incorporated. Axial CT source images, the results of 3D post-processing and colonoscopic correlation present invaluable representations in order to become familiar with different colonic pathologies and enable the radiologist to come to a precise diagnosis.

The series editors of *Medical Radiology-Diagnostic Imaging* would like to express their gratitude to the editors and authors of this book for their tremendous efforts and to Springer for publishing this outstanding atlas.

Munich M.F. Reiser

Preface

Since its introduction in 1994, CT colonography has seen a dramatic evolution that has progressively broadened the field of its diagnostic applications. In particular, the continuous improvement of CT technology and post-processing methods, the refinement of patient preparation schemes, and the growing availability of faster multislice CT scanners with submillimetric spatial resolution and greater dose efficiency have transformed CT colonography from a highly specialised imaging technique performed in a few centres into a widely accepted diagnostic tool used in community hospitals and nonacademic radiology practices as well.

The aim of this Atlas is to provide a practical reference guide for radiologists involved in the daily practice of CT colonography. It is composed of 13 independent chapters covering all the main topics related to CT colonography, with the first two chapters focused on the normal morphology and the anatomical variants of the colon, respectively, whereas Chap. 3 provides a description of the pitfalls. The most common pathological conditions of the large bowel are described in the following chapters, ranging from non-neoplastic to neoplastic diseases, with two additional special focus chapters on cancers of the ileo-cecal valve and imaging of post-surgical colon.

All topics are illustrated by CT colonography cases derived from clinical practice, preceded by a concise introduction with references to the existing literature. Of note, many images are obtained from bi- and three-dimensional reconstructions of native CT colonography datasets, reflecting the importance of post-processing for the correct evaluation of findings.

We hope that practicing radiologists will find this book helpful for their everyday activity, and encourage referring physicians to further include CT colonography in the diagnostic workup of their patients according to the current indications.

Pisa, Italy Emanuele Neri
Pisa, Italy Lorenzo Faggioni
Pisa, Italy Carlo Bartolozzi

Contents

Normal Colon

Thomas Mang, Gernot Böhm, and Wolfgang Schima

Contents

T. Mang, M.D. (✉)
Department of Radiology, Medical University of Vienna, Waehringer Guertel 18-20, 1090 Vienna, Austria
e-mail: thomas.mang@meduniwien.ac.at

G. Böhm, M.D.
Abteilung für Diagnostische und Interventionelle Radiologie, A.ö. Krankenhaus der Elisabethinen Linz, Fadingerstrasse 1, 4010 Linz, Österreich, Austria

W. Schima, M.D., M.Sc.
Abteilung für Diagnostische und Interventionelle Radiologie, KH Göttlicher Heiland, KH der Barmherzigen Schwestern Wien und Sankt Josef KH, Dornbacher Strasse 20-28, 1170 Vienna, Austria

Abstract

Aim of this chapter is to describe the normal anatomy of the colon on the basis of 2D and 3D CT colonography criteria.

In normal colon the wall thickness is thin (less than 2 mm) and may increase to 5 mm in collapsed segments.

The colon is generally recognized by three morphologic key features, which can be clearly identified in CT colonography: the semilunar folds, the taeniae, and the haustra.

The normal colon typically is divided in antegrade order into six segments: the cecum with the ileocecal valve and the appendix, the ascending colon, the transverse colon, the descending colon, the sigmoid colon, and the rectum. The splenic and the hepatic flexure should not be considered separate segments.

The ileocecal valve has a variable appearance, being classified as either labial, when it appears as a slit-like opening; papillary, when its shape is dome-like; or intermediate.

Cases showing the normal colon anatomy are presented in the chapter.

Introduction

A fundamental prerequisite for radiologists aiming to read CT colonographic examinations is a thorough knowledge of the normal anatomy of the colon. Although the large bowel has been examined by radiologists for decades with barium studies, a CT colonographic evaluation may provide a different view of the colon [1–3]. Indeed, CT colonography is quite accurate for assessing the anatomy of the colon. However, the planar 2D approach to trace the gas-distended colon may result in new challenges for some readers, since the complex intraluminal anatomy of bowel loops and haustral folds may complicate the evaluation [4]. Moreover, some radiologists may not be familiar with the "intraluminal" perspective provided by an endoluminal 3D evaluation. Thus, a combined two-dimensional and three-dimensional imaging approach is considered the best practice for

E. Neri et al. (eds.), *CT Colonography Atlas*, Medical Radiology,
DOI 10.1007/978-3-642-11149-5_1, © Springer-Verlag Berlin Heidelberg 2013

CT colonographic evaluation [5]. In this chapter the normal anatomy of the colon is described on the basis of 2D and 3D CT colonographic imaging criteria.

CT Colonography Morphology

General Two-Dimensional and Three-Dimensional CT Features of the Colonic Wall

Wall Thickness

In CT colonographic examinations, after colonic gas insufflation, the wall of the distended normal colon is very thin, measuring less than 2 mm [6]. Typically, it should be barely perceptible on 2D CT colonographic images and may be better depicted with abdominal window settings. In collapsed colonic segments, the colonic wall thickness increases physiologically to up to 5 mm or, in case of spasms, up to 8 mm (Fig. 1) [6]. The normal colonic wall itself has soft tissue attenuation on 2D CT colonographic images. It may show a slight enhancement after intravenous contrast media application. The colon is surrounded by fat tissue, which shows a homogeneous hypodense structure. On endoluminal 3D images, the normal colon presents with a smooth surface.

Morphologic Key Features of the Colon Wall

The colon is generally recognized by three morphologic key features, which can be identified on CT colonographic images: the semilunar folds, the taeniae, and the haustra (Fig. 1) [7].

The semilunar folds (plicae semilunares) are thin crescent-shaped structures. They are oriented orthogonally to the course of the colon and are located one after another in a row when passing through the coloni. Typically, the three rows of colonic folds are each separated by a taenia (see below).

On 2D CT colonographic images, normal semilunar folds are typically very thin and regular soft tissue structures. They are better recognized with wide window settings. On 3D endoluminal views, these folds are seen as crescent-shaped thin folds with a smooth surface. They can be thickened in regions of suboptimal colonic distention or form complex structures, especially at the inner parts of the flexures. The size and number of semicircular folds may vary individually and also within a single patient, due to the peristaltic activity of the colon.

The *taeniae* (taeniae coli) are three longitudinal muscular bands, which are formed from the longitudinal muscle layer of the colonic wall, each with a width of approximately 8 mm. They run along the length of the colon and are located on the anterior, dorsolateral, and dorsomedial wall section [8]. The three taeniae are most prominent in the transverse and ascending colon and, finally, coalesce at the cecum in the area of the appendiceal orifice. The taeniae are less prominent toward the descending and the sigmoid colon and disappear at the rectosigmoid junction.

Haustra are saccular outpouchings of the colonic wall, which are located in the spaces between the taeniae. The haustra are separated by the semilunar folds along the course of the colon. Haustra may vary in prominence due to the contraction of the taeniae and the peristaltic activity of the colon.

Segments of the Colon

The normal colon typically frames the abdomen. It is divided in antegrade order into six segments: the cecum with the ileocecal valve and the appendix, the ascending colon, the transverse colon, the descending colon, the sigmoid colon, and the rectum (Fig. 3). The splenic and the hepatic flexure are not considered separate segments [9].

The length and the diameter of the colon have been evaluated with CT colonography by Khasab et al. [10]. The mean total colonic length, evaluated in this study, was 189.5 cm with a range of 120–299 cm, with the transverse and sigmoid colon representing the longest and the cecum and rectum the shortest segments. The transverse diameter of the colon varied greatly. The cecum has the widest luminal diameter (7.6 cm), followed by the rectum (6.5 cm) and the ascending colon (6.1 cm). The sigmoid (3.5 cm) and descending colon (3.8 cm) have the narrowest luminal diameter [10]. Variations in the segmental or total length of the colon, as well as the length in the segmental location, are not uncommon. Some of these variations are clinically relevant. They are described in Chap. 2 (page 17, Rosa Bouzas).

The cecum is the first segment of the colon (Fig. 4). It is typically located in the right iliac fossa and represents a blind sac. At its base, the colonic taeniae converge and form the triradiate fold. Here, the appendiceal orifice can be seen on endoluminal 3D images as a small, well-circumscribed, round or oval depression of the colonic wall [1].

The *ileocecal valve* anatomically separates the cecum from the ascending colon (Fig. 5). It is located at the junction of the terminal ileum and the colon. The ileocecal valve is most commonly located on the medial side of the cecum, although anatomic variants exist. On 3D endoluminal images, the valve is typically shown with an upper lip and a lower lip [11]. The ileocecal valve has a variable appearance, being classified as either labial, when it appears as a slit-like opening, papillary, when its shape is dome-like, or intermediate. The orifice of the ileocecal valve can be seen as a tiny central depression [12]. Two-dimensional CT images demonstrate the connection of the terminal ileum to the valve. The ileocecal valve may have a wide range of attenuation values, with heterogeneous attenuation. It commonly contains fat tissue and is then referred to as a lipomatous ileocecal valve [13].

The *ascending colon* extends into the right abdomen and is located in the retroperitoneal compartment (Fig. 6). It has a triangular cross section, very similar to the transverse colon, but, typically, is greater in diameter. The semilunar folds may be slightly thicker than in the transverse colon.

The *hepatic flexure* connects the ascending colon with the transverse colon. It typically has a sharp angle (Fig. 7). The haustral folds at the inner part of colonic flexures and loops can fuse and form complex structures on 2D planar images, which are easily recognized, especially on endoluminal 3D displays [4].

The *transverse colon* extends in an intraperitoneal location from the hepatic to the splenic flexure (Fig. 8). It is the longest portion of the colon and can droop along its mesocolon into the pelvis. Therefore, it is relatively mobile. The transverse colon has a typical triangular cross section formed by the three taeniae. It typically has a distinct haustration.

The *splenic flexure* connects the transverse with the descending colon. It is located below the left diaphragm and is the highest point of the colon. The splenic flexure is often more tortuous than the hepatic flexure and contains, at worst, a series of complex twists (Fig. 9).

The *descending colon* extends into the left abdomen and is located within the retroperitoneal compartment. It is characterized by a straight, tubular shape, with a less triangular to oval cross section (Fig. 10). The haustration is less pronounced than in the proximal colonic segments.

The *sigmoid colon* normally lies within the pelvis and, ideally, has an S-shaped course connecting the descending colon with the rectum (Fig. 11). It is a relatively narrow, mobile, and tortuous segment of the colon with a typically round or oval cross section. The degree of haustration is variable. Due to its intraperitoneal location, there may be a considerable range of movement in the central portion.

The *rectum* is the most distal segment of the colon and has the second largest diameter (Fig. 12) [10]. The upper rectum begins intraperitoneally, but its distal two-thirds are located extraperitoneally. Typically, three distinct semilunar folds are found in the rectum (also referred as Houston's valves or transverse folds). The middle fold, typically the largest one, is more often located at the right side of the rectum [14]. The rectum ends at the anorectal junction (anatomically "linea dentata") and extends to the anal canal. At the anorectal junction, radiating folds are often observed, which are caused by the contraction of the anal sphincter muscles. The anal channel itself cannot be evaluated with CT colonography.

Case 1. Normal Wall Thickness of the Colon

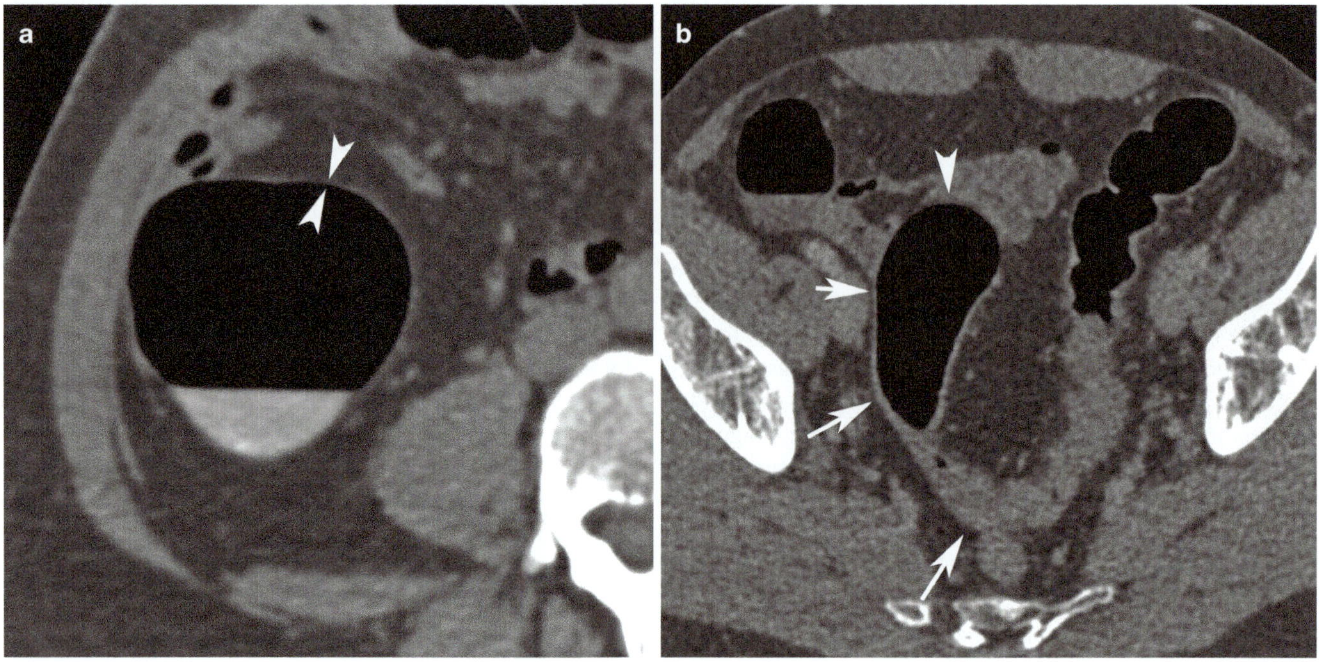

Fig. 1 (**a**) Axial 2D CT image shows the well-distended ascending colon. The colonic wall (*arrowheads*) is barely perceptible. (**b**) Axial 2D CT image shows the partially distended (*arrowheads*) and partially collapsed sigmoid colon. The colonic wall thickness increases gradually (*arrows*) in the collapsed segment

Case 2. CT Morphologic Key Features of the Colon

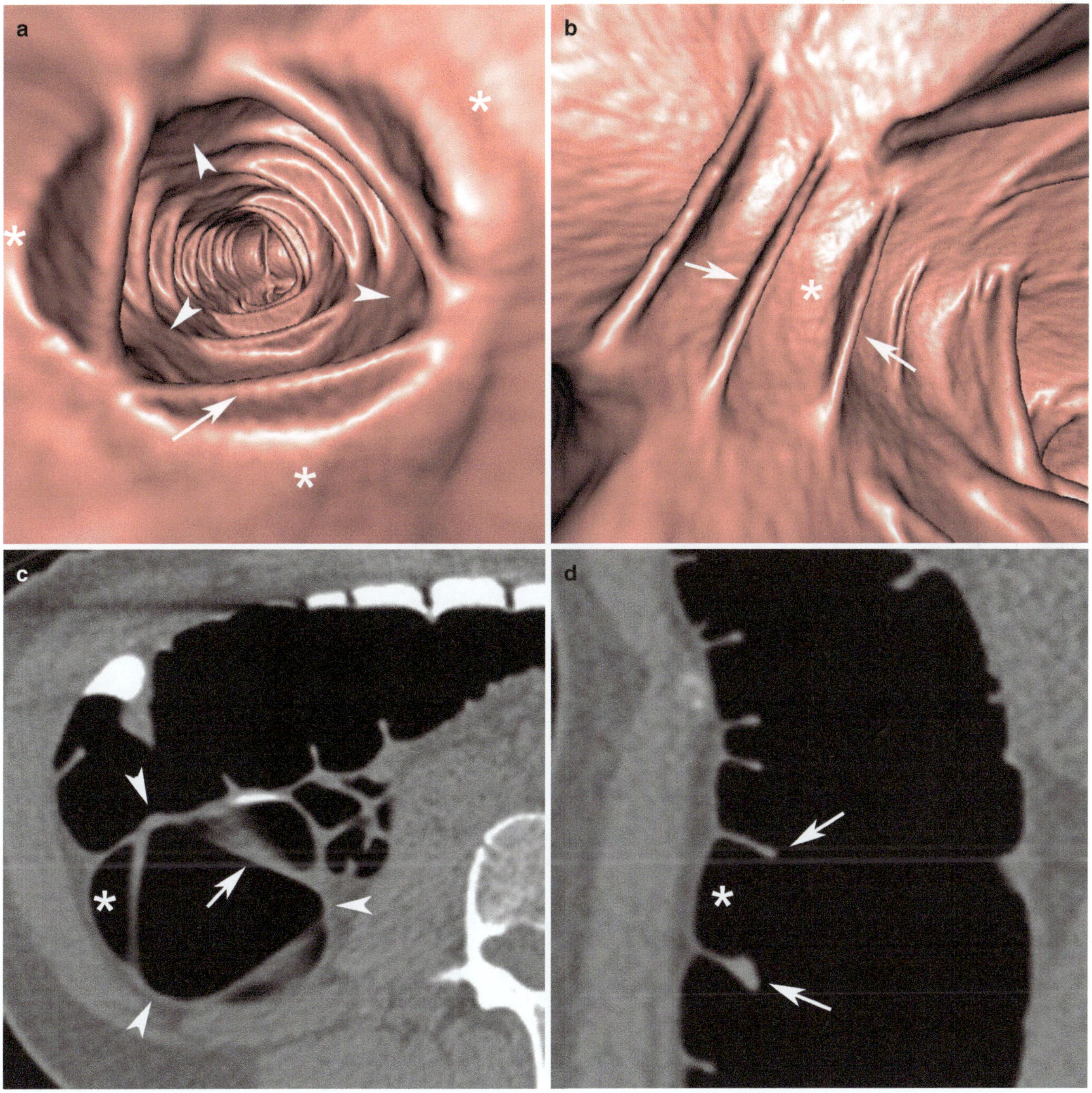

Fig. 2 (**a**) Endoluminal 3D CT image of the ascending colon. Three taeniae are shown as longitudinal bands running along the length of the colon (*arrowheads*). Haustra are located in the spaces between the taeniae (*). (**b**) Endoluminal 3D CT image shows haustra (*) separated by thin semilunar folds (*arrows*). The semilunar folds appear as very thin crescent-shaped structures (*arrows*) (**a**, **b**). (**c**) Axial 2D CT image of the same colonic segment shows corresponding taeniae (*arrowheads*), semilunar folds (*arrow*) as thin soft tissue dense structures, and the haustra (*). Note the triangular cross section of the ascending colon. (**d**) Coronal 2D CT image showing haustra (*) separated by thin semilunar folds (*arrows*)

Case 3. Six Segments of a Normal Colon

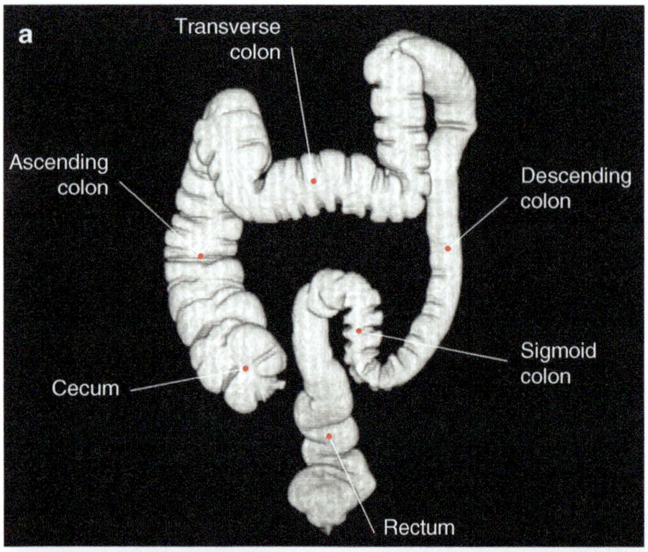

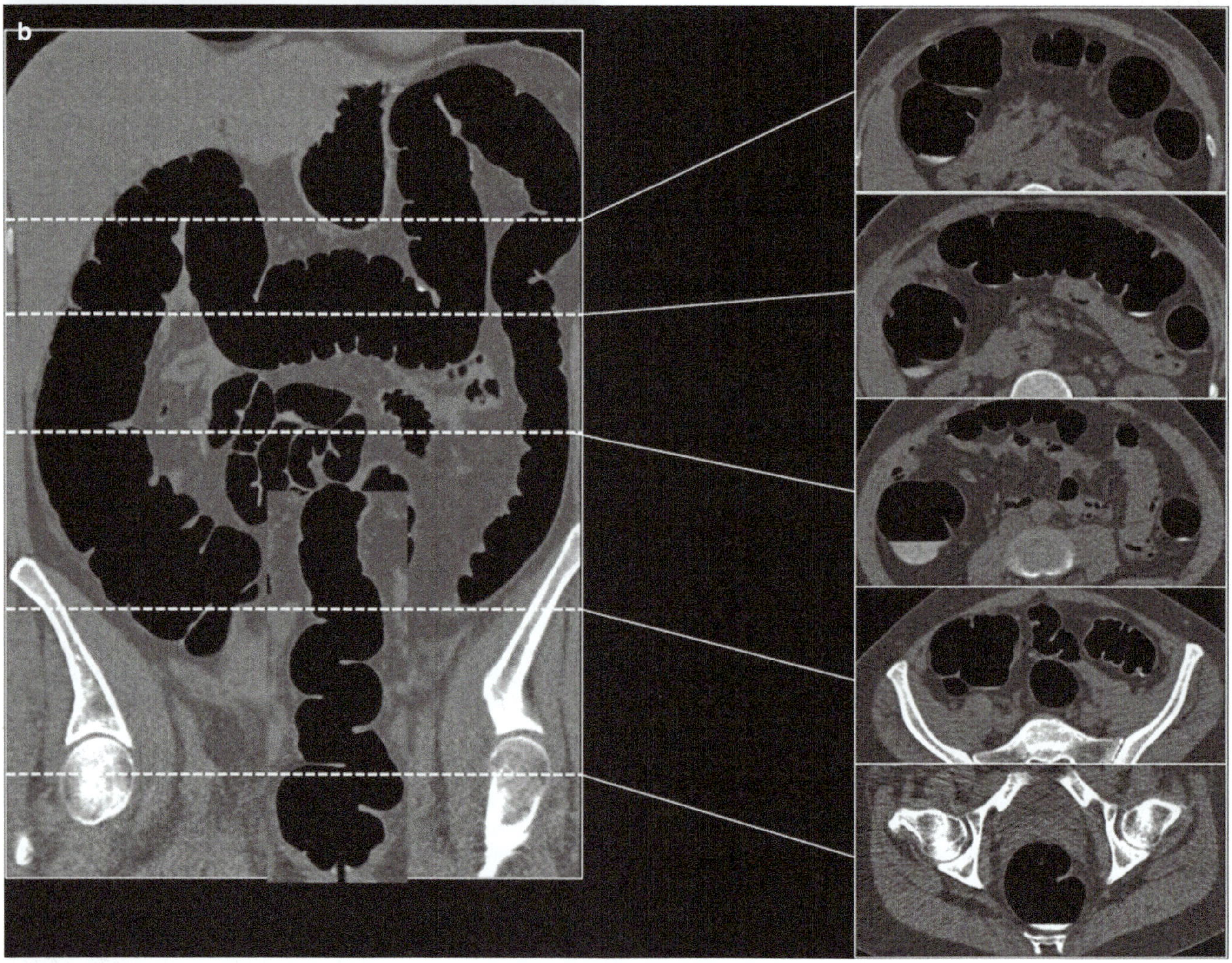

Fig. 3 (**a**) Global surface-rendered 3D view shows the cecum, ascending colon, transverse colon, descending colon, and the rectum. All segments are of normal location, length, and diameter. (**b**) Coronal 2D CPR illustrates the course of the colon and rectum (inlay) (*left*). Corresponding axial 2D CT images show the location of the colonic segments (*right*)

Case 4. Cecum: Triradiate Fold and Appendiceal Orifice

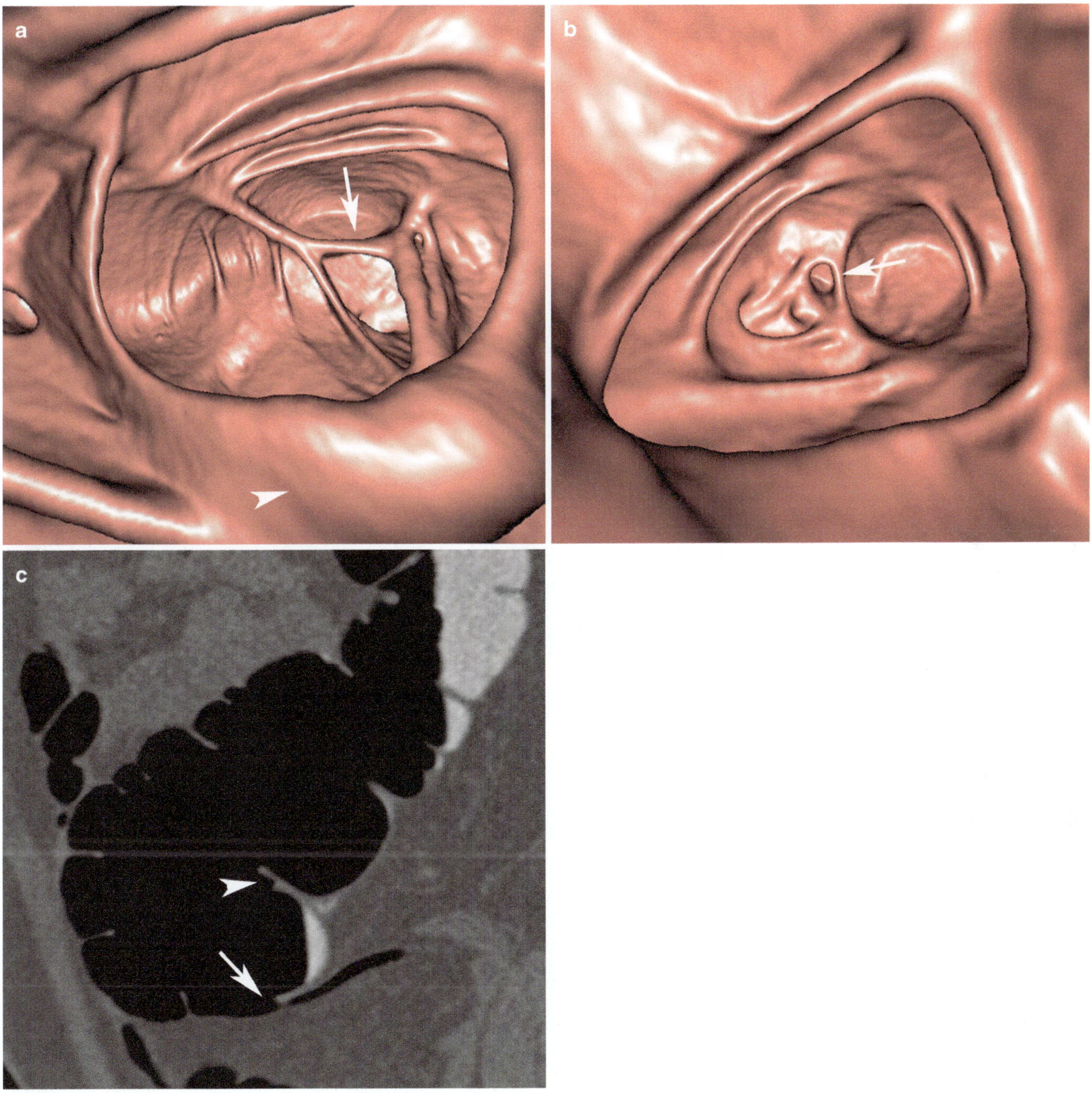

Fig. 4 (**a**) Retrograde endoluminal 3D CT image of the cecum, showing the three colonic taeniae converging and forming the triradiate fold (*arrow*). Note the papillary ileocecal valve (*arrowhead*). (**b**) Retrograde endoluminal 3D CT image of the cecum in another patient, showing the appendiceal orifice at the area of the triradiate fold (*arrow*), appearing as a small, well-circumscribed, round depression. (**c**) Coronal 2D image showing the blind end of the cecum in the right iliac fossa. Note the labial ileocecal valve (*arrowhead*) on the medial aspect of the cecum and the appendiceal orifice (*arrow*) at the cecal base. The appendix is filled with air

Case 5. Cecum: Normal Labial Ileocecal Valve

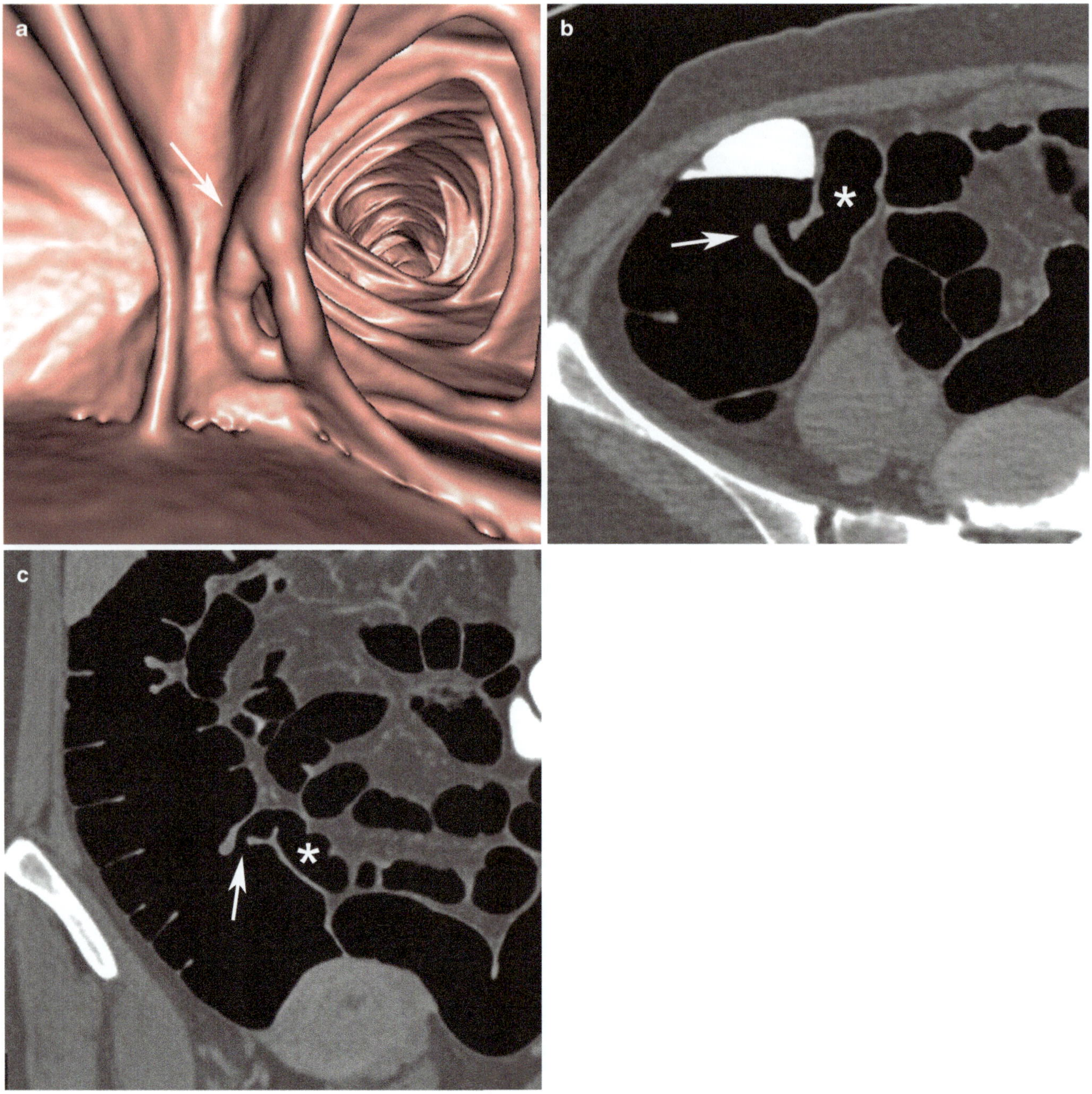

Fig. 5 (**a**) Antegrade endoluminal 3D CT view from the cecum into the ascending colon, showing the ileocecal valve (*arrow*) with an upper and lower lip and, in between, the opened orifice. (**b**, **c**) Axial and coronal 2D CT image showing the blind-ending cecum in the right iliac fossa. The ileocecal valve is located on the medial side of the cecum and shows the open orifice with an upper and a lower lip (*arrow*). Note the connection of the terminal ileum (*) to the valve

Case 6. Ascending Colon

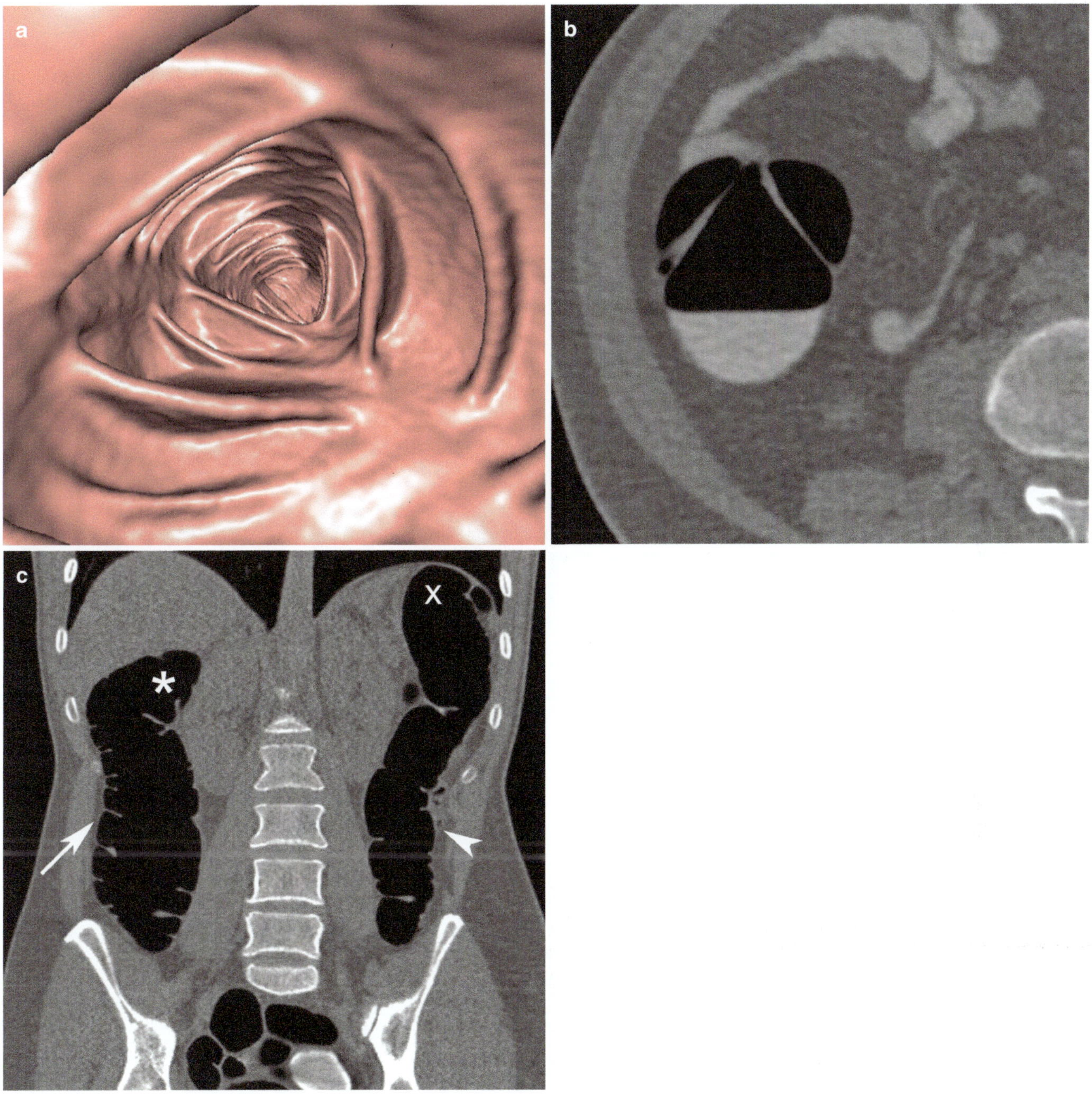

Fig. 6 (**a**) Antegrade endoluminal 3D CT view and (**b**) axial 2D CT image of the ascending colon, showing a triangular cross section and distinct haustration. (**c**) Coronal 2D CT image showing the ascending colon (*arrow*) extending retroperitoneally into the right abdomen. Note the right (*) and left (X) flexure and the descending colon (*arrowhead*)

Case 7. Right Flexure

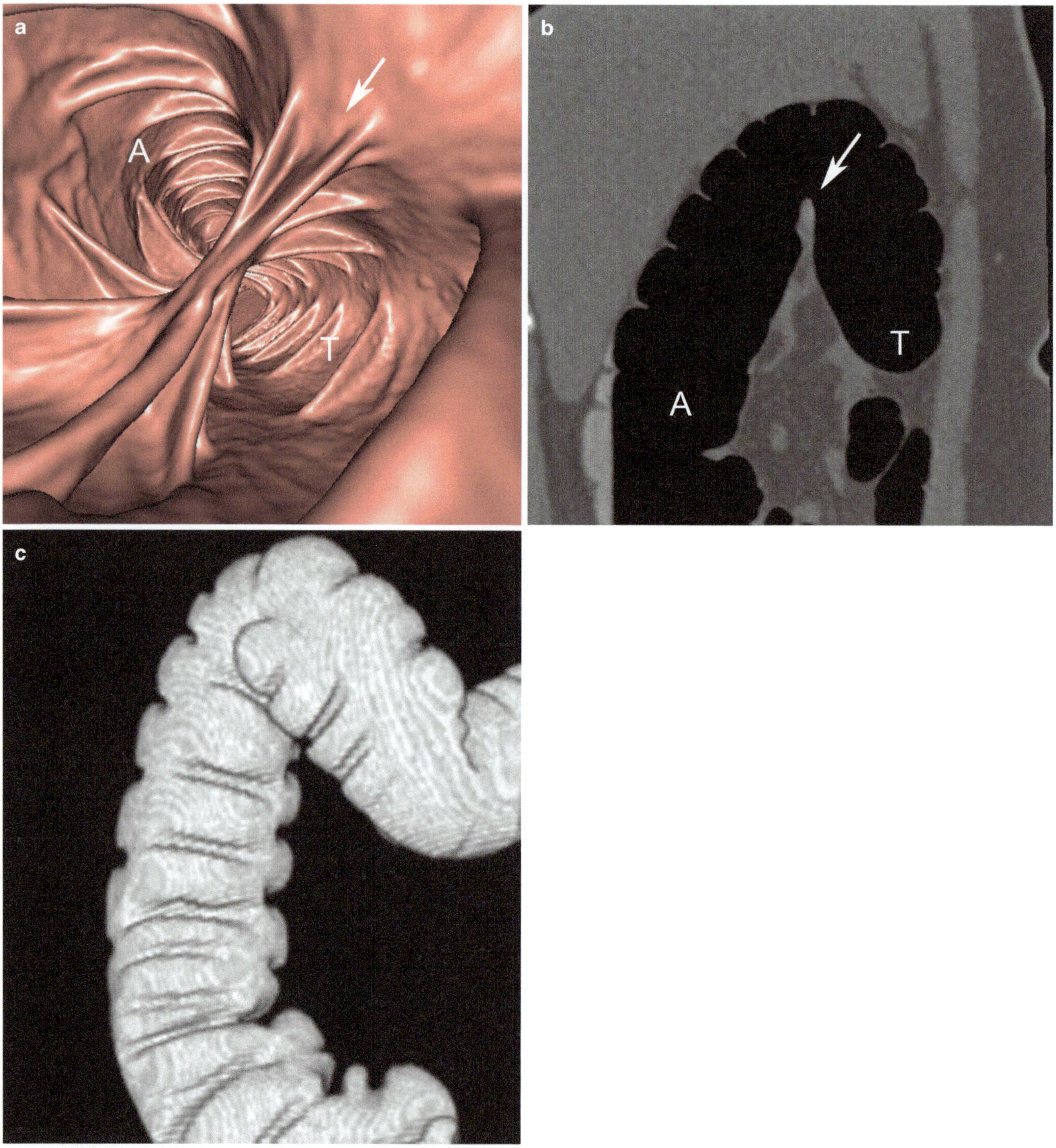

Fig. 7 (**a**) Endoluminal 3D CT view and (**b**) sagittal 2D image showing the right flexure (*arrow*) connecting the ascending (*A*) with the transverse (*T*) colon and forming a relatively sharp angle. (**b**) Sagittal 2D CT image showing the thickened fold pattern at the inner part of the right flexure (*arrow*), which is easily realized on endoluminal 3D views. *A* ascending colon, *T* transverse colon. (**c**) Global surface-rendered 3D view shows the course of the right flexure

Case 8. Transverse Colon

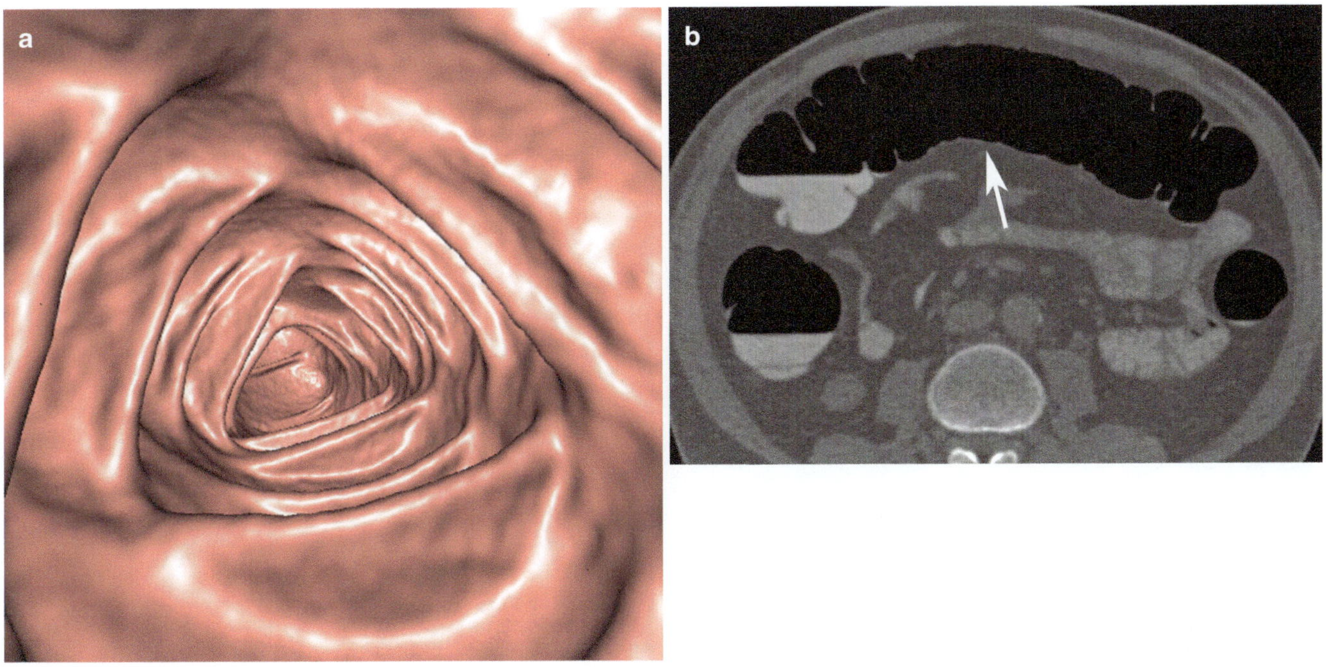

Fig. 8 (**a**) Endoluminal 3D CT image of the transverse colon with a typical triangular lumen formed by the three taeniae and with a distinct haustration. The diameter is slightly smaller than in the ascending colon. (**b**) Axial 2D CT image showing the course of the transverse colon (*arrow*) connecting the ascending colon on the *right side* and the descending colon on the *left side*

Case 9. Left Flexure

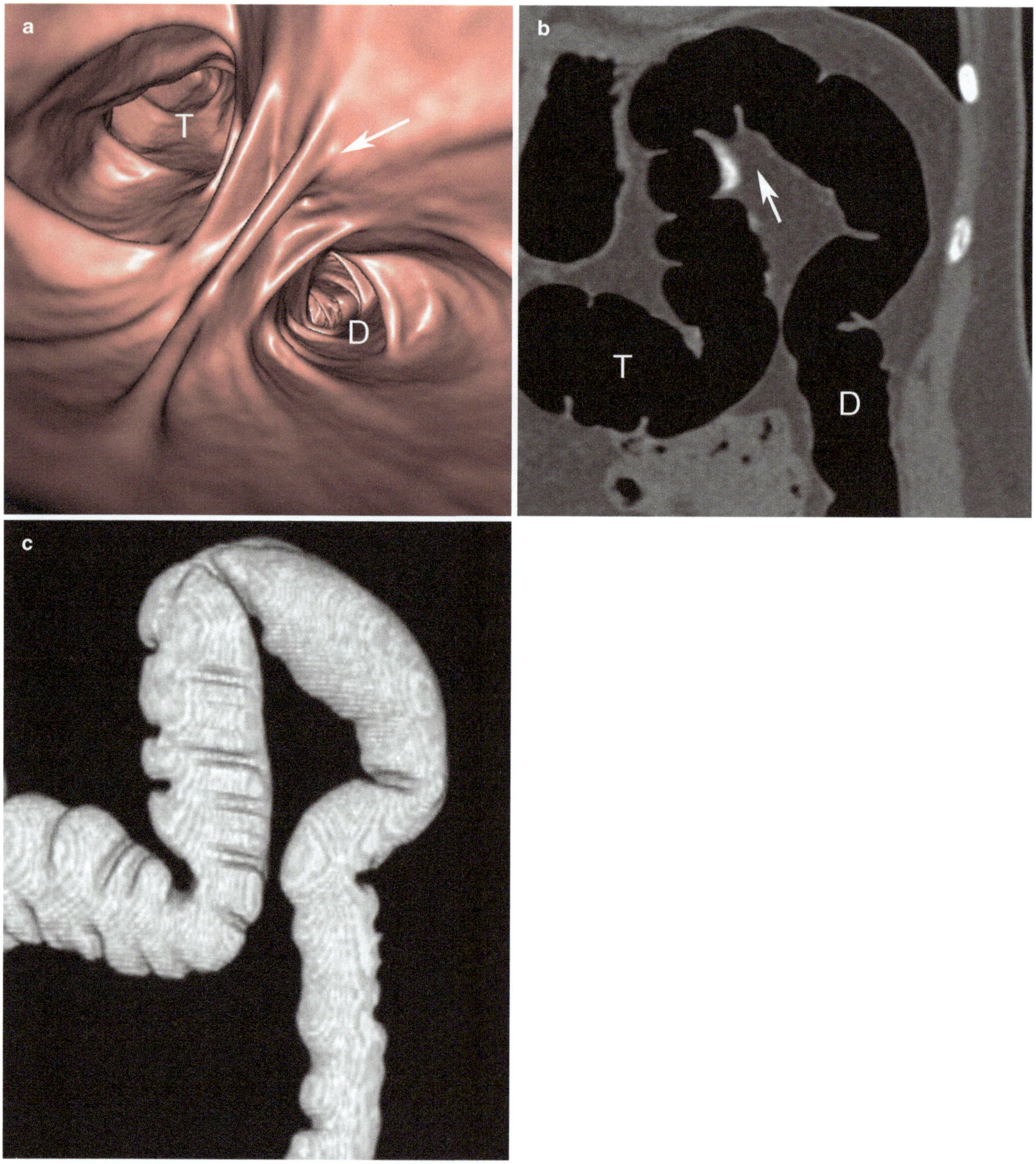

Fig. 9 (**a**) Endoluminal 3D CT view and (**b**) sagittal 2D image showing the left flexure (*arrow*) connecting the transverse (*T*) with the descending (*D*) colon. (**b**) Sagittal 2D CT image showing the complex fold pattern at the inner part of the left flexure (*arrow*), being more tortuous than the hepatic flexure. *T* transverse colon, *D* descending colon. (**c**) Global surface-rendered 3D view shows the course of the left flexure

Case 10. Descending Colon

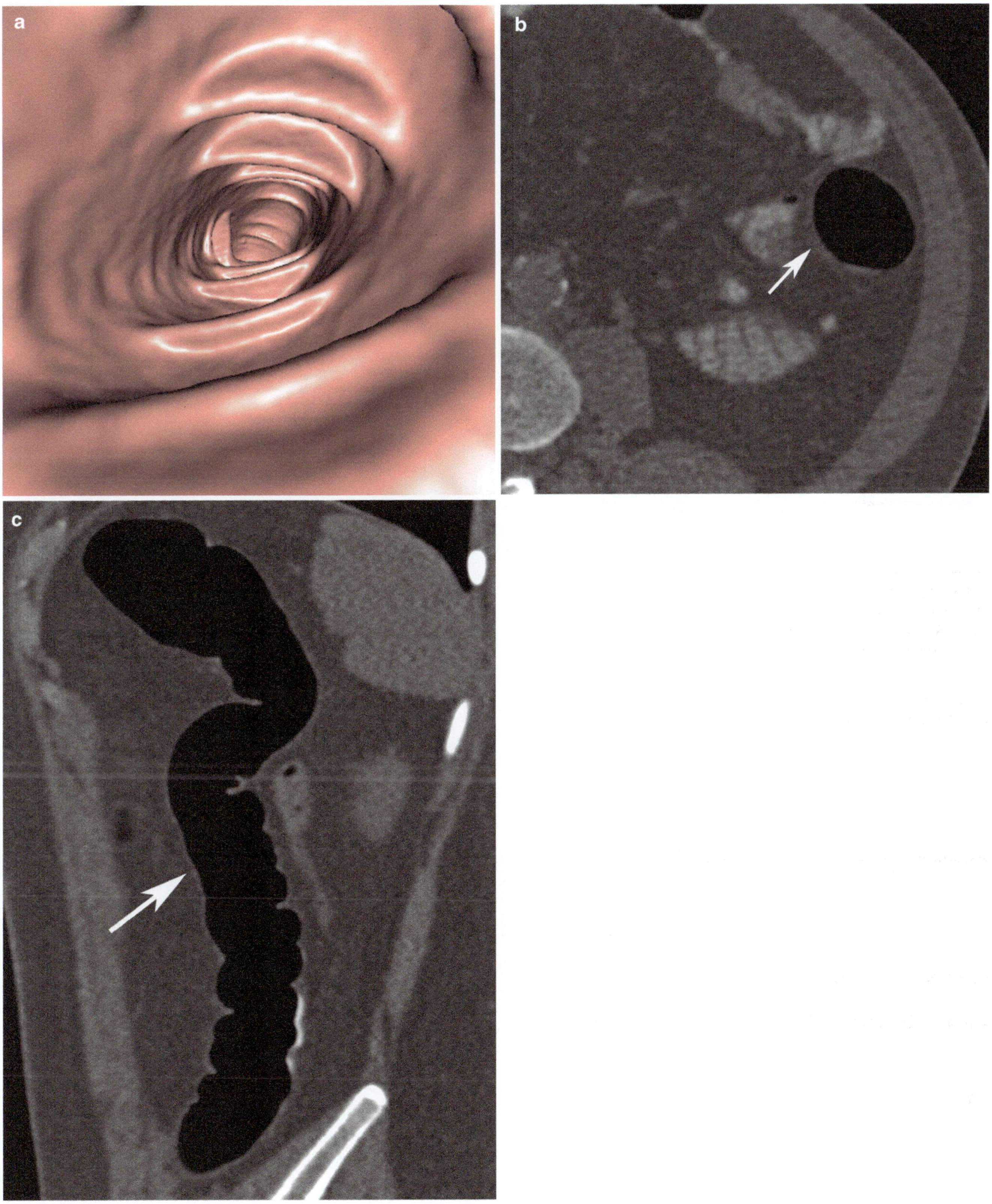

Fig. 10 (**a**) Antegrade endoluminal 3D CT view and axial 2D CT image of the descending colon, showing a round lumen compared to the triangular lumen in the transverse colon (see Fig. 8a). Note that the diameter is smaller in comparison to the upper colonic segments. (**b**) Axial 2D CT image showing the descending colon located in the left abdomen with a round cross section of (*arrow*). (**c**) Sagittal 2D view showing the straight and tubular shape of the descending colon (*arrow*)

Case 11. Sigmoid Colon

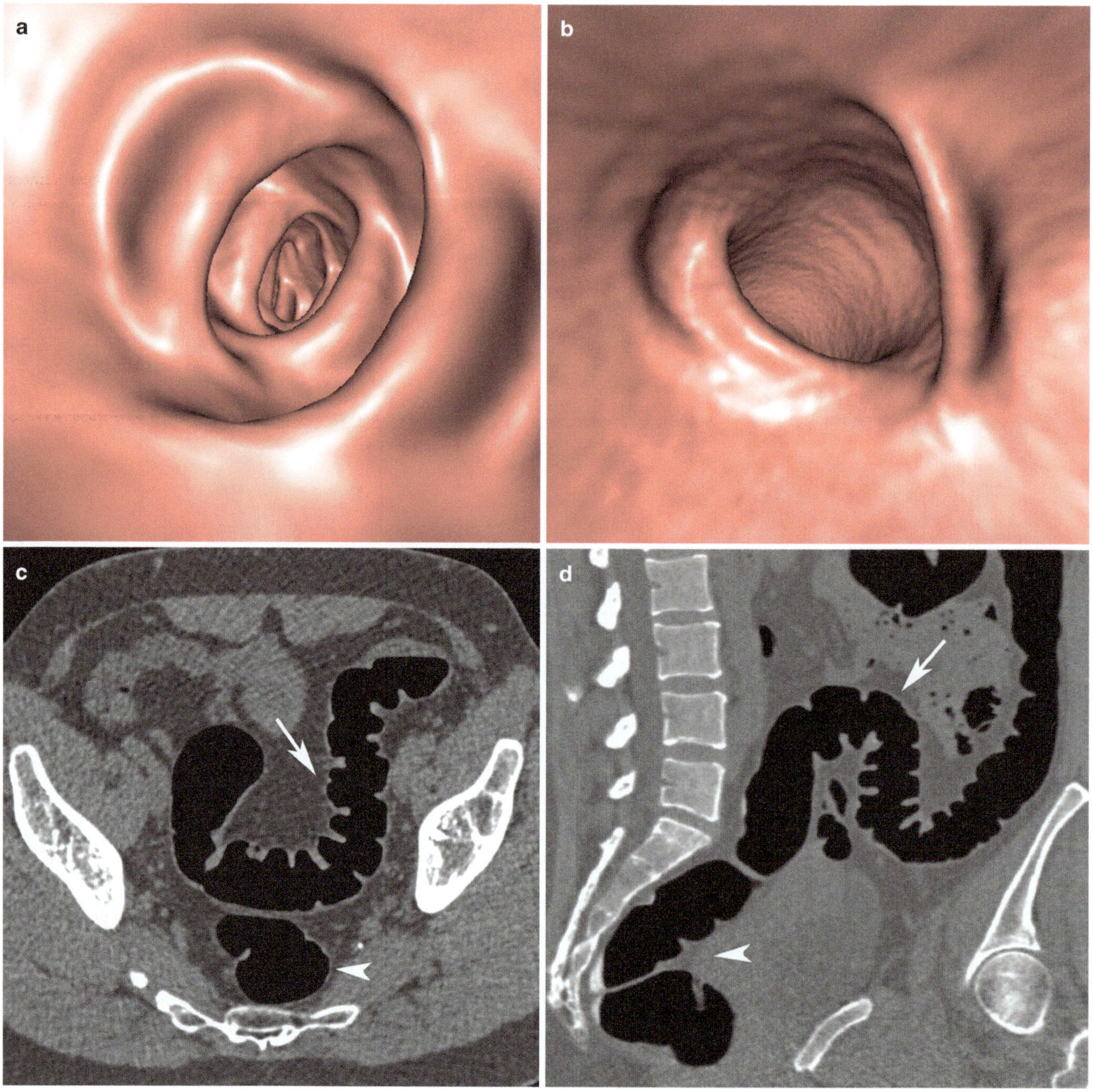

Fig. 11 Sigmoid colon. (**a**, **b**) Endoluminal 3D views from two different patients show a relatively narrow lumen with a typically round or oval cross section. The degree of haustration is variable and can be pronounced (**a**) or low (**b**). (**c**) Axial unenhanced prone 2D CT image and (**d**) sagittal 2D CPR show the typical S-shaped course of the sigmoid colon (*arrow*), connecting the descending colon with the rectum (*arrowhead*)

Case 12. Rectum

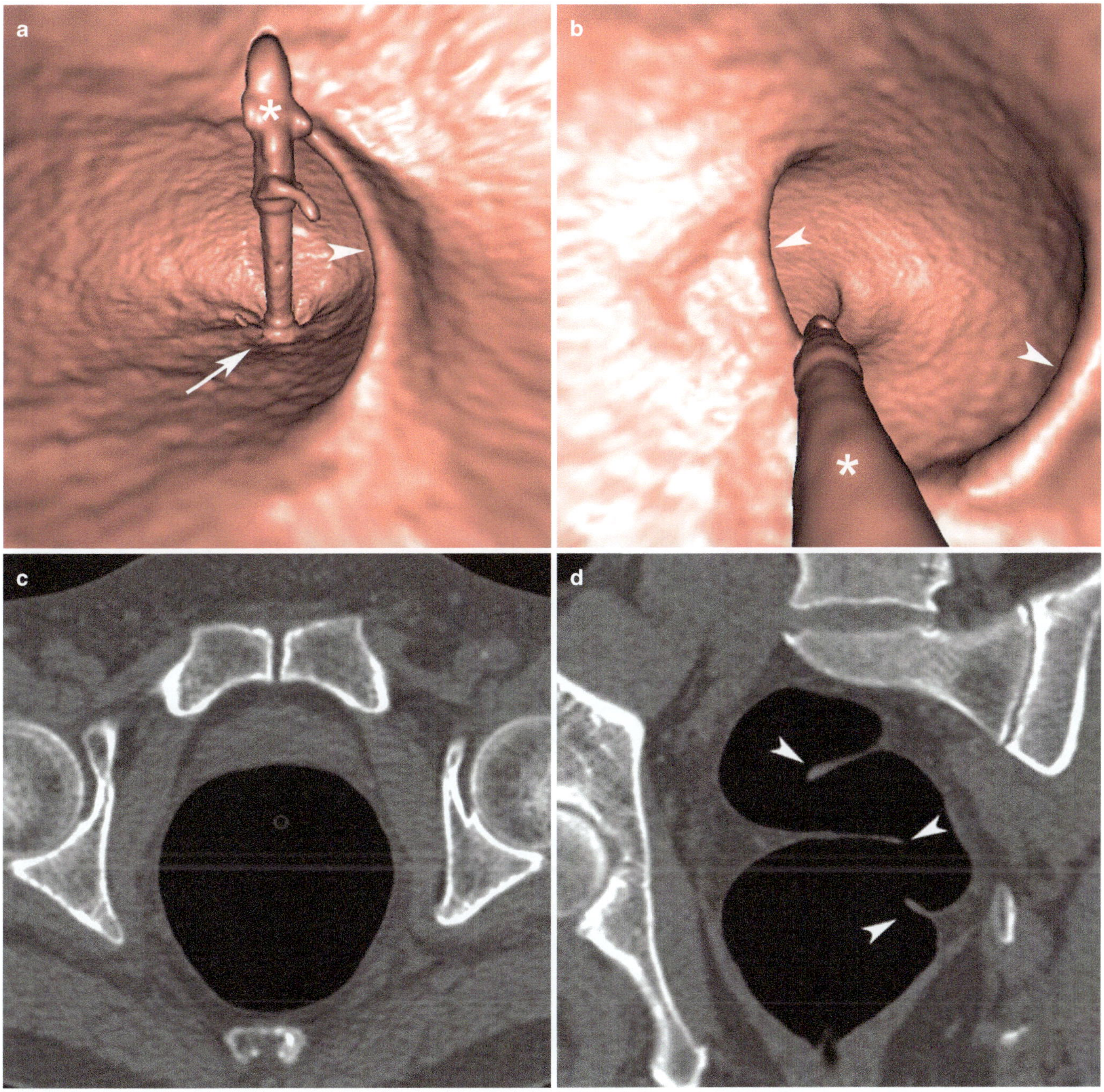

Fig. 12 (**a**) Antegrade endoluminal 3D view shows small radiating folds (*arrow*) at the anorectal junction caused by contraction of the anal sphincter muscles. Distal transverse rectal fold (*arrowhead*) and rectal tube (*). (**b**) Retrograde endoluminal 3D view showing two transverse rectal folds (*arrowheads*) and the rectal tube (*). (**c**) Axial 2D CT image shows a well-distended rectum with a large diameter will provide ane fig with 3 arrowheads and without the arrow. (**d**) Coronal 2D CT image shows three distinct semilunar rectal folds (*arrowheads*) that were found in the rectum (Houston's valves)

References

1. Fenlon HM, Clarke PD, Ferrucci JT (1998) Virtual colonoscopy: imaging features with colonoscopic correlation. AJR Am J Roentgenol 170(5):1303–1309
2. Macari M, Megibow AJ (2001) Pitfalls of using three-dimensional CT colonography with two-dimensional imaging correlation. AJR Am J Roentgenol 176(1):137–143
3. Silva AC, Wellnitz CV, Hara AK (2006) Three-dimensional virtual dissection at CT colonography: unraveling the colon to search for lesions. Radiographics 26(6):1669–1686
4. Mang T, Maier A, Plank C, Mueller-Mang C, Herold C, Schima W (2007) Pitfalls in multi-detector row CT colonography: a systematic approach. Radiographics 27(2):431–454
5. Neri E, Halligan S, Hellström M (2012) ESGAR CT Colonography Working Group. Eur Radiol. Sep 15. [Epub ahead of print] PMID: 22983280
6. Wiesner W, Mortele KJ, Ji H, Ros PR (2002) Normal colonic wall thickness at CT and its relation to colonic distension. J Comput Assist Tomogr 26(1):102–106
7. Mang T, Schima W (2009) CT-Kolonographie, 1st ed. Georg Thieme Verlag, Stuttgart
8. Horton KM, Corl FM, Fishman EK (2000) CT evaluation of the colon: inflammatory disease. Radiographics 20(2):399–418
9. Zalis ME, Barish MA, Choi JR et al (2005) CT colonography reporting and data system: a consensus proposal. Radiology 236(1):3–9
10. Khashab MA, Pickhardt PJ, Kim DH, Rex DK (2009) Colorectal anatomy in adults at computed tomography colonography: normal distribution and the effect of age, sex, and body mass index. Endoscopy 41(8):674–678
11. Silva AC, Beaty SD, Hara AK et al (2007) Spectrum of normal and abnormal CT appearances of the ileocecal valve and cecum with endoscopic and surgical correlation. Radiographics 27(4):1039–1054
12. Iafrate F, Rengo M, Ferrari R, Paolantonio P, Celestre M, Laghi A (2007) Spectrum of normal findings, anatomic variants and pathology of ileocecal valve: CT colonography appearances and endoscopic correlation. Abdom Imaging 32(5):589–595
13. Regge D, Gallo TM, Nieddu G et al (2005) Ileocecal valve imaging on computed tomographic colonography. Abdom Imaging 30(1):20–25
14. Silva AC, Vens EA, Hara AK, Fletcher JG, Fidler JL, Johnson CD (2006) Evaluation of benign and malignant rectal lesions with CT colonography and endoscopic correlation. Radiographics 26(4): 1085–1099

Anatomical Variants

Rosa Bouzas

Contents

R. Bouzas, M.D.
Diagnostic Radiology, Complexo Hospitalario
Universitario de Vigo/ES (CHUVI),
Vigo, Spain
e-mail: mrbouzas@telefonica.net

Abstract
Variants in the position of the colon or segments of colon are often observed during CTC; although most of these anomalies have no clinical importance, a significant number are related factors to explain an incomplete colonoscopy ,mild abdominal pain or unsual clinical presentations. Positional abnormalities could be divided on two groups, due to external displacement or congenital anomalies either positional anomalies related to the process of intestinal rotation or the process of intestinal fixation of colon, normally named as intestinal malrotation. Several clinical examples of variants in position of the colon and their clinical relevance are discussed.

Introduction

Variants in the position of the colon or its segments are often observed at CT colonography (CTC). Although most of these anomalies have no clinical importance, a significant number of them may be responsible for an incomplete colonoscopy. Positional abnormalities of the colon can be divided into two groups:

1. Those due to external displacement of the large bowel (e.g., by enlargement or abnormal position of solid organs, vessels, and other neighboring structures)
2. Those due to congenital anomalies (mainly related to the process of colonic rotation and fixation), grouped as intestinal malrotation

The incidence of colonic malrotation in the general population is not well known. It is estimated to range between 1:6,000 and 1:200 of live births [1]; most cases are diagnosed in the first years of life, and only a small percentage of adults are asymptomatic or do not receive a diagnosis of colonic malrotation [2].

During the normal embryological development of the gastrointestinal tract, the midgut takes its place into the peritoneal cavity and both the duodenojejunal and the ileocolic segments rotate 270° counterclockwise around the

E. Neri et al. (eds.), *CT Colonography Atlas,* Medical Radiology,
DOI 10.1007/978-3-642-11149-5_2, © Springer-Verlag Berlin Heidelberg 2013

omphalomesenteric vessels to reach their final normal position. The duodenum is the first portion to rotate, and the cecum is the last one; the complete rotation of the gut allows the cecum to descend into the right lower abdominal quadrant. Peritoneal fixation of the bowel is the last stage of development.

The most important anomalies of rotation and fixation are nonrotation, malrotation, and reverse fixation [2]. In nonrotation, the midgut rotates only 180° instead of 270°, and the colonic limb reenters the abdomen first, thus leaving the whole colon and cecum in the left position with a right small bowel. Malrotation means that rotation is incomplete: the degree of malrotation is indicated by the position of the cecum in the left, higher than normal in the right side or in an intermediate position. In reversed rotation, the migration of the cecum unwinds the normal counterclockwise rotation, and the transverse colon finally lies behind the duodenum, from which it is separated by the superior mesenteric artery. Abnormal bowel position does not cause symptoms in itself; however, the abnormal fixation of the gut may cause it to twist, leading to formation of a midgut volvulus. Between asymptomatic nonrotation and midgut volvulus, intermediate condition may occur that may result in nonspecific mild abdominal complaints [1].

CT Colonography Pattern

After air or CO_2 insufflation of the colon, a 3D map of the large bowel can be generated that allows fast and direct evaluation of the position of the whole colon. Variants of the colonic morphology are diverse and numerous, and their early detection can usually explain atypical [3] and mild abdominal complaints or, in a few patients, even suggest surgery to prevent volvulus formation [1].

On the other hand, external colonic compression by surrounding structures can simulate colonic pathology, such as polyps or submucosal masses as seen in endoluminal views. In those cases, endoluminal findings must be correlated with MPR in order to clearly reveal the external compression.

Case 1. Colonic Nonrotation

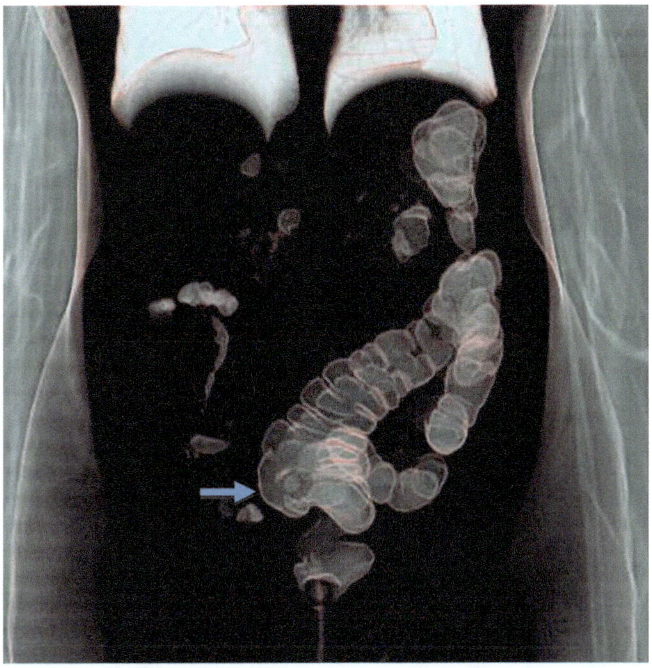

Fig. 1a Double contrast-like 3D colon map

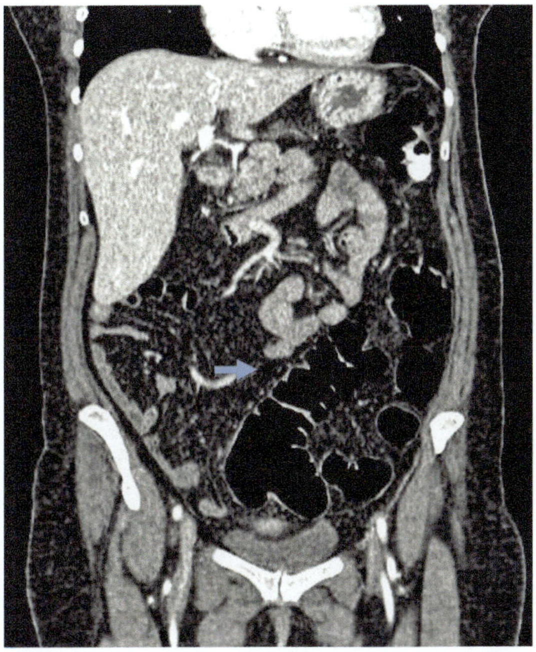

Fig. 1b CTC examination, coronal MPR

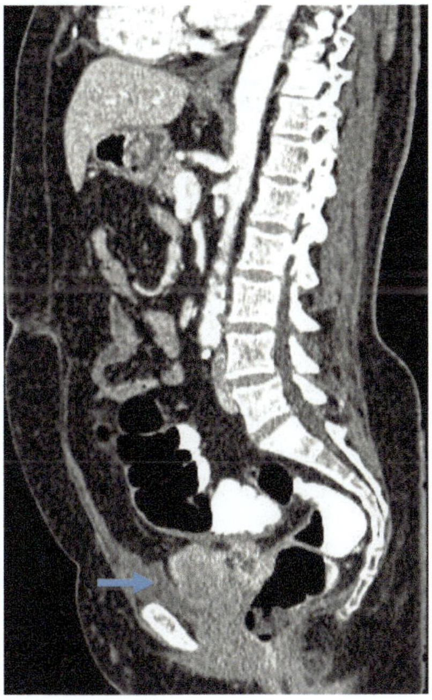

Fig. 1c CTC examination, sagittal MPR

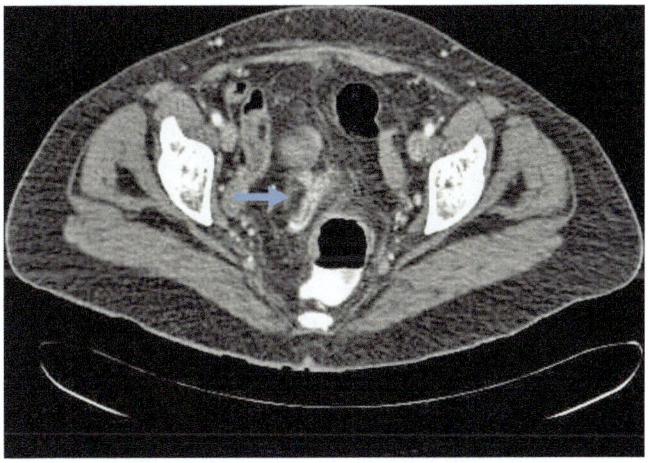

Fig. 1d CTC examination, axial image

Description

A 40-year-old female with recurrent abdominal pain.

3D reconstruction of the CTC dataset shows abnormal position of the right colon on the left of the midline (Fig. 1a), with the whole colon lying in the left hemiabdomen due to intestinal nonrotation. Coronal MPR shows small bowel in the right fossa (Fig. 1b). The cecum lies very close to the rectum in the pelvis; the sagittal MPR view shows a mass below the cecum (Fig. 1c), while the source axial CT image shows a distended appendix (Fig. 1d). A diagnosis of left appendicitis complicated with abscess was made; however, there was no peritoneal reaction and appendicitis was not suspected before CTC.

Case 2. Undescended Cecum with Malrotation

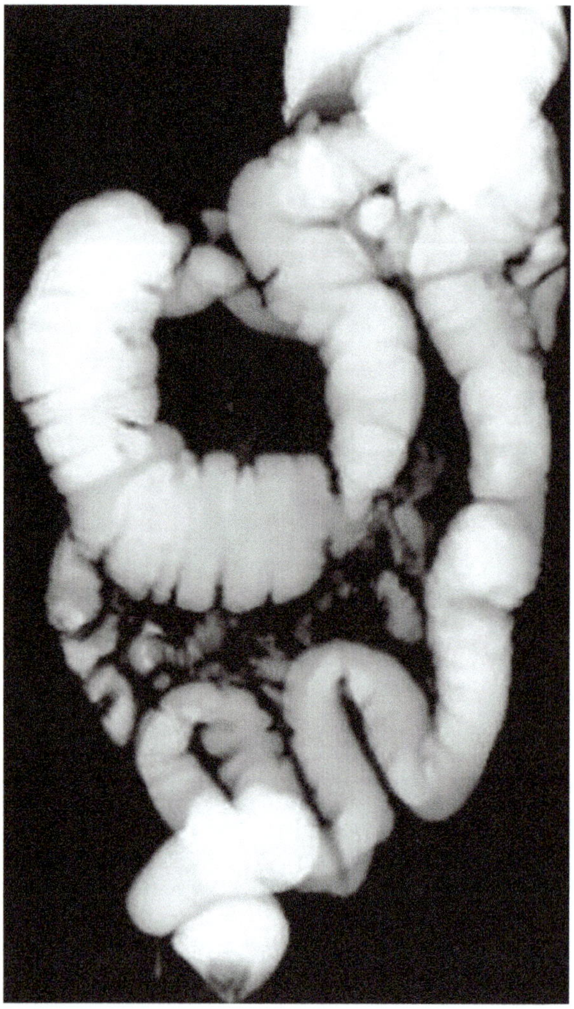

Fig. 2a 3D colon map

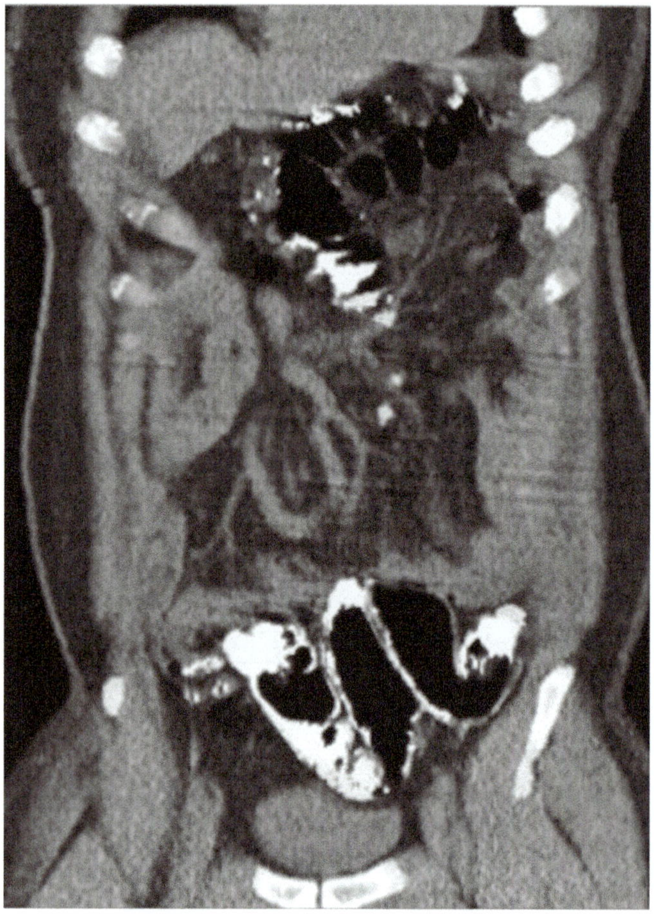

Fig. 2b Coronal MPR

Description

A 45-year-old man with recurrent cramp-like abdominal pain. The 3D map shows an undescended cecum lying in the upper right abdomen (Fig. 2a). Coronal MPR shows torsion of mesenteric vessels (Fig. 2b). Malrotation with a movable cecum secondary to a defect of intestinal attachment was demonstrated. Such situation is at risk for development of a midgut volvulus, and abdominal surgery was performed to properly fix the intestinal mesentery. Of note, two optical colonoscopies carried out before CTC had shown no abnormalities.

Case 3. Medial Cecum

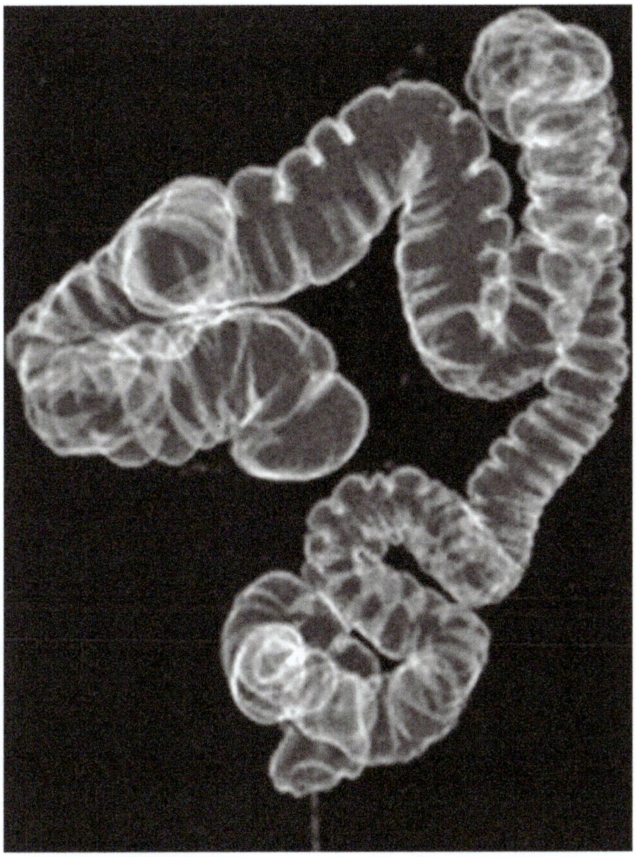

Fig. 3a 3D colon map

Description

Medially placed cecum in an asymptomatic patient who underwent CTC for CRC screening (Fig. 3a). This is a common finding that is usually accepted as a non-pathological anatomical variant.

Case 4. Chilaiditi Syndrome

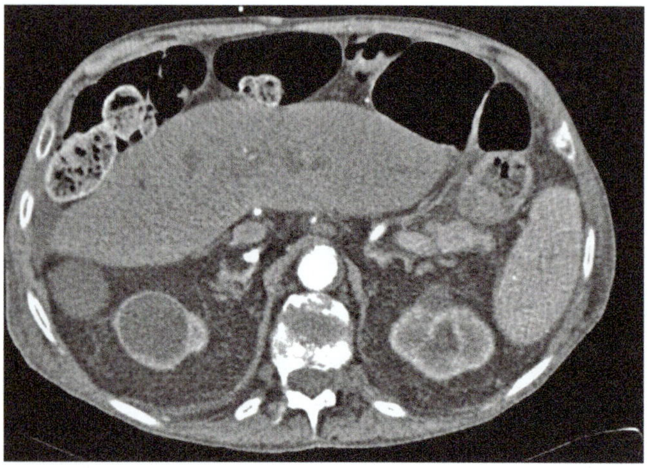

Fig. 4a Axial CT image

Description

Hepatodiaphragmatic interposition of the colon (Chilaiditi syndrome) with the transverse colon located between the liver and the diaphragm (Fig. 4a). This is an incidental finding in abdominal CT that is mostly related to colon redundancy rather than to faulty fixation.

Case 5. Defective Fixation of the Ascending Colon

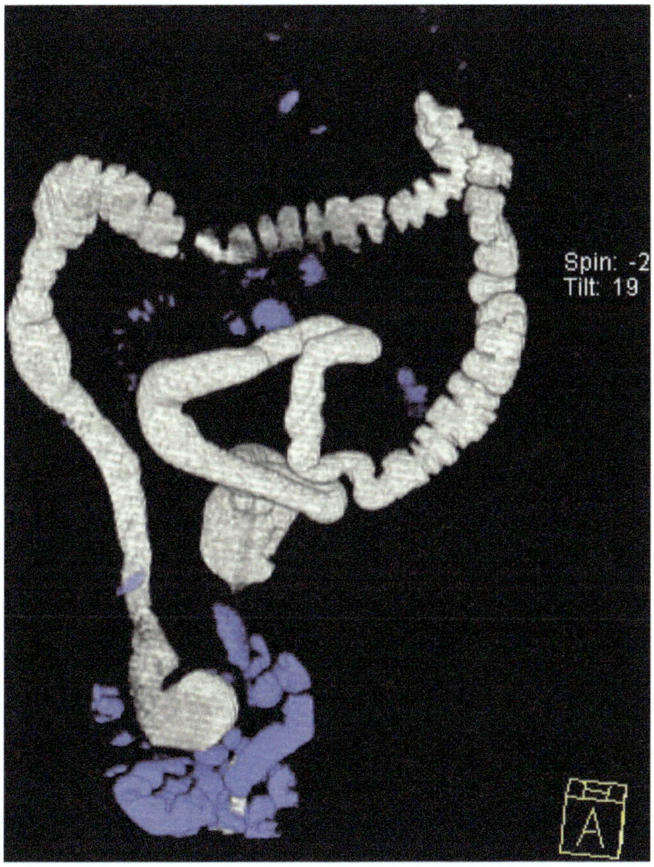

Fig. 5a 3D colon map

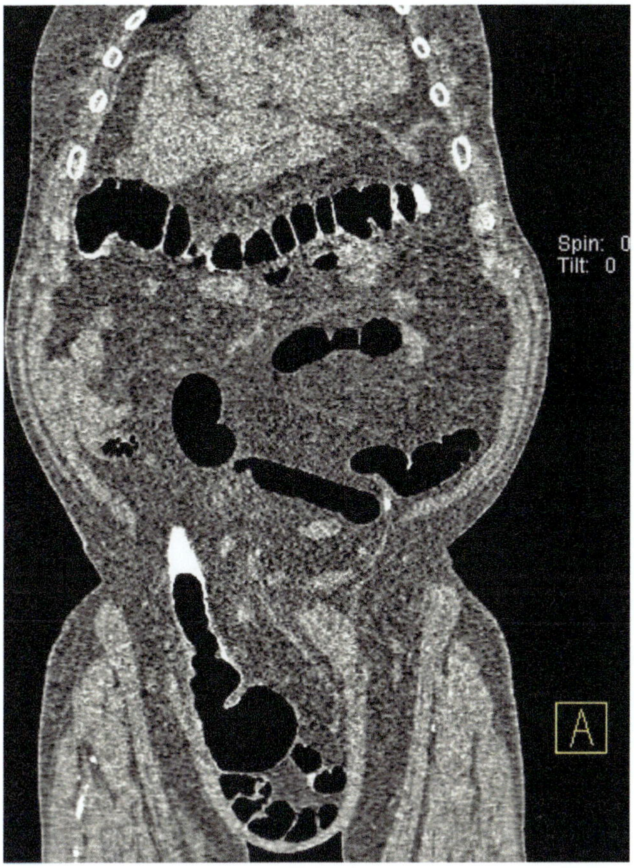

Fig. 5b CTC examination, coronal MPR

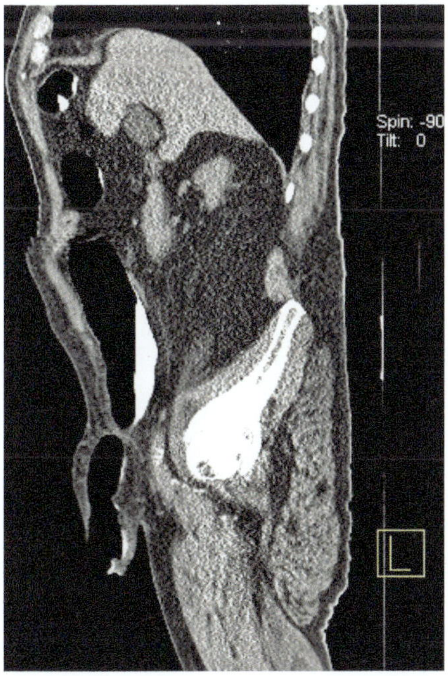

Fig. 5c CTC examination, sagittal MPR

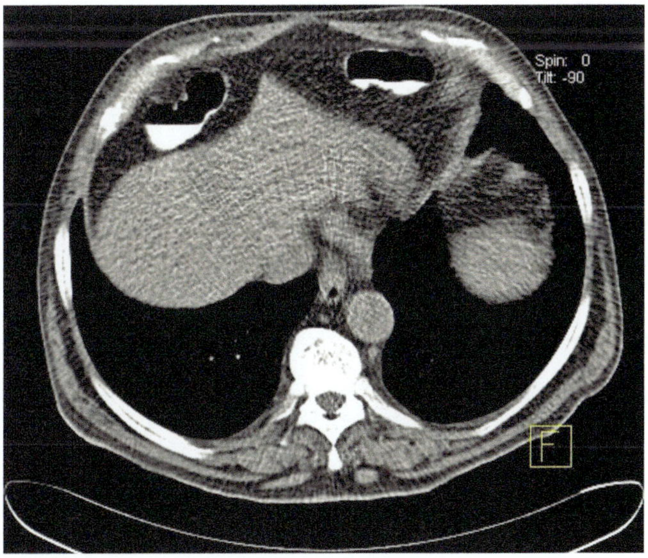

Fig. 5d CTC examination, axial image

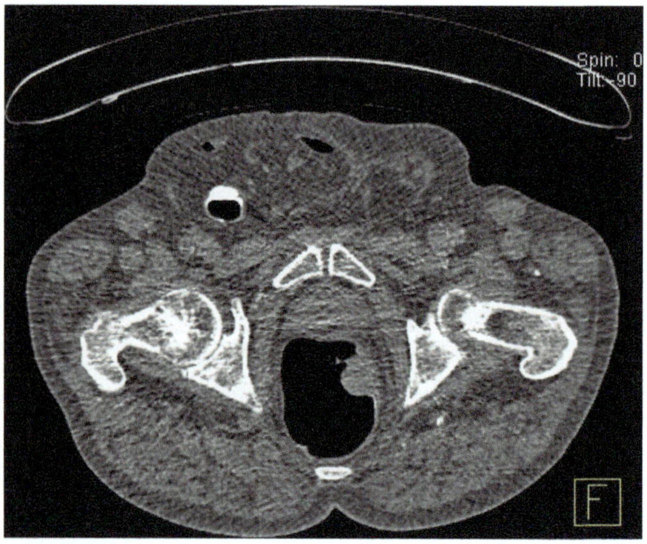

Fig. 5e Axial CTC rectum level

Description

Adult male with rectal advanced adenoma and CTC performed after incomplete colonoscopy.

3D volume rendering of the colon shows a large right colon with the cecum and small bowel placed in a very low position, lower than the rectum (Fig. 5a). MPR images show the cecum and ascending colon inside a right inguinoscrotal hernial sac (Fig. 5b); note the very high position of the hepatic flexure, located below the diaphragm at the same level of the upper surface of the liver, together with a very long and tense ascending colon (Fig. 5c) and a segment of transverse colon between liver and diaphragm (Chilaiditi syndrome) (Fig. 5d). These findings are related to the mobility of the entire ascending colon secondary to defective fusion, an abnormal fixation that may cause the right colon to be located virtually anywhere in the abdomen. Axial CTC image (Fig. 5e) shows a large sessile rectal polyp.

Case 6. Medial Flexures and Persistence of Descending Mesocolon

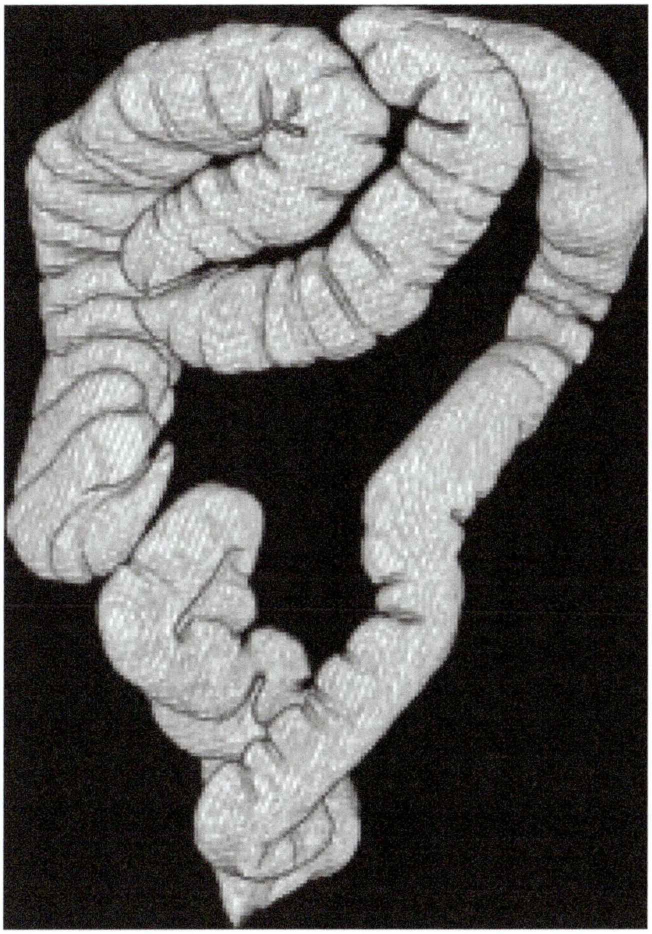

Fig. 6a 3D colon map (supine CTC acquisition)

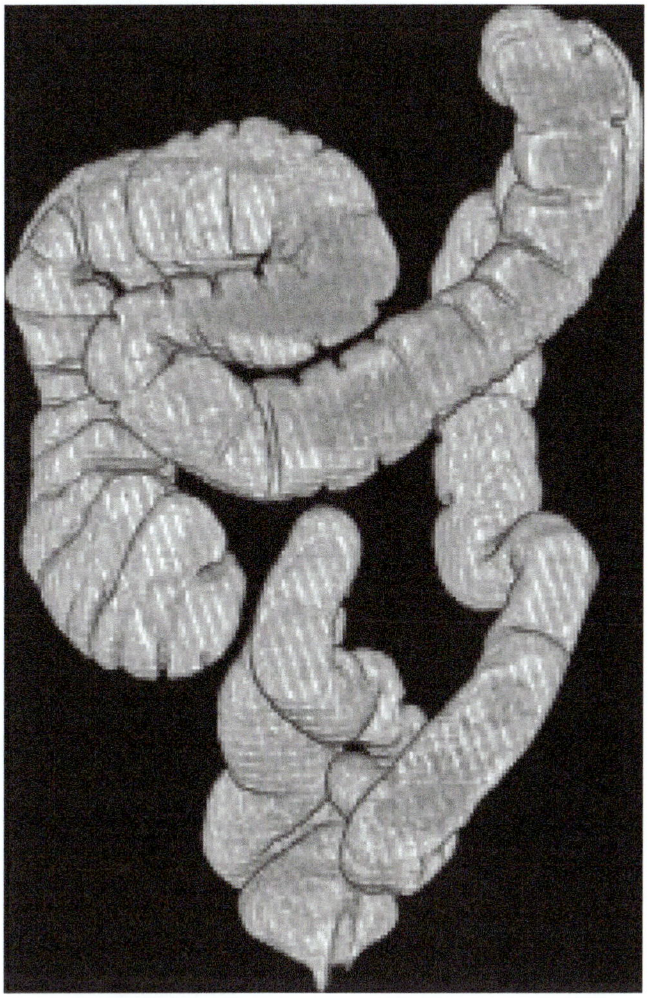

Fig. 6b 3D colon map (prone CTC acquisition)

Description

Screening CTC examination in an asymptomatic patient.

Abnormal position of hepatic and splenic flexures. Note the different position of the left descending colon in the supine (Fig. 6a) and prone acquisition (Fig. 6b); in the latter the splenic flexure lies in a slightly reverse position (Fig. 6b), and the descending colon is located more medially than in the supine decubitus (Figs. 6a and 6b). The upper segment of the left colon is the only movable one in this patient, indicating persistence of a descending mesocolon, while its caudal segment and the sigmoid colon are on the right side (close to the cecum) due to a low attachment of the left colon (Figs. 6a and 6b).

Case 7. Variant of Splenic Flexure

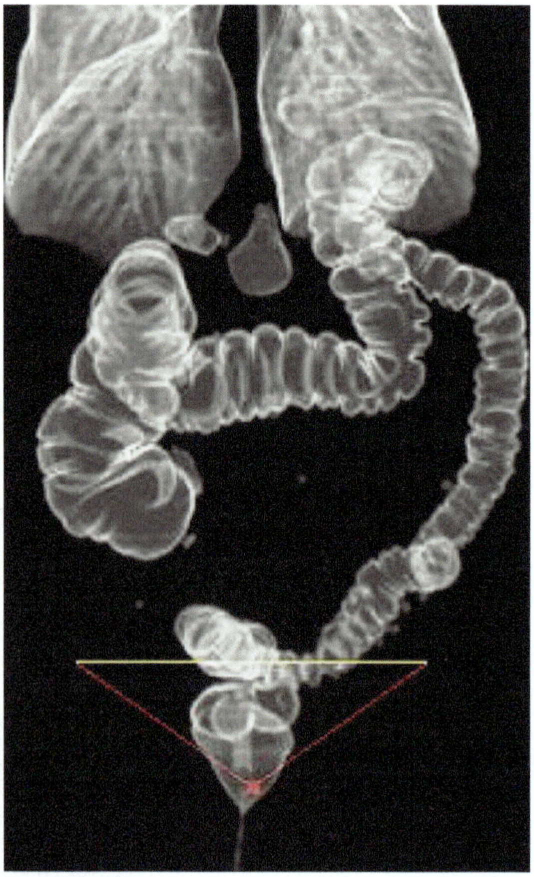

Fig. 7a 3D colon map

Description

Incomplete colonoscopy. Slightly reversed splenic flexure with normal position of the descending colon. Fixed and very close colonic angles are well-known causes of incomplete colonoscopy, yet all colonic segments are well distended at CTC, thus enabling its optimal exploration. The final position of the splenic flexure depends on the rotation of the distal midgut, the return of the jejunal loops to the left upper quadrant, the development of an open colonic angle, and the mesenteric fixation following the rotation process.

Case 8. Abnormal Transverse Colon

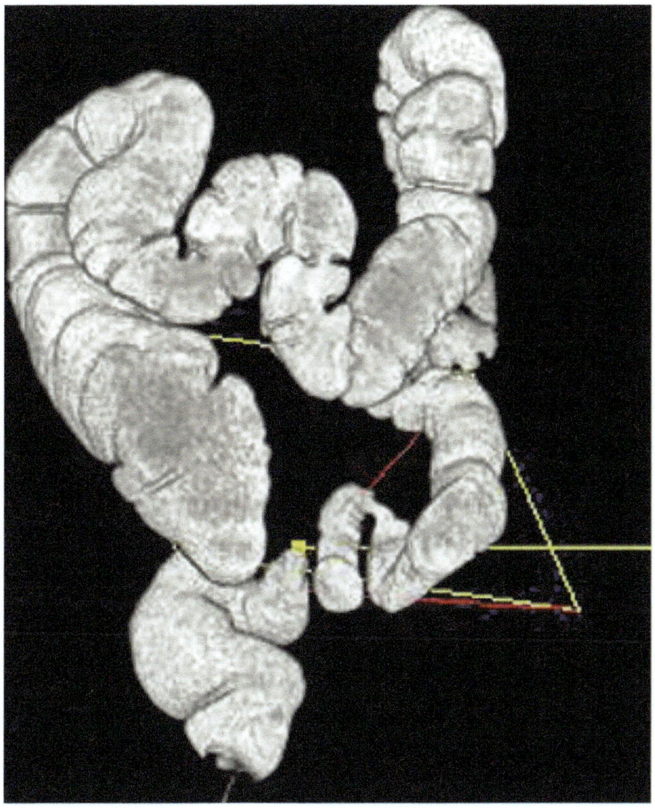

Fig. 8a Rotated 3D colon map in the supine position

Description

CTC for CRC screening shows a redundant transverse colon with a supernumerary flexure in the middle transverse colon (Fig. 8a). This anatomical variant may lead to confuse this loop with the hepatic flexure at optical colonoscopy if the real colonic anatomy of the patient is unknown.

Case 9. Abnormal Transverse Colon and Flat Rectal Lesion

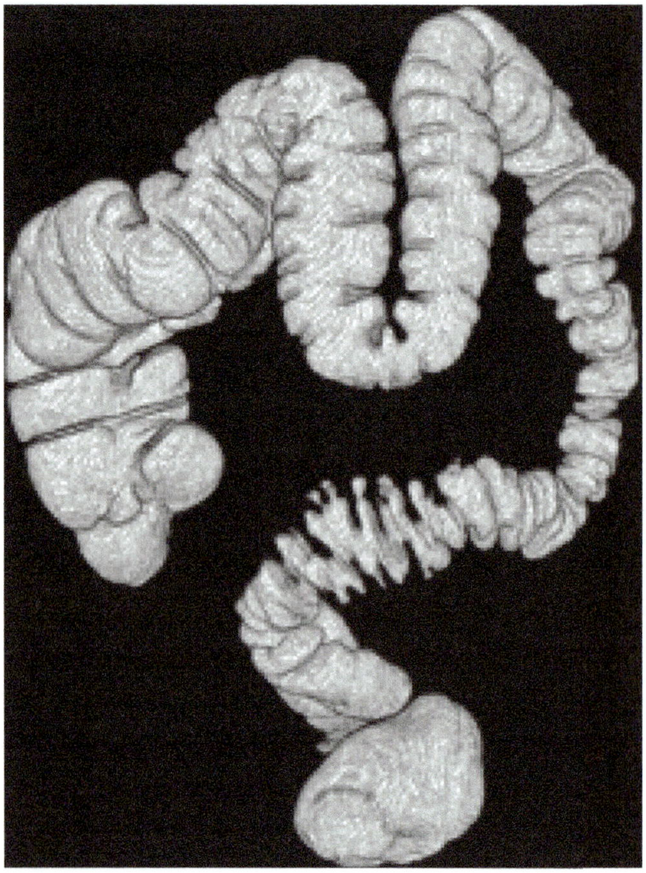

Fig. 9a 3D colon map (supine acquisition)

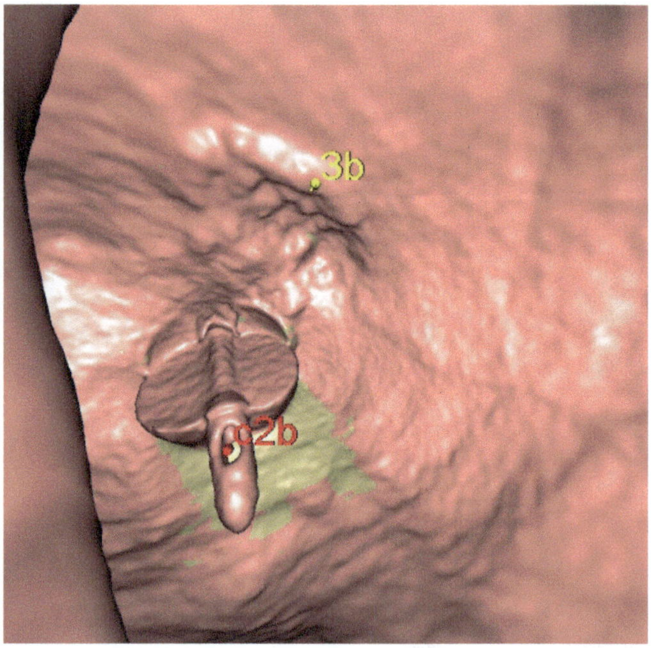

Fig. 9b CTC, virtual endoscopy of the rectum

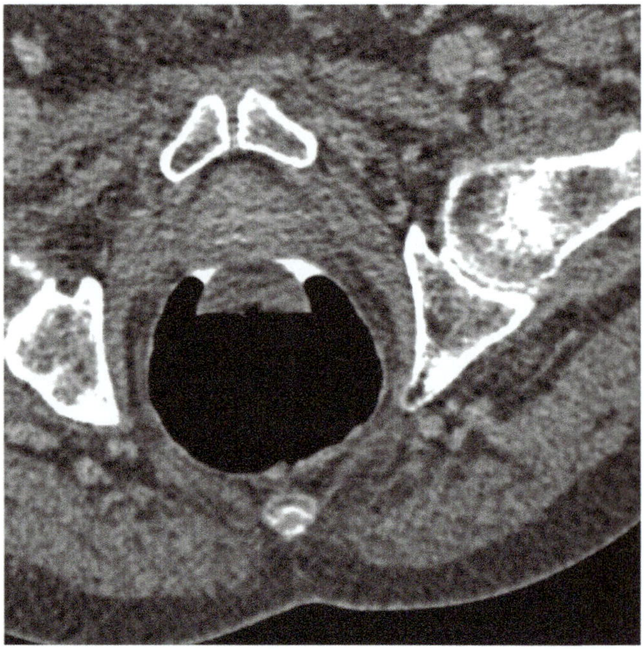

Fig. 9c Axial CTC at rectal level

Description

A 45-year-old man with moderate risk of CRC complaining about intermittent abdominal pain. Two previous incomplete optical colonoscopy examinations performed within the last 5 years revealed diverticular disease of the sigmoid colon without further abnormalities.

The 3D colon map (Fig. 9a) shows a redundant transverse colon with a caudally oriented U-shaped close angle of its mid portion (note the difference against Fig. 8a, underscoring the variability in the process of colonic rotation and fixation). Typical diverticular disease of the sigmoid colon (Fig. 9a). Optical colonoscopy performed 6 months before did not detect the rectal flat carpet lesion that is shown on CTC virtual endoscopic views (Fig. 9b) close to the rectal tube; notice the irregularity of the inner colonic surface with a carpet morphology marked as "3b." Axial CTC image shows a circumscribed thickening of the posterior rectal wall (less than 3 mm) (Fig. 9c). Second-look optical colonoscopy confirmed the presence of a flat villous adenoma without dysplasia.

Case 10. Paracolic Left Fossa

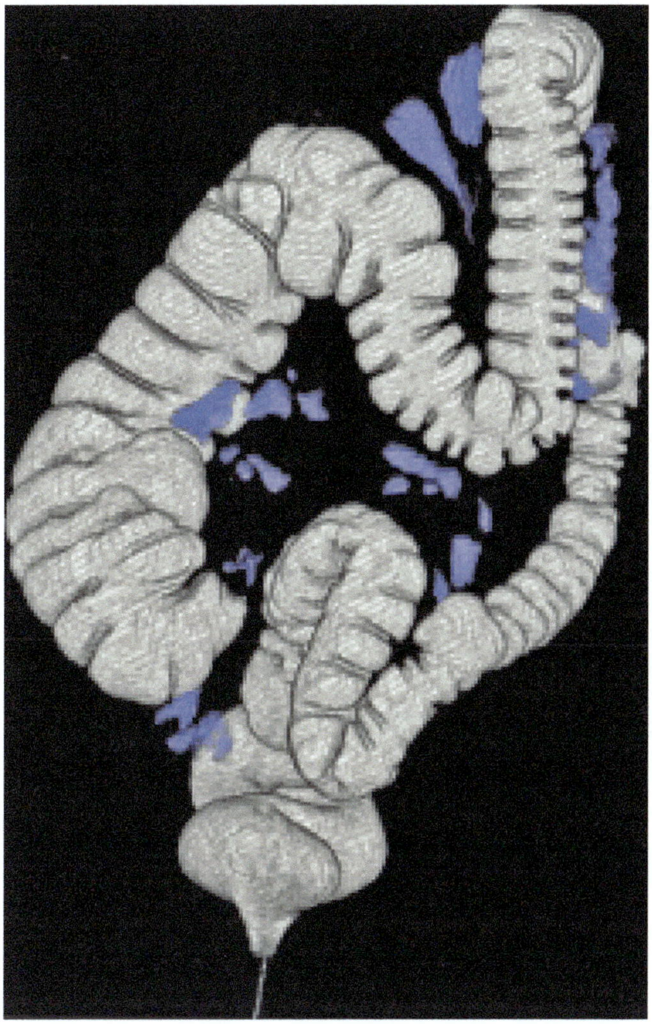

Fig. 10a 3D colon map (supine acquisition)

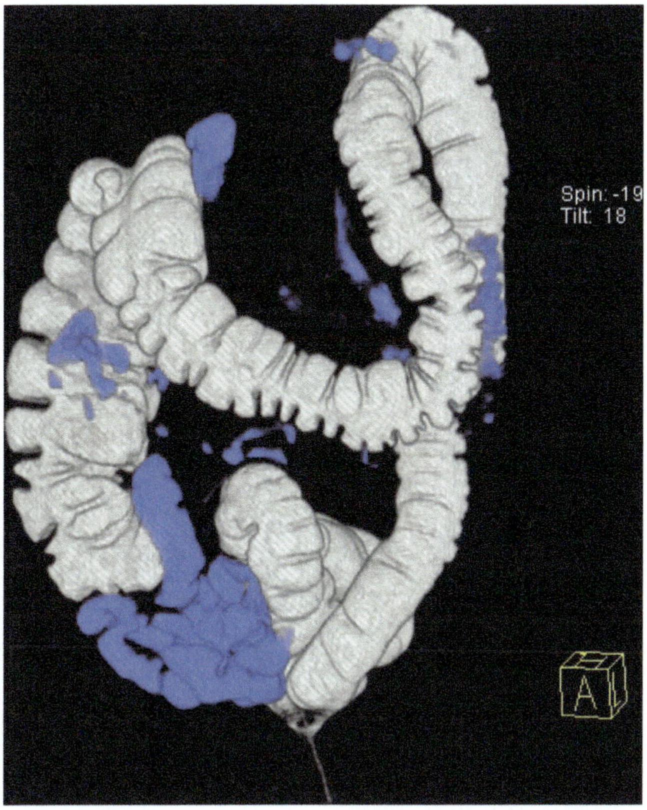

Fig. 10b 3D colon map (prone acquisition)

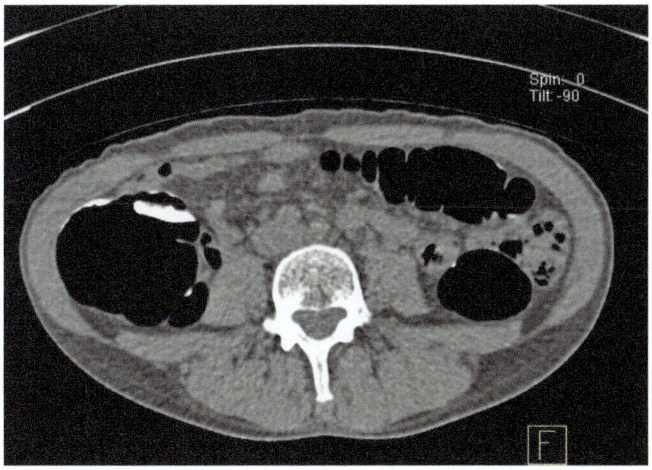

Fig. 10c Axial CTC image acquired in the prone position

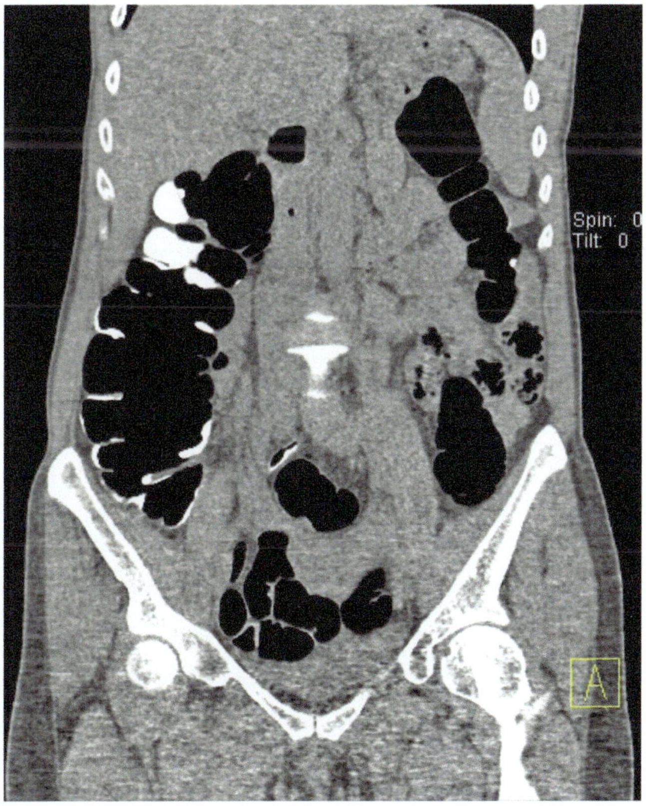

Fig. 10d Coronal MPR

Description

CTC performed for CRC screening after incomplete colonoscopy.

Note the low fixation of the splenic flexure (Fig. 10a) and the position of the descending colon, which is slightly displaced medially in a short segment just above the iliac bone. This latter finding is more evident in the prone position, with a highly movable distal left colon descending into the lower pelvis (Fig. 10b), suggesting a persistent descending mesocolon with a fixed point between those two segments. Axial CTC in the prone decubitus shows small bowel loops placed lateral to the descending colon, outside the colonic frame (Fig. 10c). Coronal MPR shows a paracolic left small fossa occupied by small bowel loops (Fig. 10d). Presence of the paracolic fossa is associated to persistent mesocolon, probably related to adhesions and free space due to movable left colon. The abdominal compression induced by the prone position helped demonstrate the atypical location of the small bowel.

Case 11. Movable Right Colon and Paracolic Right Fossa

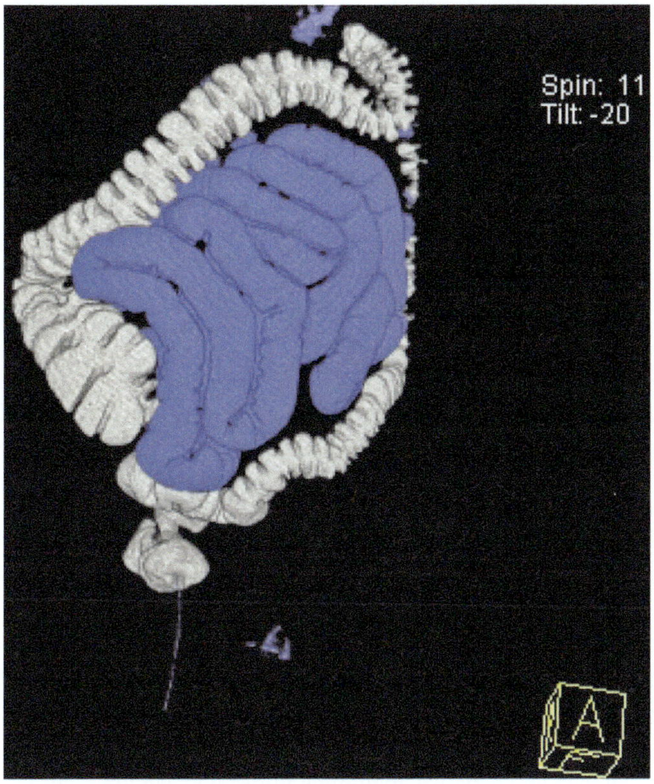

Fig. 11a 3D colon map (supine acquisition). Anterior view

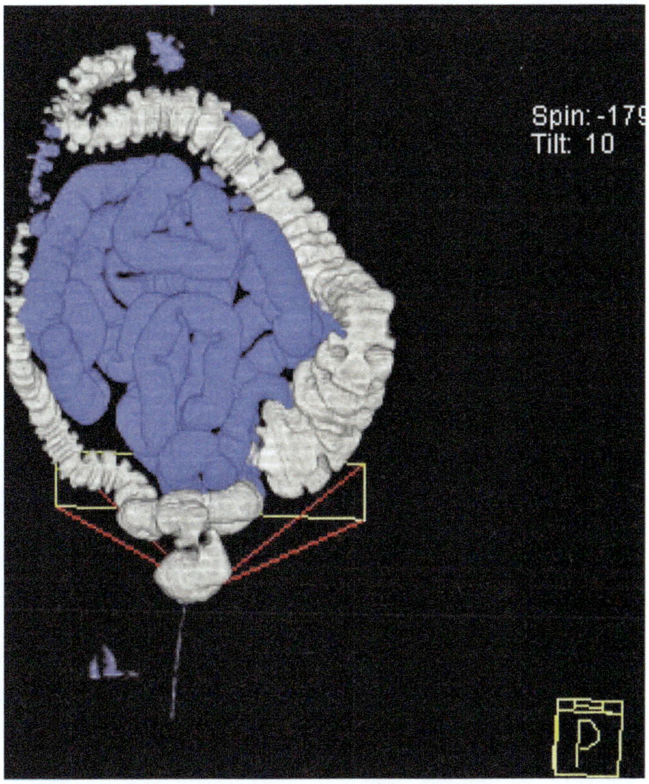

Fig. 11b 3D colon map (supine acquisition). Posterior view

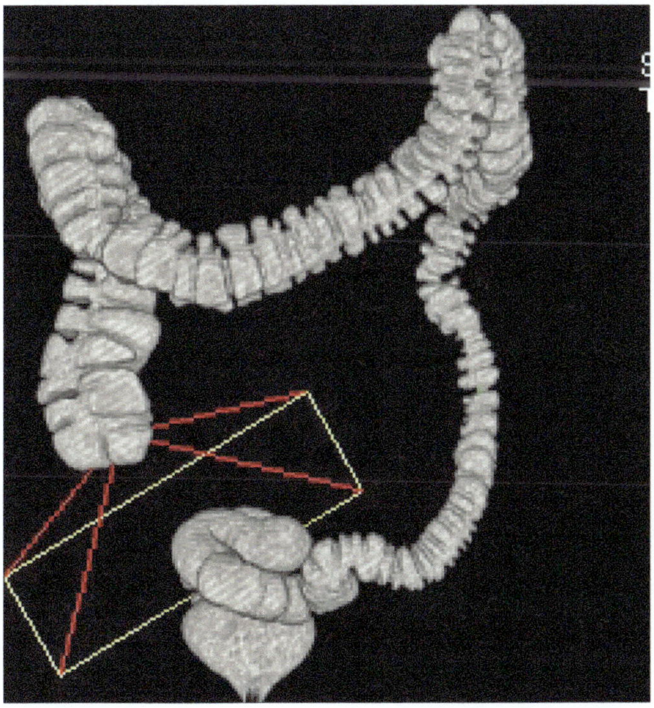

Fig. 11c 3D colon map (prone position). Anterior view

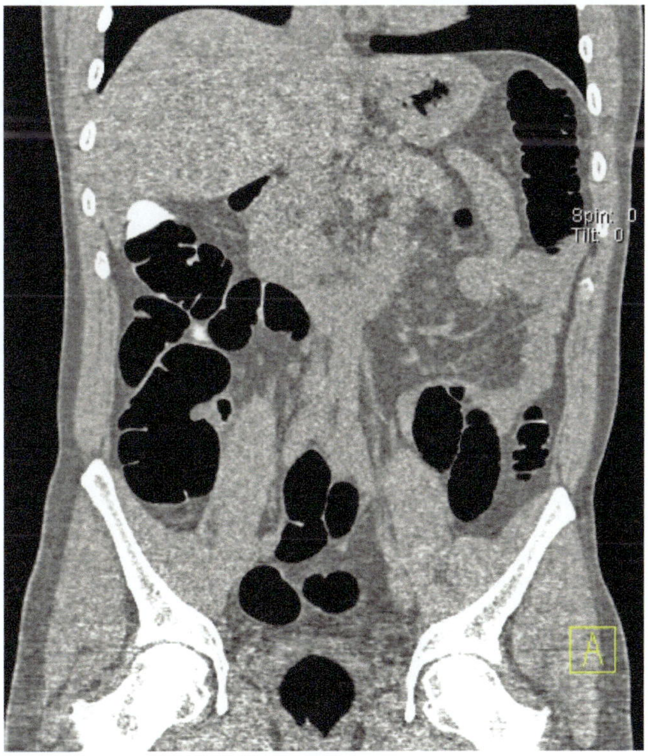

Fig. 11d Coronal MPR image (prone acquisition)

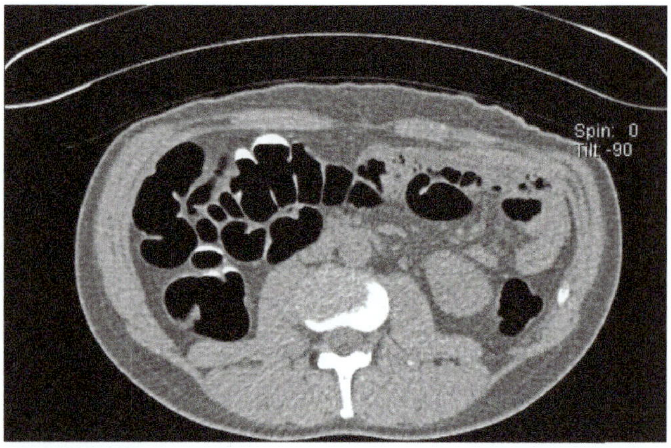

Fig. 11e Axial CTC (prone position)

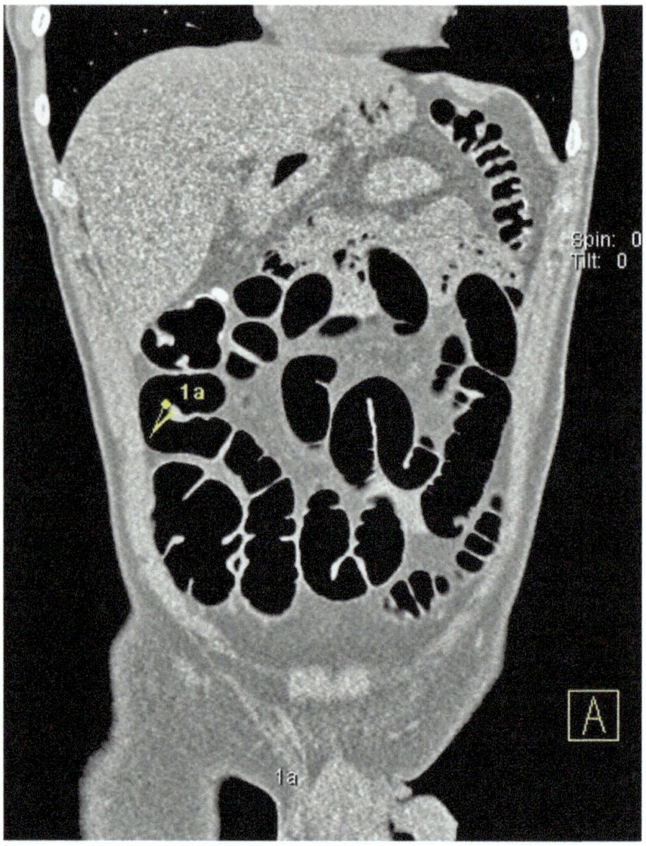

Fig. 11g Coronal MPR (supine acquisition)

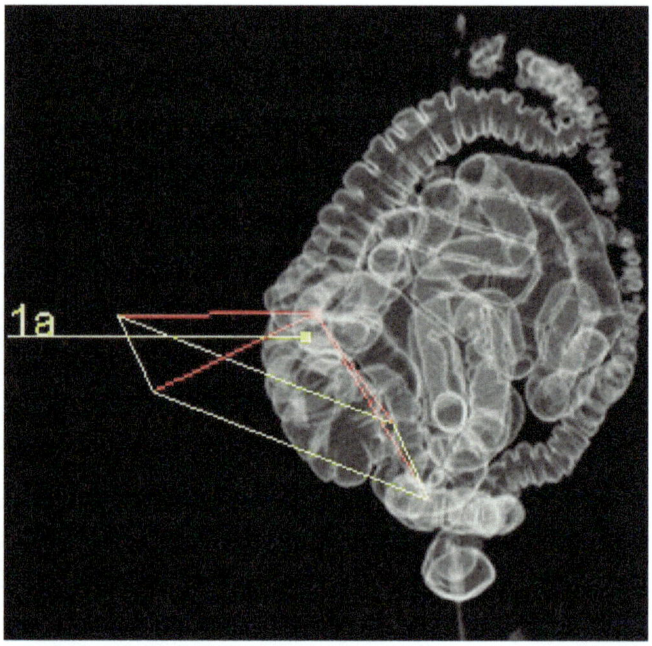

Fig. 11f Double contrast CTC (supine acquisition)

Description

Adult male with acute, intermittent onset of upper right abdominal pain and negative abdominal ultrasound examination.

In the supine 3D colon map, the ascending colon and the cecum have an anterior and slightly medial location (Fig. 11a); note that small bowel loops are very close to the hepatic flexure also in the posterior supine view (Fig. 11b). The hepatic flexure forms an open angle in the supine position and a very close one in the prone decubitus, in which the right colon is partially rotated and shows a reverse hepatic flexure (Fig. 11c). Coronal MPR in the prone position (Fig. 11d) shows a small bowel loop outside the colonic frame; axial CTC image in the prone position (Fig. 11e) clearly shows the right paracolic fossa. Note that the latter is less evident in the supine decubitus due to the position of the right colon (Figs. 11f and 11g). Right mesocolon persistence is a risk factor for the development of a full or partial volvulus of the cecum and the right colon, depending on the degree of mesocolon laxity.

Case 12. Colonic Malrotation and Compression by Iliac Vessels

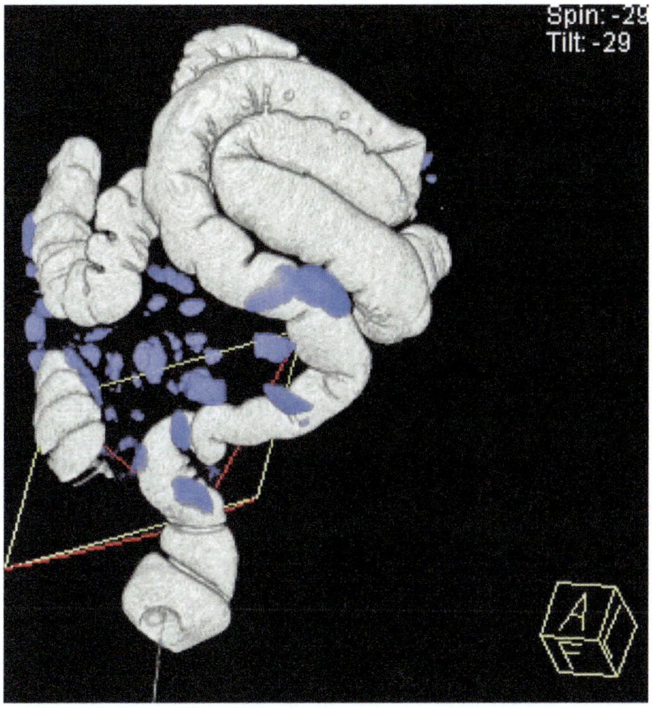

Fig. 12a 3D map of colon

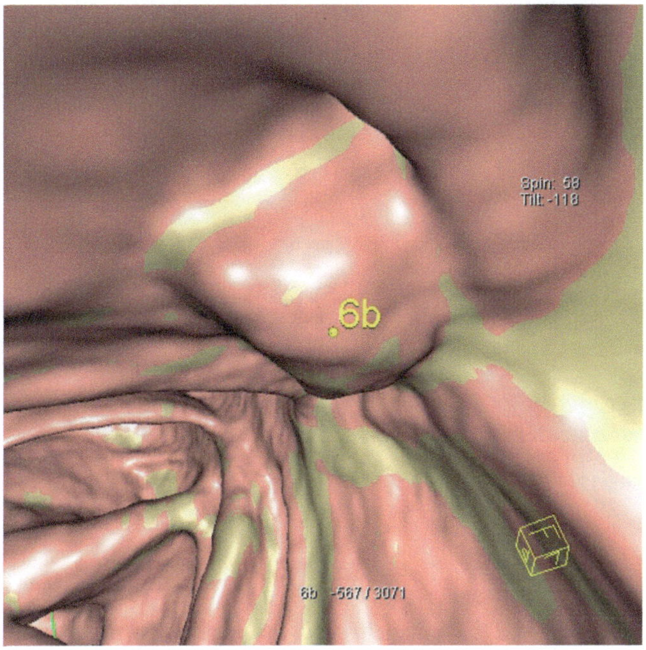

Fig. 12b Endoscopic view

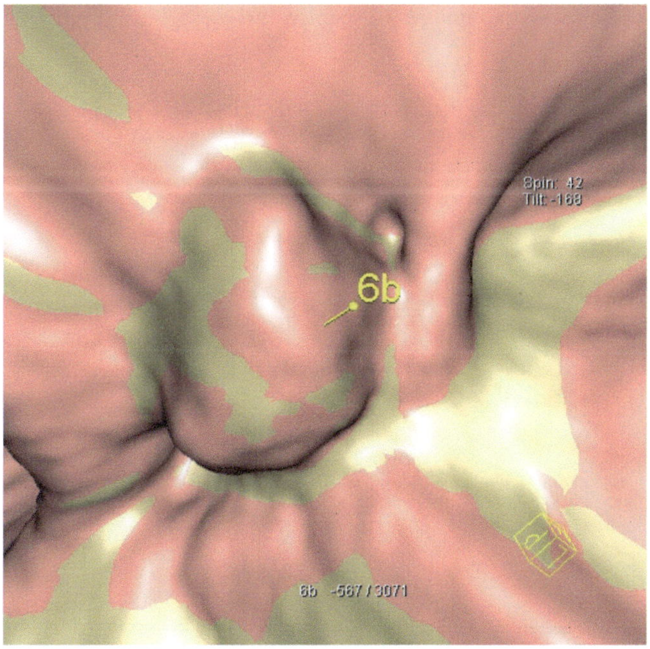

Fig. 12c Endoscopic view

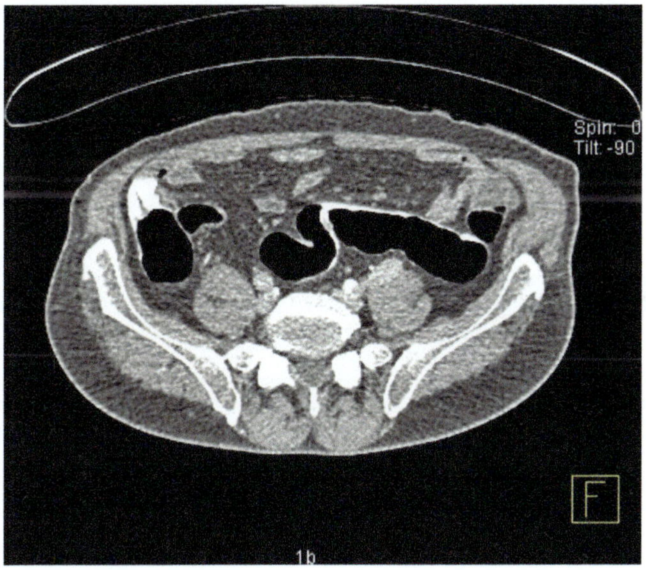

Fig. 12d Axial imagen

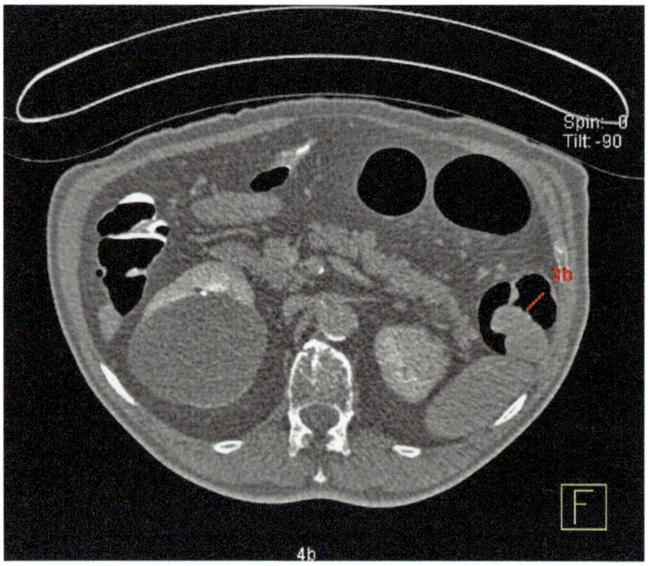

Fig. 12e Axial imagen

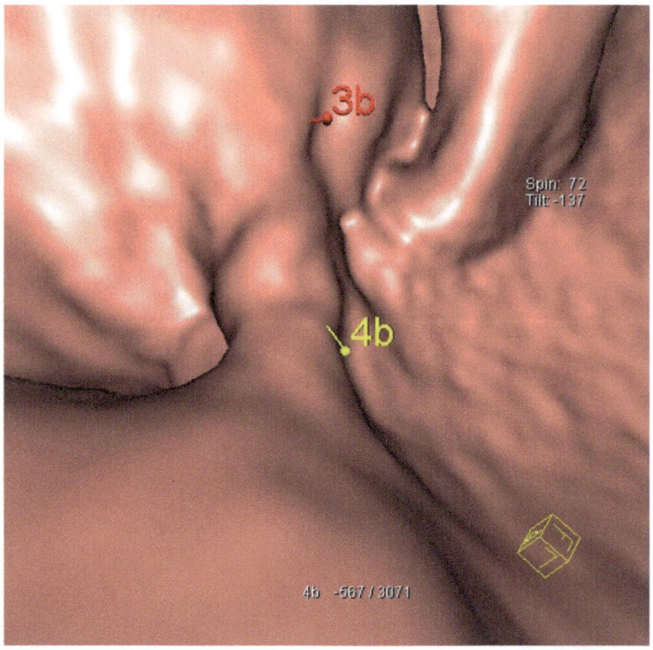

Fig. 12f Endoscopic view

Description

Screening CTC in patient with average CRC risk. Note extreme redundancy of the left colon characterized by an apparently double splenic flexure with reverse and non-reverse angles and a descending colon placed in a nearly medial position (Fig. 12a), which are related to partial malrotation and abnormal fixation of the left mesocolon. The inner view shows a mass protruding in the lumen of the sigmoid colon (Figs. 12b and 12c, marked as 6b), notice presence of a straight border (Fig. 12b), suggesting a pseudopolyp. Axial CTC image clearly shows compression of the transverse tract of the sigmoid colon by the iliac vessels (Fig. 12d). There is a true polyp with a large stalk in the left descending colon (Figs. 12e, 12f, polyp marked as "3b" and "4b" in the axial and endoscopic images, respectively).

Case 13. Colonic Compression by Ribs

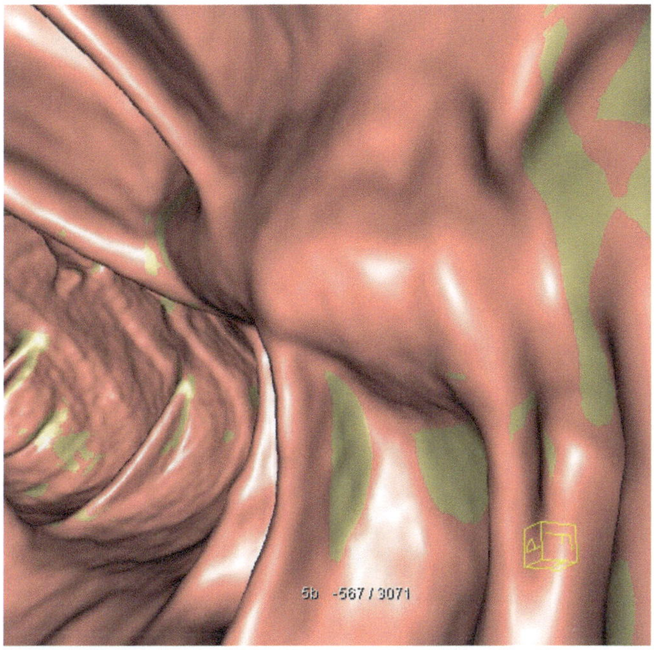

Fig. 13a Endoscopic view

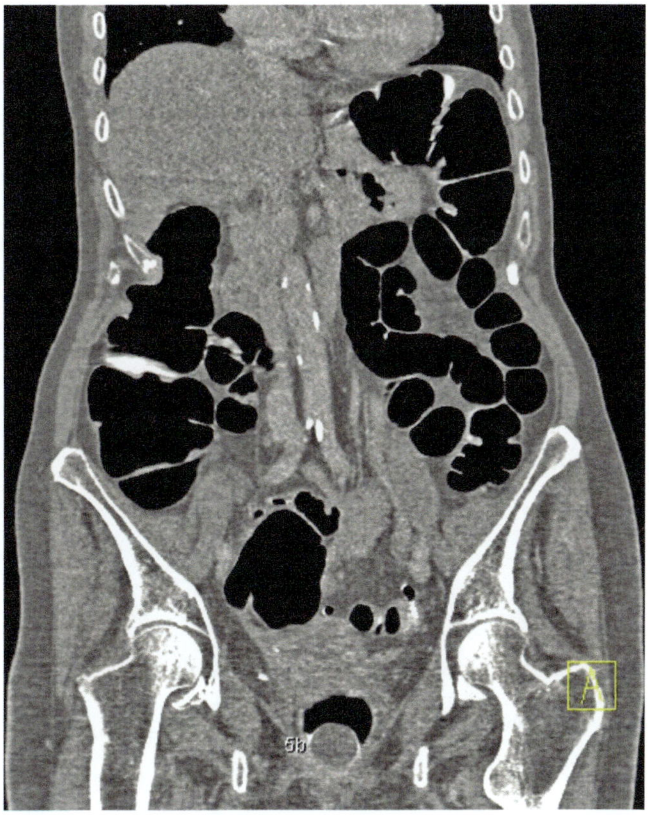

Fig. 13b Coronal MPR

Description

An elongated mass protruding toward the right colonic lumen (Fig. 13a) is due to external compression by a floating rib, as nicely shown by the coronal MPR view (Fig. 13b).

Case 14. Bilateral Renal Compression of the Colon

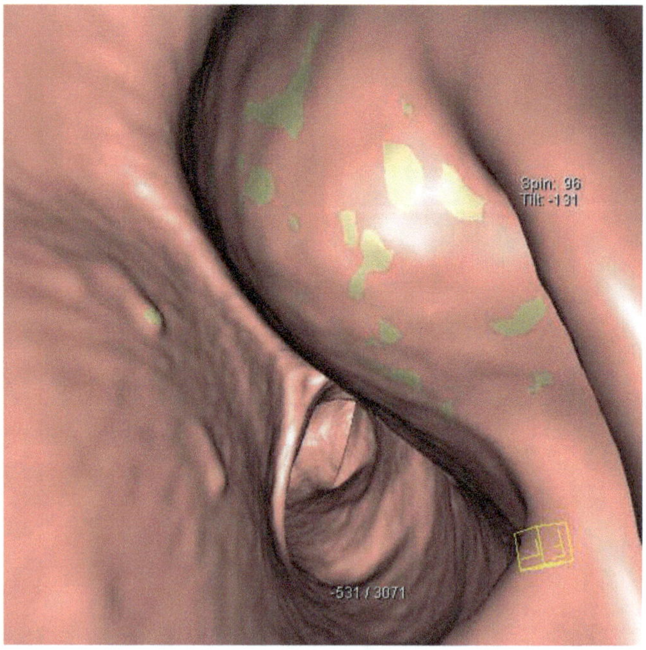

Fig. 14a Inner view of left colon

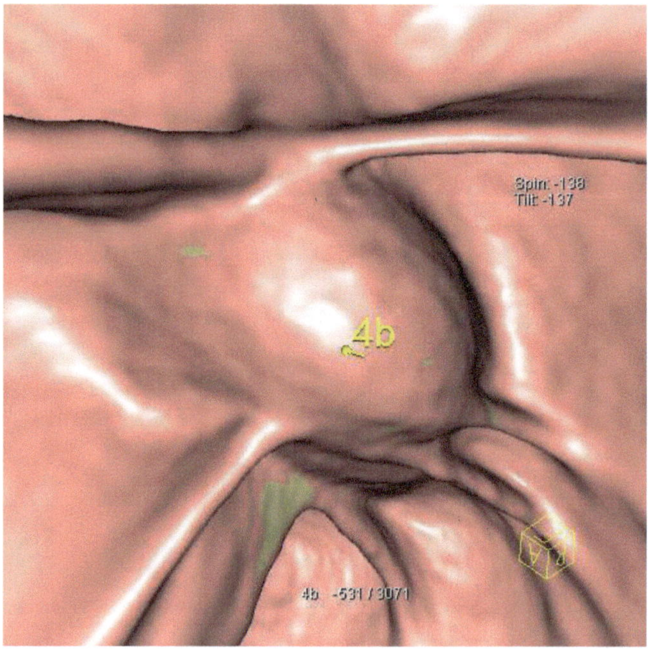

Fig. 14b Inner view of the right colon

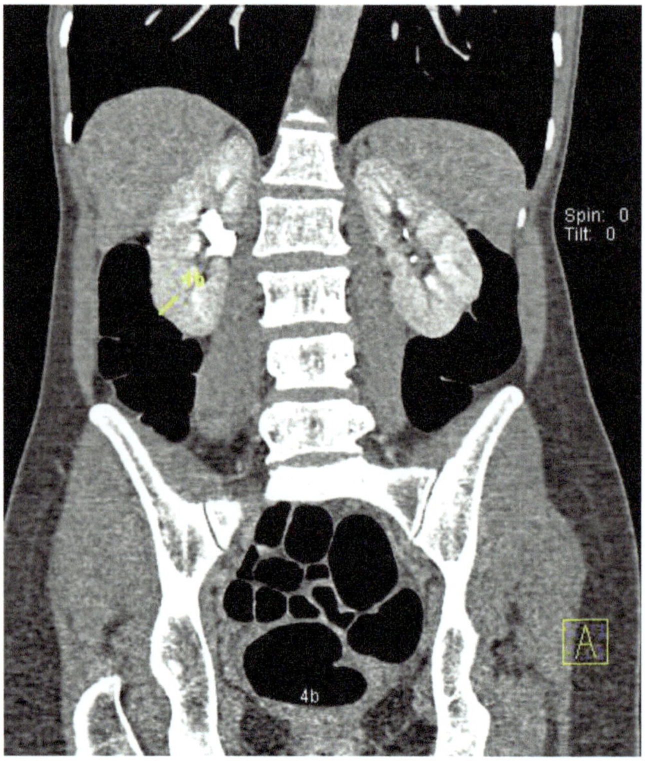

Fig. 14c Coronal MPR in prone position

Description

Bilateral masses with smooth borders impressing the left (Fig. 14a) and right colonic walls (Fig. 14b) due to bilateral renal compression, as shown by MPR views (Fig. 14c).

Case 15. Colon Redundancy and Multiple Polyps

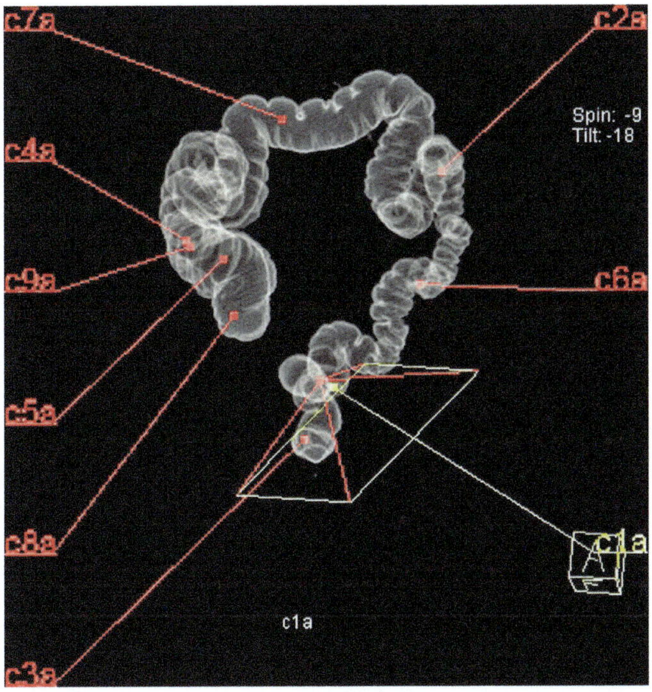

Fig. 15a Double contrast-like 3D colon map with several polyp markings

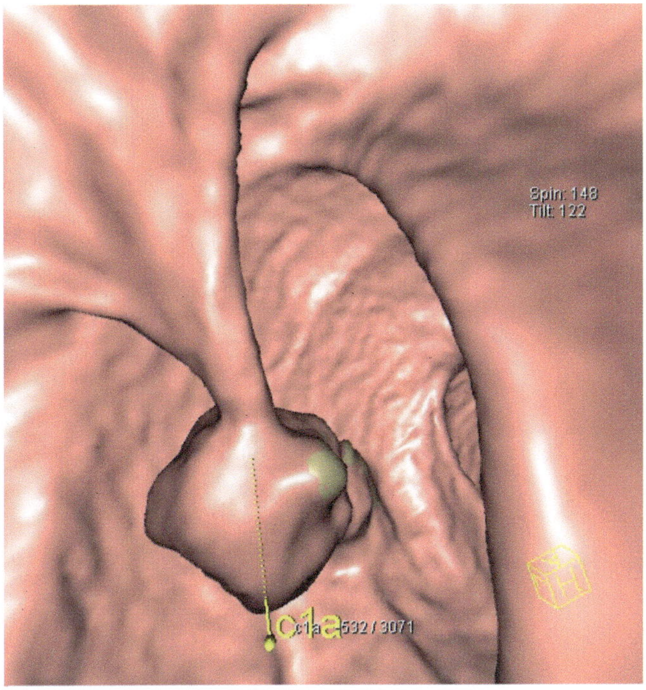

Fig. 15b Inner view of the sigmoid colon

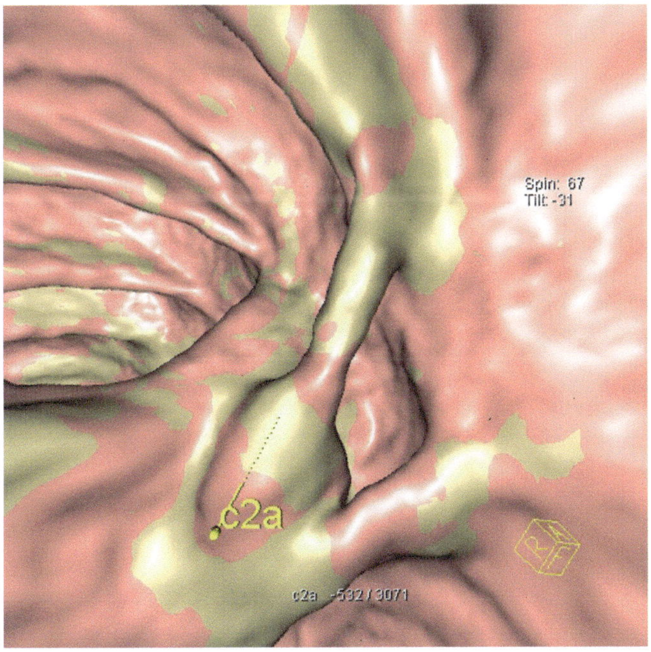

Fig. 15c Inner view of the descending colon distal to the splenic flexure

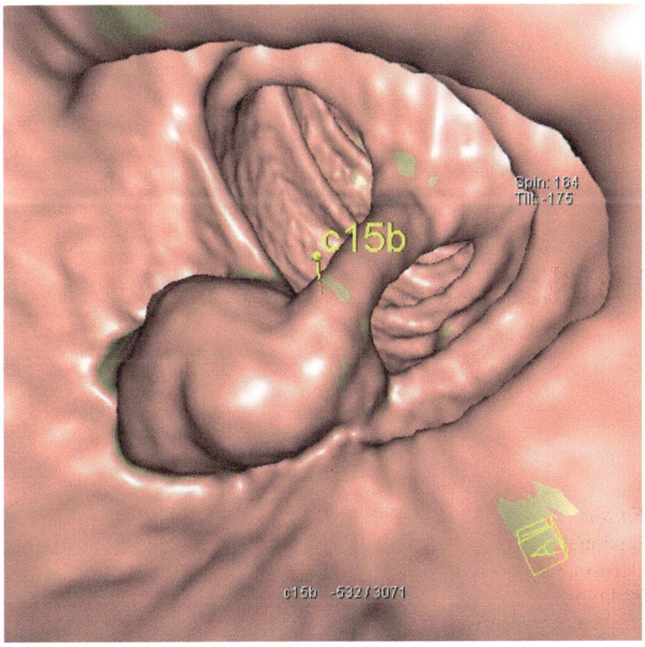

Fig. 15d Inner view of the descending colon (prone position)

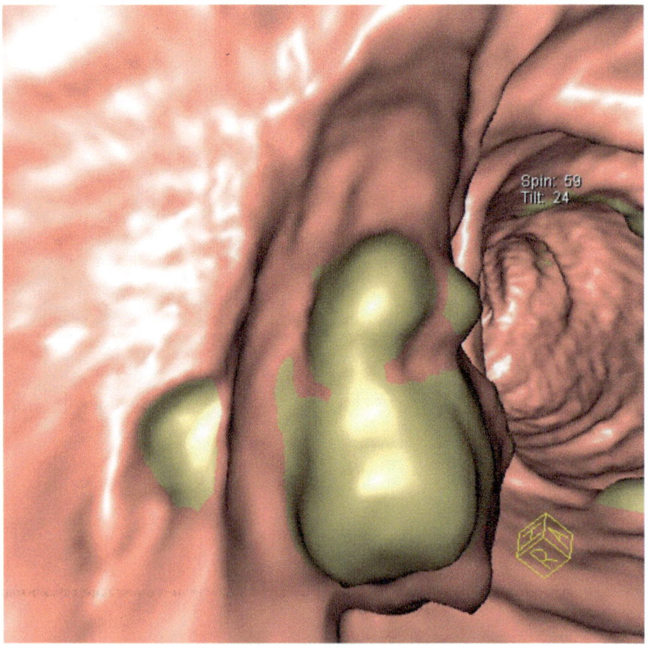

Fig. 15e Inner view of the proximal hepatic flexure

Description

Screening CTC shows a peculiar morphology of flexures with redundancy of the left flexure (a short horizontal segment of the transverse colon has a high position in the abdominal cavity) and a reverse hepatic flexure (Fig. 15a). CAD marks several polyps with head diameter larger than 1 cm, nearly all of which with large stalks (Figs. 15b, 15c, and 15d). A broad-based mass with nodular surface partially covered with tagged residual stool (yellow) was detected at the hepatic flexure (Fig. 15e). Biopsy revealed adenocarcinoma.

References

1. Vaos G, Misiakos EP (2010) Congenital anomalies of the gastrointestinal tract diagnosed in adulthood – diagnosis and management. J Gastrointest Surg 14(5):916–925
2. Berrocal T, Lamas M, Gutieerrez J, Torres I, Prieto C, del Hoyo ML (1999) Congenital anomalies of the small intestine, colon, and rectum. Radiographics 19(5):1219–1236
3. Bider K, Kaim A, Wiesner W, Bongartz G (2001) Acute appendicitis in a young adult with midgut malrotation: a case report. Eur Radiol 11(7):1171–1174

Pitfalls in Imaging

Philippe Lefere and Stefaan Gryspeerdt

Contents

Abstract

Interpretation of CT colonography frequently is difficult because of imaging pitfalls. These pitfalls may be a source of false negative and false positive findings. The pictorial review in this chapter focuses on some important issues of colonic imaging with CT colonography and at each time proposes a solution.

P. Lefere (✉) • S. Gryspeerdt
Virtual Colonoscopy Teaching Centre (VCTC),
Akkerstraat 32c, B-8830 Hooglede, Belgium
e-mail: radiologie@skynet.be, www.vctc.eu

E. Neri et al. (eds.), *CT Colonography Atlas*, Medical Radiology,
DOI 10.1007/978-3-642-11149-5_3, © Springer-Verlag Berlin Heidelberg 2013

Case 1. Preparation

Problem

For adequate interpretation of CT colonography, the patient needs a preparation leaving the colon as clean and dry as possible. This can be achieved with a 1-day preparation. However, despite intensive colonic cleansing, frequently colonic residue remains in the colon. This residue is sometimes easy to characterise because of air inclusions and positional shift between the supine and prone acquisition. However, in case of sticky solid colonic residue, there is no positional shift nor is there any air inclusion. This may result in a false-positive interpretation with pseudopolypoid images (Fig. 1a, b).

Solution

To perform state-of-the-art CT colonography, the preparation should include a combination of a low-residue diet, laxative or cathartic products, and faecal tagging the day before CT colonography. Catharsis can be obtained with sodium phosphate or magnesium citrate. Faecal tagging is performed with barium and/or iodine. Faecal tagging consists of drinking positive contrast material during the meals the day before CT colonography. This results in labelling the colonic contents in the colon and is called stool and fluid tagging. Stool tagging allows for easy differentiation between hyperdense solid stool and a true polyp (Fig. 2). Fluid tagging allows for detecting polyps in hyperdense fluid (Figs. 3a, b and 8a, b).

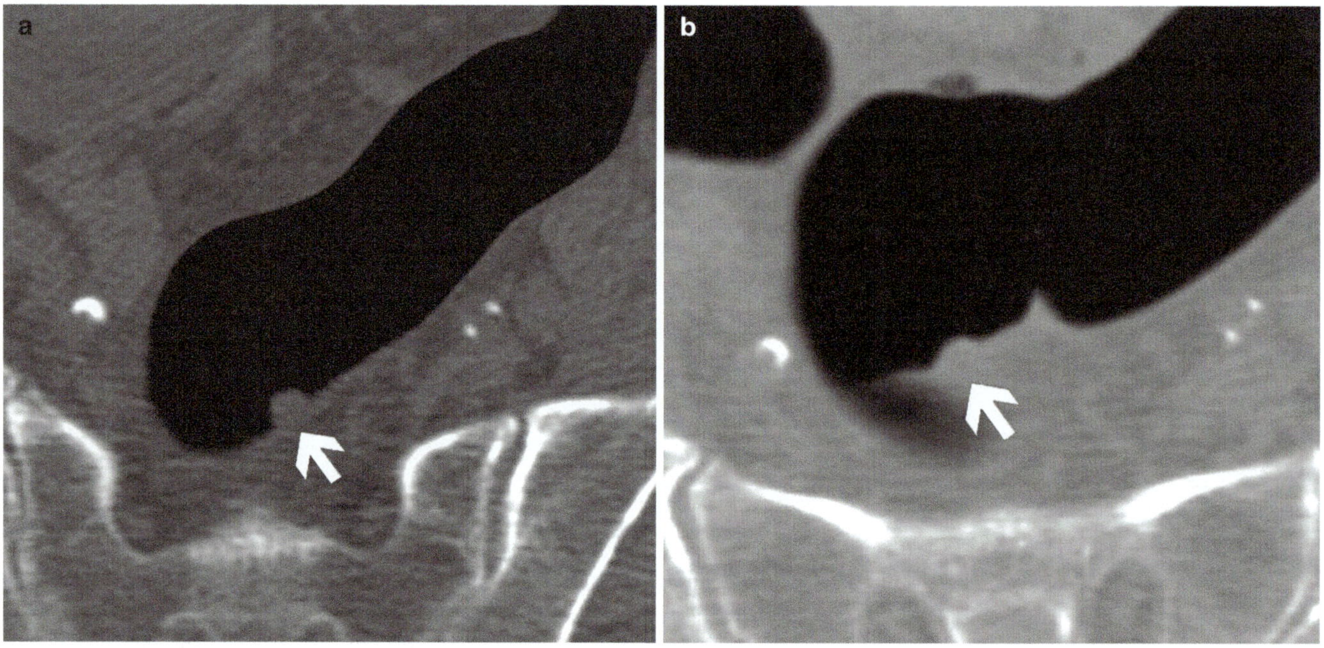

Fig. 1a and b Patient prepared without faecal tagging: 8-mm sessile defect in the distal sigmoid in supine (**a**) and prone (**b**) acquisition (*white arrow*): no air inclusion, no positional shift, slight change in shape. Polyp? Residual stool? The exact diagnosis cannot be made on these images. Optical colonoscopy is necessary to confirm or exclude a lesion. No lesion was detected. Faecal tagging would have avoided optical colonoscopy in this patient

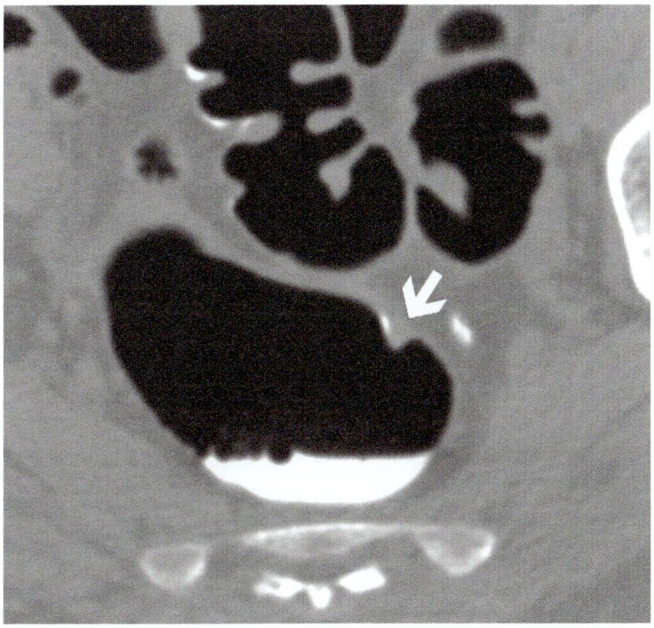

Fig. 2 Rectum: 7-mm sessile polyp with some tagged residue

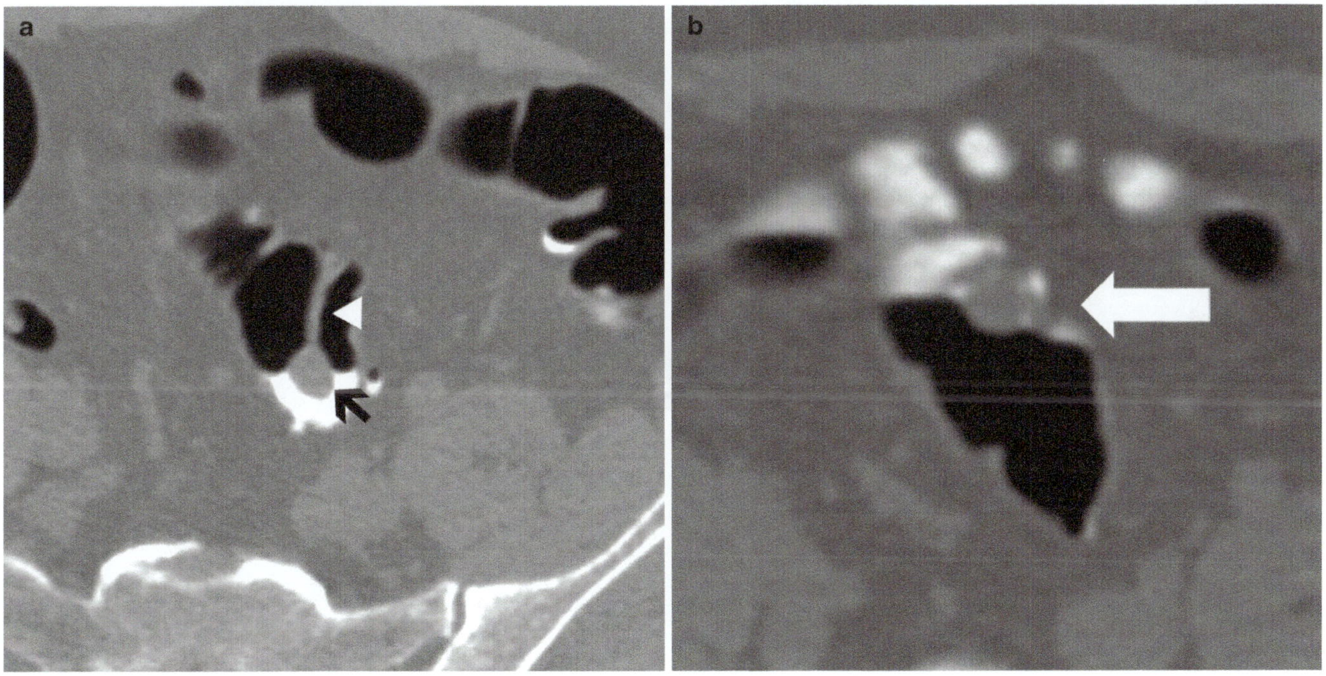

Fig. 3a and b Sigmoid: pedunculated polyp with thin stalk and 11 mm head (*black arrow*), partially submerged in tagged fluid in supine (*white arrowhead*, **a**) and totally submerged in prone position (*white arrow*, **b**)

Case 2. The Rectum

Problem

The colon starts at the anal margin. Being a closed structure with a wide lumen, the rectum is difficult to examine and needs our particular attention. Furthermore, visualisation of the rectum is hampered by the rectal catheter needed to insufflate the colon with carbon dioxide. The catheter is provided with an inflatable balloon preventing dislocation. The balloon may compress luminal defects against the rectal wall reducing their conspicuity significantly (Fig. 4a) and making inspection of the rectum more complicated.

Solution

Meticulous inspection, combining 3D and 2D visualisation techniques, with close inspection of the anal margin around the entrance point of the rectal tube is mandatory. This can be done by turning the virtual camera in retrograde direction to inspect the "peri-catheter" segment. To avoid compression of lesions by the balloon of the catheter, it is necessary to deflate the balloon immediately before starting the prone acquisition (Fig. 4b).

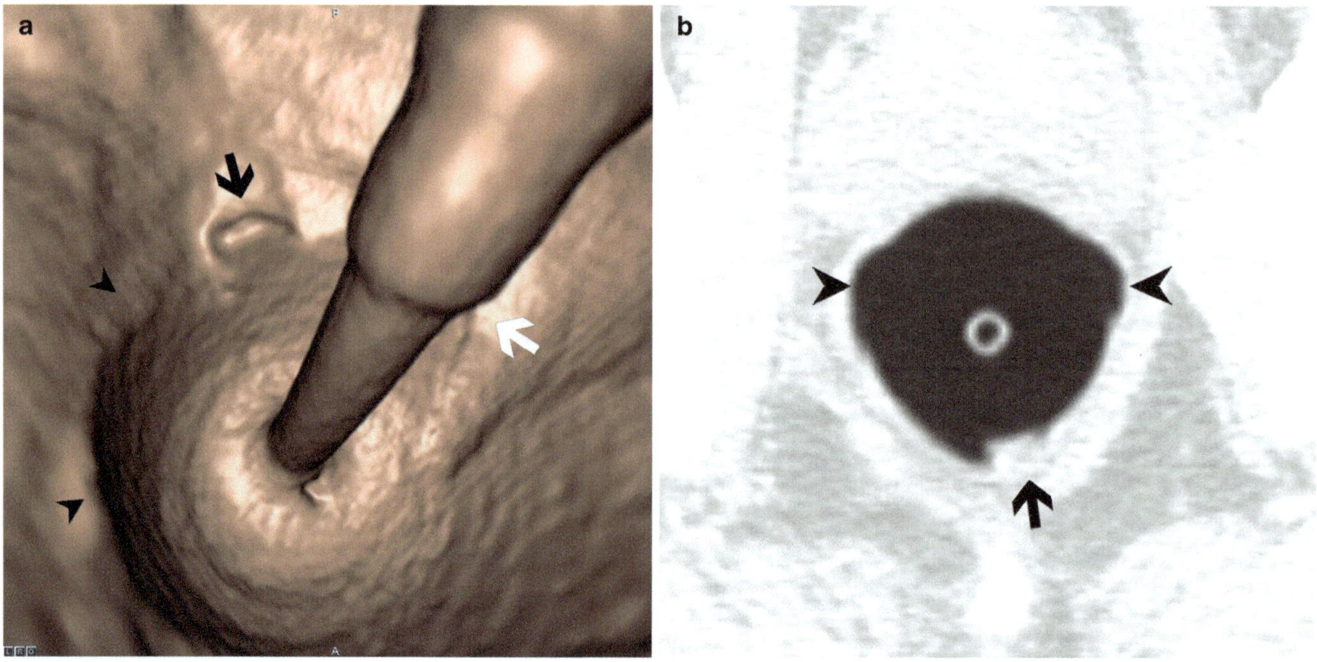

Fig. 4a and b Retrograde view (looking from cecum to rectum) of the rectum in supine position showing the rectal catheter (*white arrow*). As the balloon of the rectal catheter is inflated, its impression on the rectal wall is easily appreciated (*black arrowheads*). The balloon is also partly compressing a small luminal defect (*black arrow*)

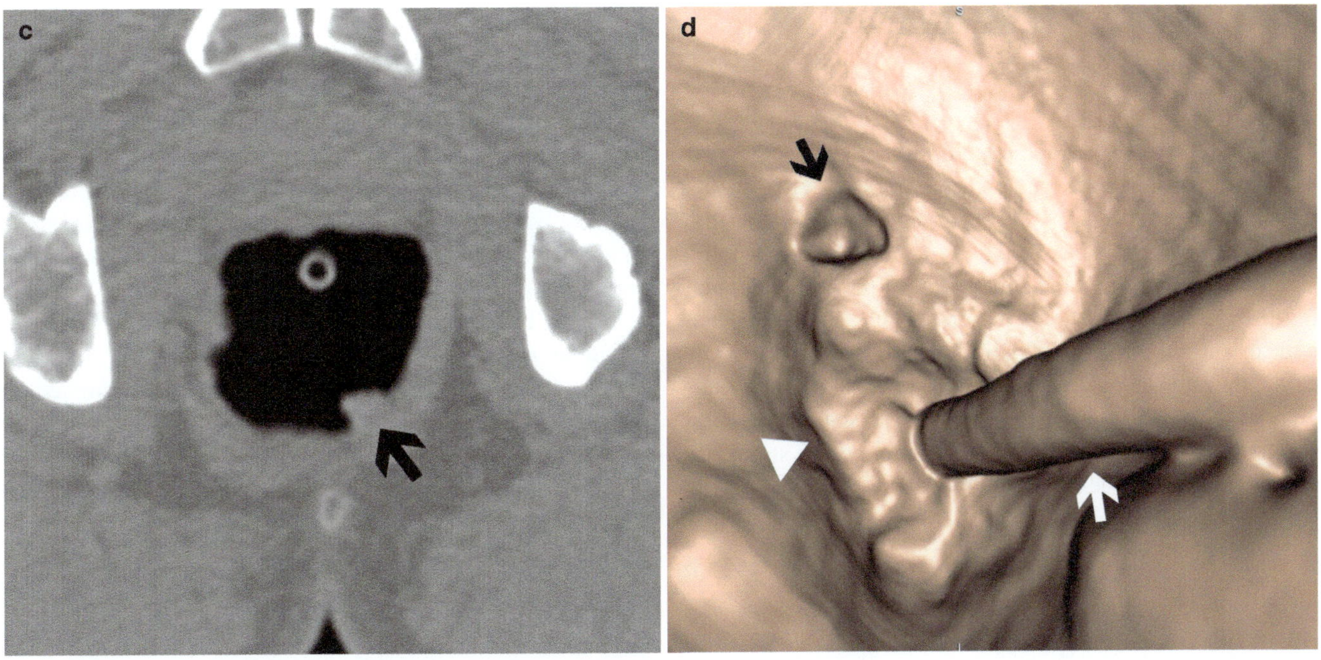

Fig. 4c and d In prone position, the balloon is deflated allowing better visualisation of the "peri-catheter" segment and revealing an 8-mm polyp (*black arrow*) and internal haemorrhoids (*white arrowhead*). Catheter (*white arrow*). Conclusion: always deflate the balloon before the second acquisition

Case 3. Spasm

Problem

The appearance of the colonic lumen is defined by 3 longitudinal external muscular bands, the taenia coli. They start at the sigmoid and end in the cecum where they converge towards the appendicular orifice. Being less prominent in the sigmoid, they give a round appearance of the colonic lumen. In the descending colon, the lumen also has a tubular aspect with more, although mostly subtle, folds. In the transverse colon, the taeniae become prominent and give a typical triangular aspect of the colonic lumen. This is also the case in the ascending colon. According to their contraction status, the colonic lumen will be more or less distended.

Solution

Optimal colonic distension is mandatory for correct interpretation of the CT colonography images. This can be obtained by combining smooth muscle relaxation, colonic insufflation with a CO_2 injector and dual positioning (i.e., acquisition in supine and prone position). Good distension flattens the semilunar folds and improves the visibility of the colonic wall. In case a spasm occurs, the shape of the colonic lumen is defined by the taenia coli: round in the sigmoid (Fig. 5a), round or slightly triangular in the descending colon, and clearly triangular in the transverse and ascending colon (Fig. 9a–d). In case of spasm, the folds mostly have a smooth and slightly thickened appearance. In 2D, they come closely together, appearing as "kissing folds" (Fig. 5b).

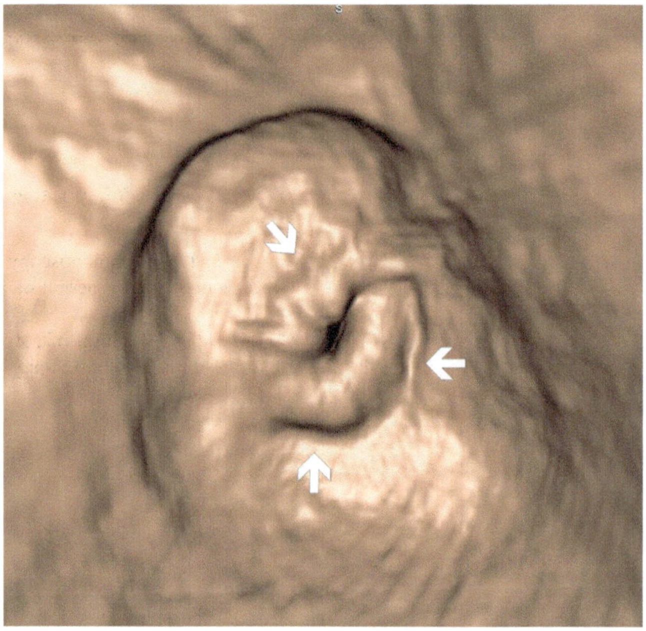

Fig. 5a Sigmoid colon: luminal narrowing with round appearance. Thickened folds with smooth aspect (*white arrows*)

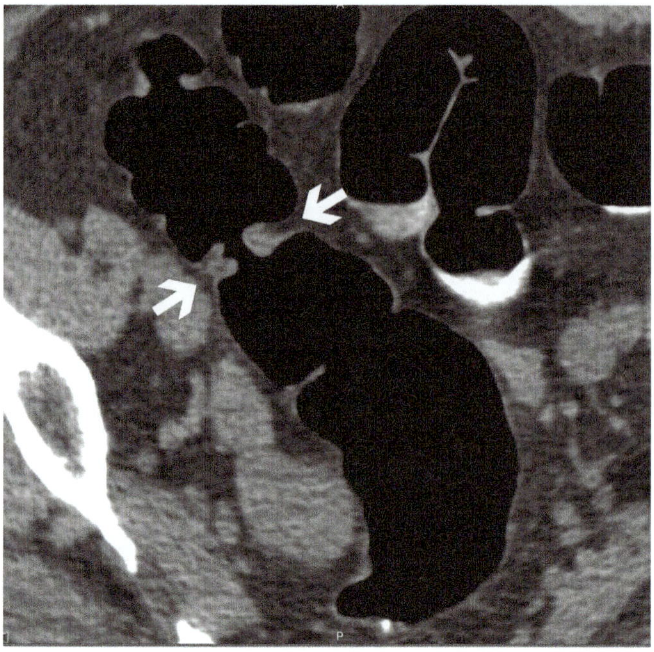

Fig. 5b The corresponding axial image shows the typical aspect of kissing folds: the slightly thickened folds are abutting each other (*white arrows*)

Case 4. Flexural Pseudotumour

Problem

Semilunar folds may mimic tumoral lesions. This is especially the case when they are located at the inner part of acute flexures. This thickening is called a flexural pseudotumour (Fig. 6a, b). The most typical locations are the hepatic and splenic flexures. However, as the colon varies in length, these thickened folds may occur wherever the colon makes an acute flexure. When this occurs, the pericolonic structures at the inner part of the flexure are compressed and cause a thickening of the fold. The thickening frequently presents with a lipomatous density representing the pericolonic structures. This thickening may have a pseudotumoral aspect and is sometimes very difficult to differentiate from a real malignant tumour (Fig. 7a–d).

Solution

It is important to know that the pericolonic structures are compressed at the inner part of a flexure causing thickening of the semilunar fold. In 3D, this thickening is regular and smooth. Frequently the thickened fold has a different aspect between the supine and prone acquisition (Fig. 6c).

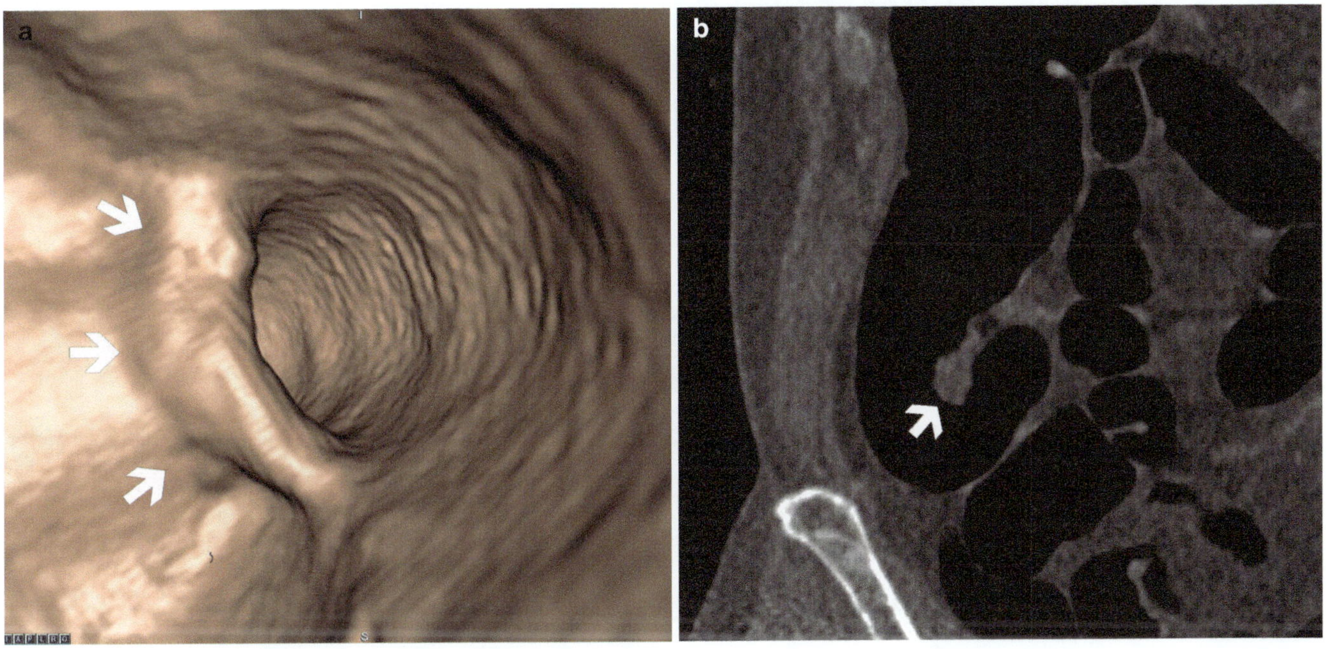

Fig. 6a and b Supine acquisition: antegrade view (from rectum to cecum) in the transverse colon showing thickening of a fold with a possible tumoral aspect (*white arrows*). The corresponding coronal reformat shows the fold is located at the inner part of an acute flexure of the transverse colon. It has a slightly hypodense texture

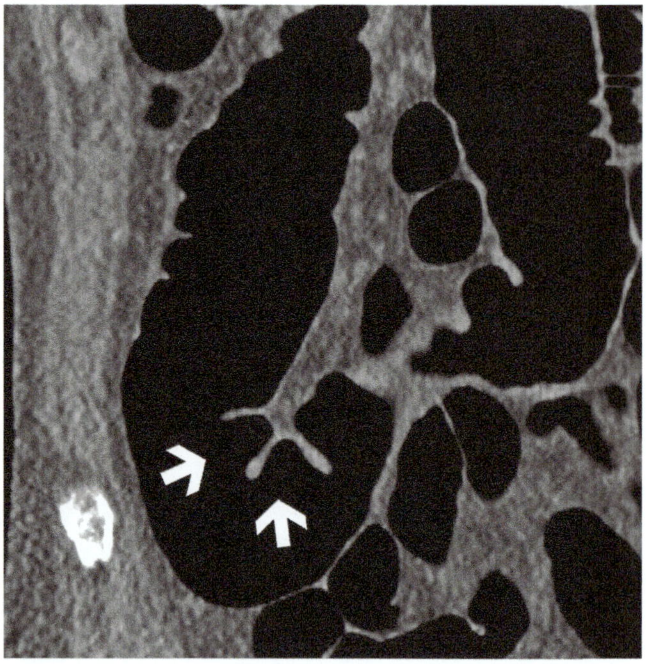

Fig. 6c The corresponding coronal reformat of the prone acquisition shows normal folds at the same flexure excluding any tumoral lesion

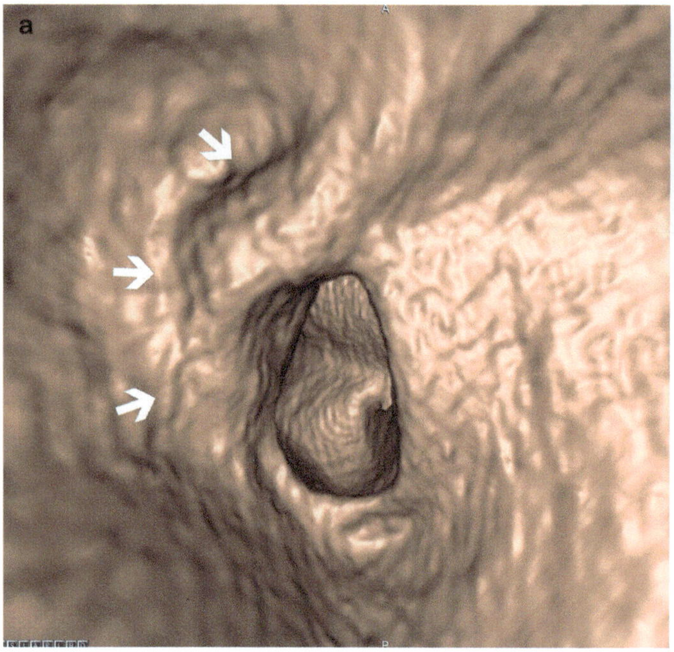

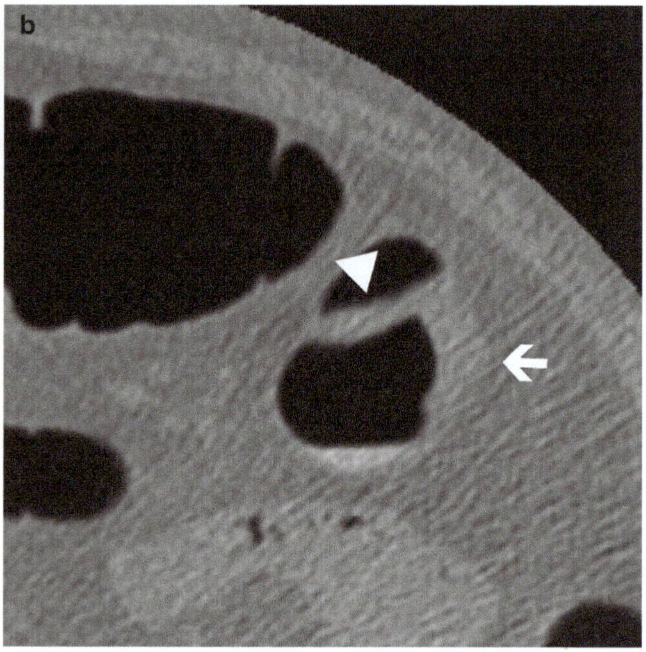

Fig. 7a and b Transverse colon, antegrade view: thickened semilunar folds (*white arrows*) corresponding to the white arrow on the axial image. The axial image also suggests thickening of the adjacent fold (*white arrowhead*)

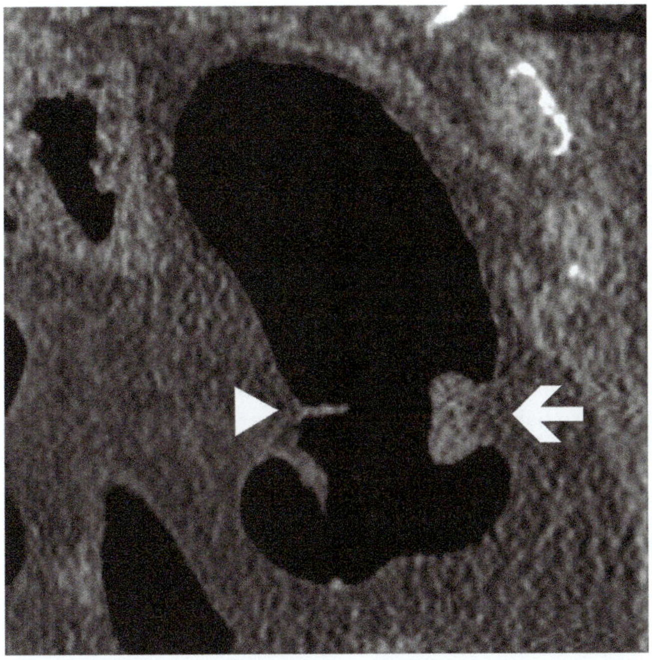

Fig. 7c The corresponding coronal reformat shows focal wall thickening which is not located at a flexure (*white arrow*). The other fold (*white arrowhead*) is normal

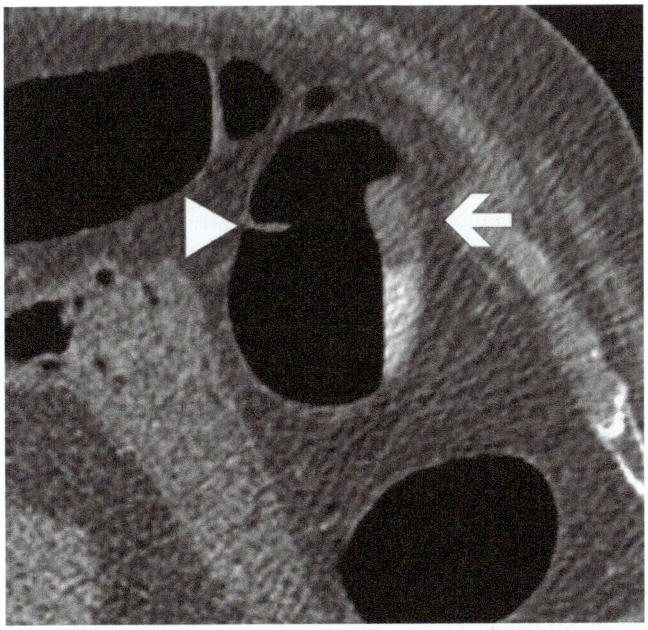

Fig. 7d The aspect does not change in left decubitus. The wall thickening (*white arrow*) corresponds to a malignant tumour with horse saddle aspect. *White arrowhead*: normal semilunar fold

Case 5. Segmental Mobility

Problem

Because of the different length of the mesenteric attachments of the colon to the posterior abdominal wall, the colonic segments are more or less mobile in the abdomen. This may cause a change in position of these segments between the supine and prone acquisition. When detecting a polyp on one acquisition, it is always mandatory to detect this polyp on the same location in the other acquisition. In case of segmental mobility, the polyp may appear at a different location in the abdomen complicating matching between the 2 acquisitions. Because of this change in position, a lesion may appear as moving solid residue and have a "pseudo-stool" appearance resulting in a false-negative diagnosis (Fig. 8a, b).

Solution

This problem can be solved by comparing both acquisitions with the different imaging tools available: scout views, reformatted images. Comparing the scout view is already helpful in detecting obvious positional changes (Fig. 8c, d). For more subtle positional changes, comparing both acquisitions on the coronal and sagittal reformats may solve the problem. It is also helpful to localise the lesion with reference to other structures which in case of segmental mobility shows the same positional change (folds, diverticula, ileocecal valve).

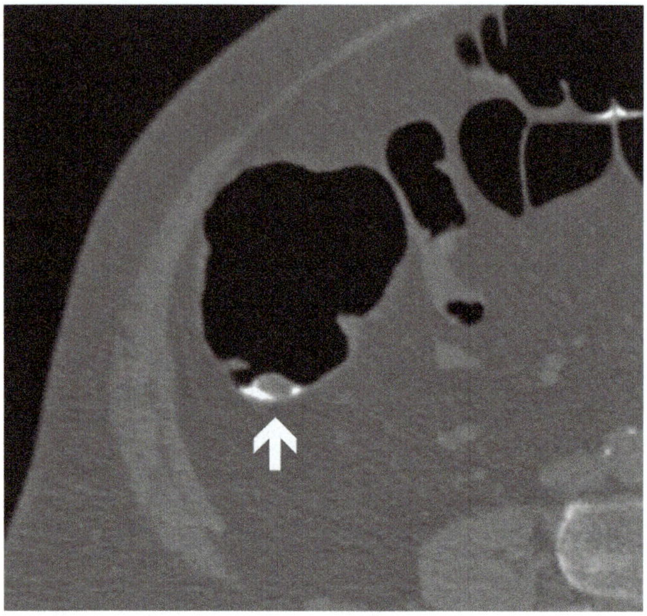

Fig. 8a Ascending colon, supine acquisition: 1-cm luminal defect on the posterior wall surrounded by tagged fluid (*white arrow*)

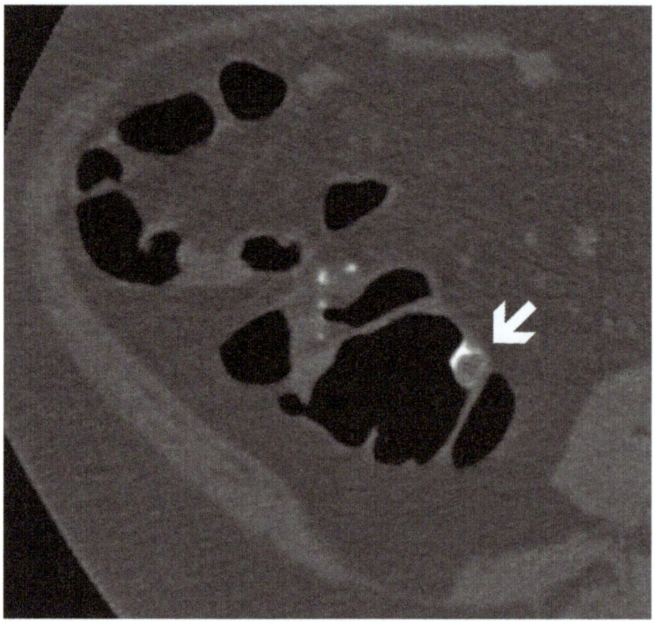

Fig. 8b The corresponding prone view shows the ascending colon in a more posterior-medial position in the abdomen with the luminal defect on the anterior colonic wall (*white arrow*)

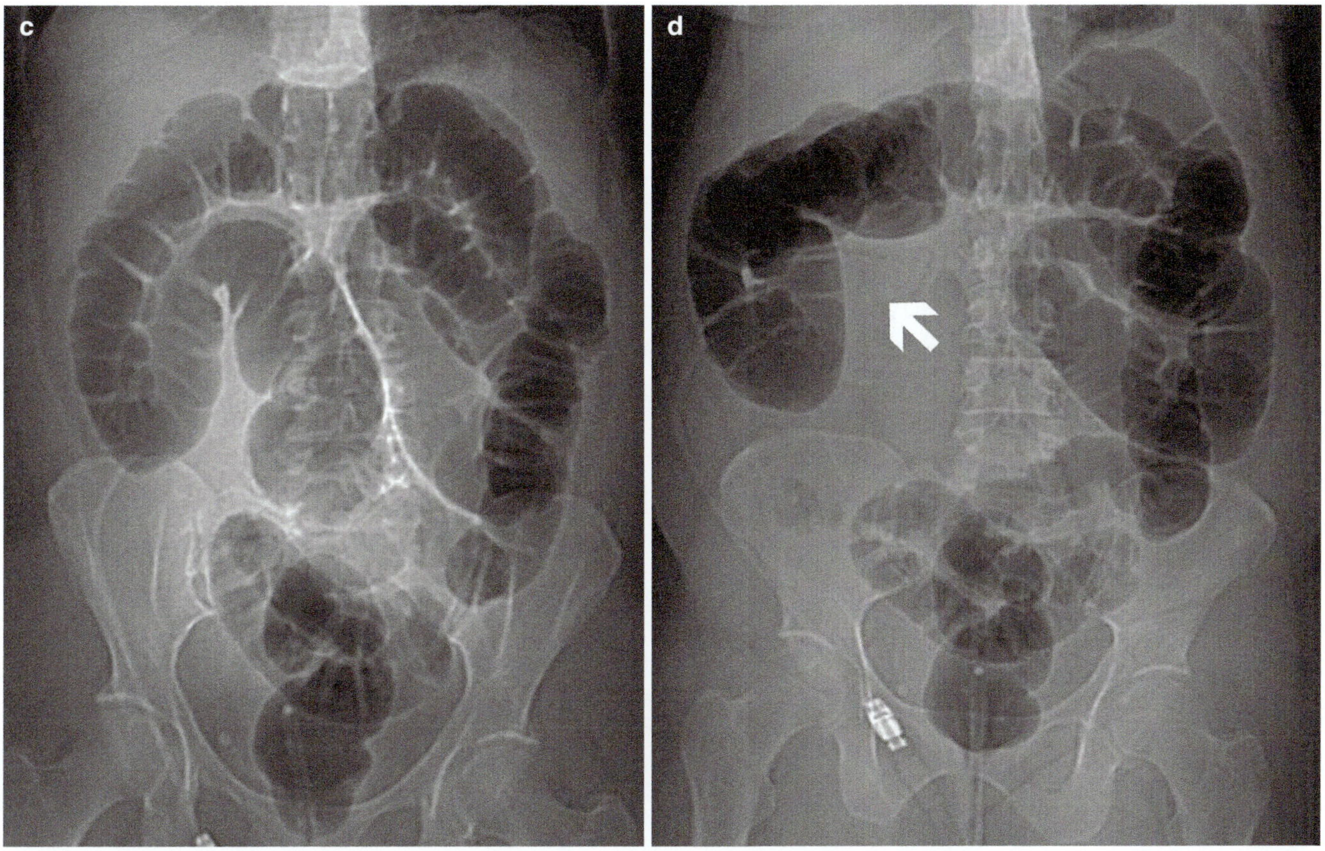

Fig. 8c and d The segmental mobility is confirmed on the scout view with an obvious positional change of the ceco-ascending colon (*white arrow*). Based on these findings, diagnosis of a 1-cm polyp was made and confirmed

Case 6. The Cecum

Problem

Being the terminal part of the colon, the cecum presents as a large pouch making it difficult to examine. It is very important to meticulously scrutinise the entire cecal wall going from the ileocecal valve to the cecal tip. It is also important localising both the ileocecal valve and, if visible, the appendicular orifice. Both structures may give rise to pitfalls in imaging. The ileocecal valve may be enlarged and have a pseudotumoral aspect (Fig. 9a–d). The appendicular orifice may present as a slightly elevated luminal defect (Fig. 10a–c).

Solution

It is mandatory to define the structure of the ileocecal valve by assessing the frenulum and both upper and lower lip of the ileocecal valve with a slit in between, corresponding to the last ileal loop. Comparing 3D with 2D images to assess its texture is also mandatory. The ileocecal valve may be lipomatous (density between 0 and −100 H.U.) or papillary (mixed density: lipomatous and/or soft tissue density). The papillary ileocecal valve is a normal physiological status consisting of a protrusion of the terminal ileal loop into the valve preventing reflux of colonic contents into the ileum. The papillary ileocecal valve may have a pseudotumoral appearance. It can be recognised by defining both lips of the valve. The papillary valve has a mixed density with lipomatous and soft tissue contents. Frequently there is change in aspect between supine and prone acquisition.

If a polypoid defect is detected at the cecal tip, the lesion needs of course to be characterised. Sometimes these defects are caused by an impression the appendiceal base on the cecal tip or by a prolapsing appendix. This can be confirmed by localising the appendix on the coronal and sagittal reformats.

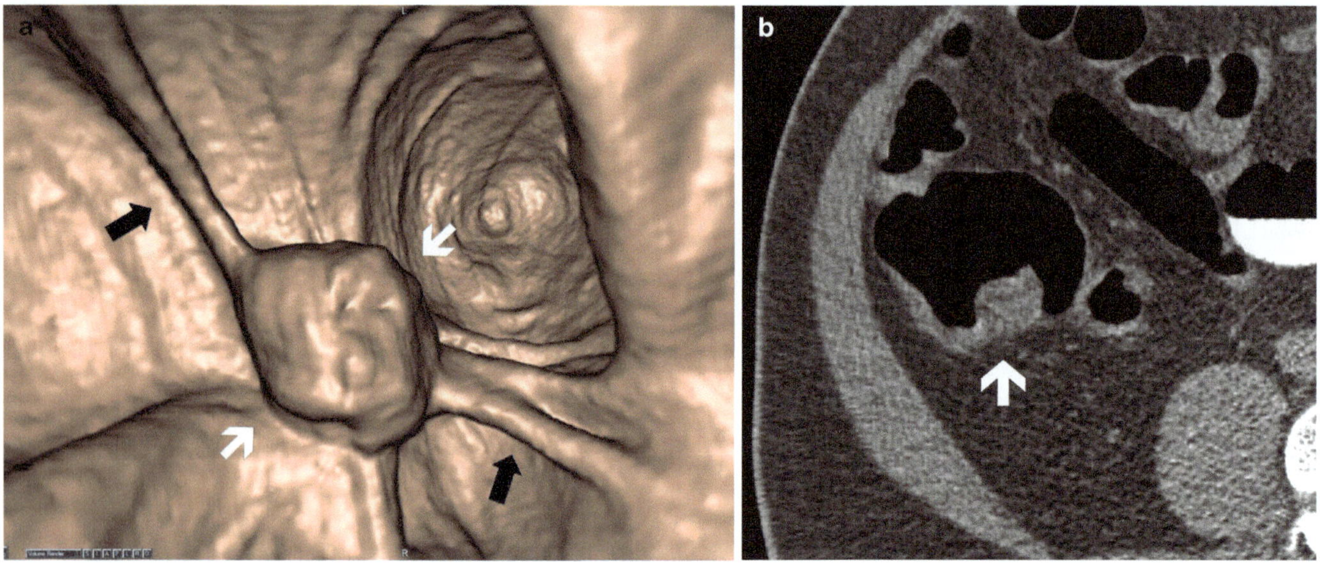

Fig. 9a and b Antegrade view of the cecum in supine position, showing a large nodular structure (*white arrows*), confirmed on the corresponding axial image (*white arrow*). Two large folds are in contact with this structure: frenulum (*black arrows*)? This "tumoral" structure has a mixed density with fatty and soft tissue components

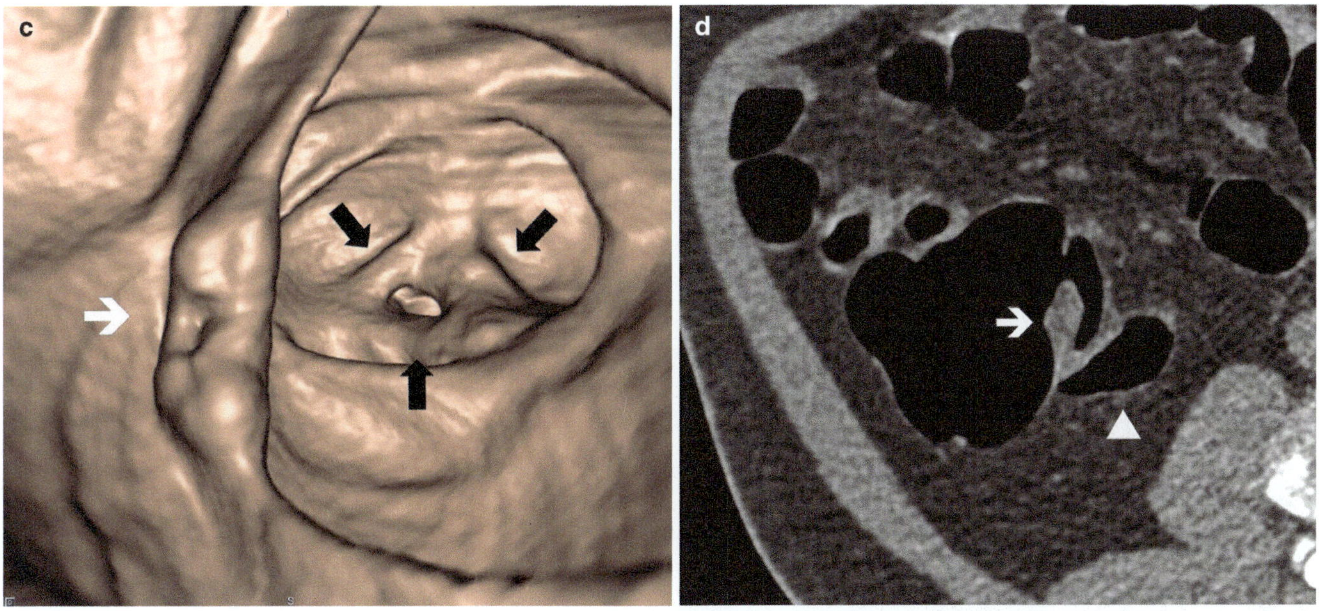

Fig. 9c and d Retrograde view of the cecum in prone position shows a normal ileocecal valve with the upper and lower lip converging to the frenulum on both sides (*white arrow*). The small nodules correspond to lipomatous tissue. The corresponding axial image shows a normal sized ileocecal valve with mainly fatty components. There is a spasm more distally in the ascending colon with the typical triangular aspect and slightly thickened folds (*black arrows*). There some air in the terminal ileal loop (*white arrowhead*)

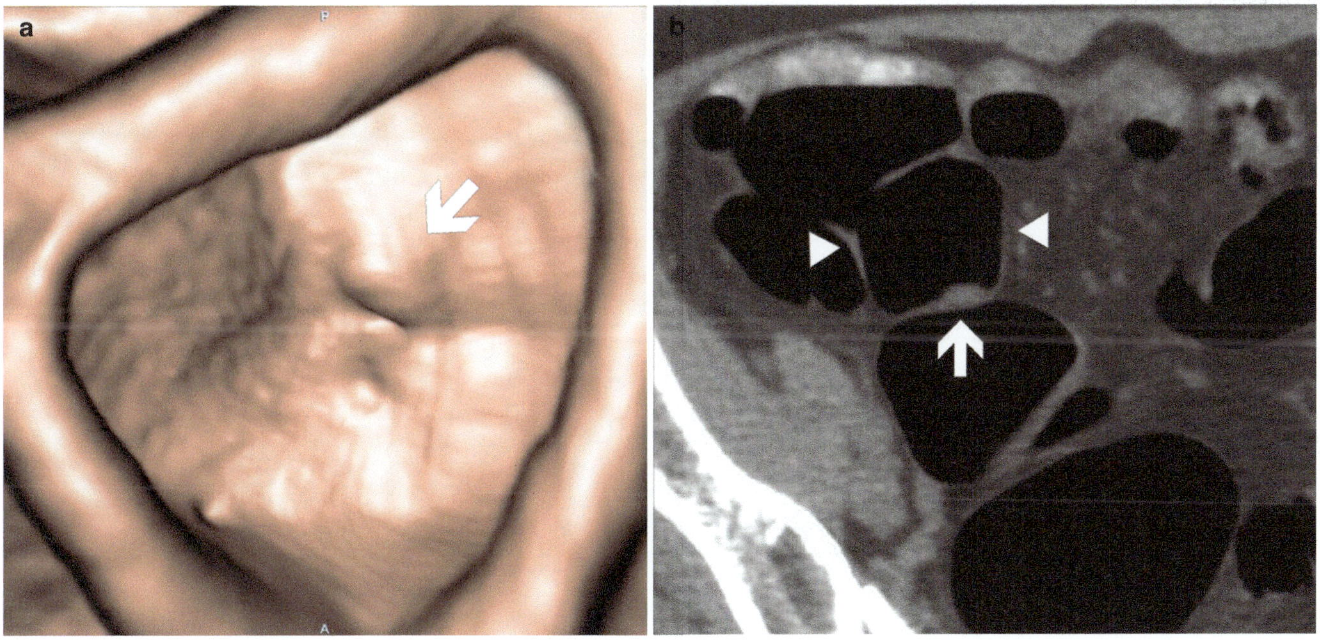

Fig. 10a and b Antegrade view of the cecum (*white arrowheads*, axial image) showing a small polypoid defect at the cecal tip (*white arrow*), corresponding with an 8-mm flat defect on the axial image

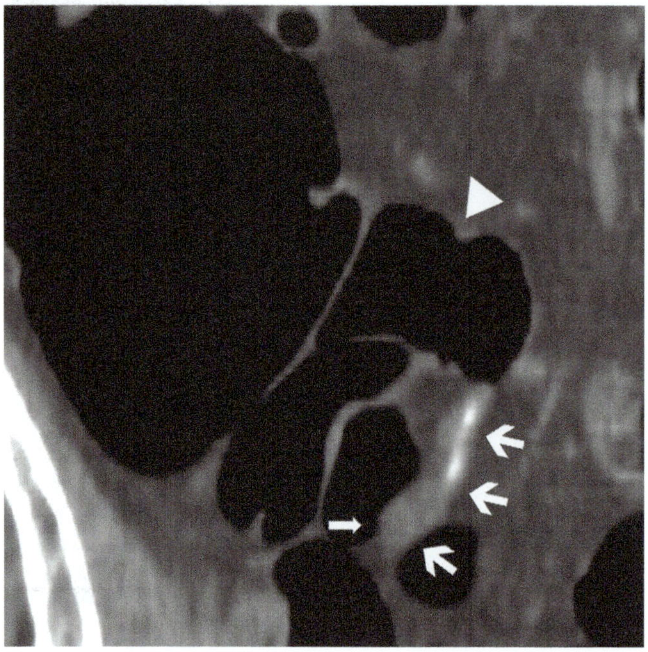

Fig. 10c The coronal reformat shows the appendix prolapsing in the cecal lumen (*large white arrows*) and causing the luminal defect (*small white arrow*). Last ileal loop (*white arrowhead*)

Case 7. Lesion Characterization

Problem

Interpretation of CT colonography consists of 2 important steps: lesion detection and lesion characterization. When detecting a luminal defect in 3D, it is indeed mandatory to confirm the luminal defect is a true lesion.

Solution

When detecting a luminal defect, it is always necessary to assess the nature of this defect by comparing the 3D findings with the 2D images. If the luminal defect corresponds to a soft tissue structure (most typically with muscular density), it is a polyp until proven otherwise. The luminal defect may present as: a hyperdense structure (tagged stool), isodense with air inclusion (non-tagged stool, mostly in tagged fluid), a hyperdense ring with hypodense centre (diverticular faecalith), and hypodense with density varying between 0 and −100 H.U. (lipoma, inverted diverticulum) (Fig. 11a, b).

Luminal defects may also be caused by extrinsic impressions. Again, comparing 3D with the 2D images provides the solution (Figs. 12a, b and 13a, b).

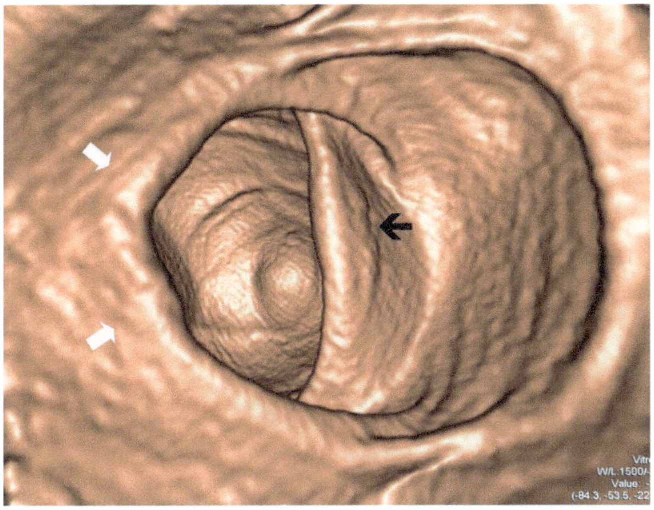

Fig. 11a Cecum: view in antegrade direction, showing the ileocecal valve as a flattened bilobated fold (*white arrows*) and slightly thickened fold appearing as a possible flat polyp (*black arrow*)

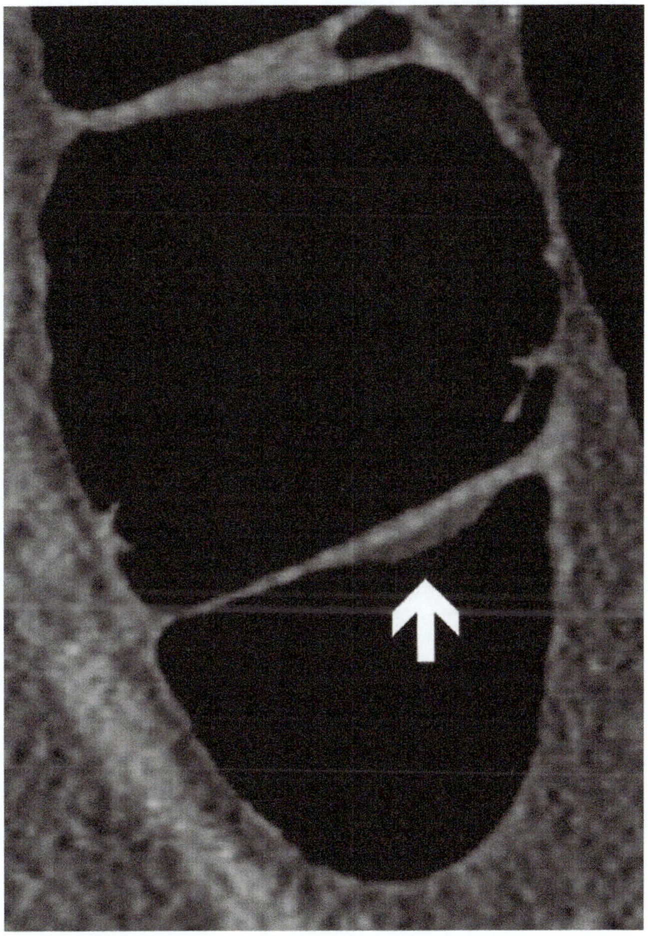

Fig. 11b The corresponding coronal reformat allows for lesion characterization, showing a flat structure with negative density: lipoma with flat morphology (*white arrow*)

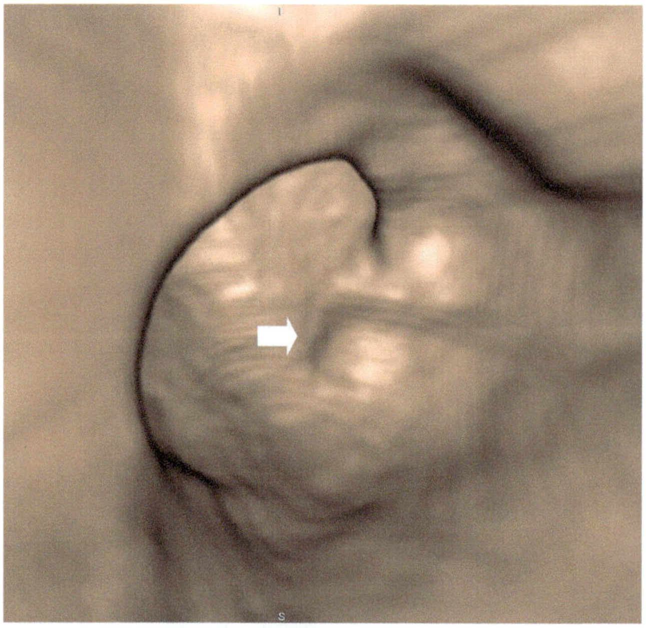

Fig. 12a Antegrade view of the descending colon showing the round aspect of the colonic lumen. A 1-cm flat defect is detected (*white arrow*)

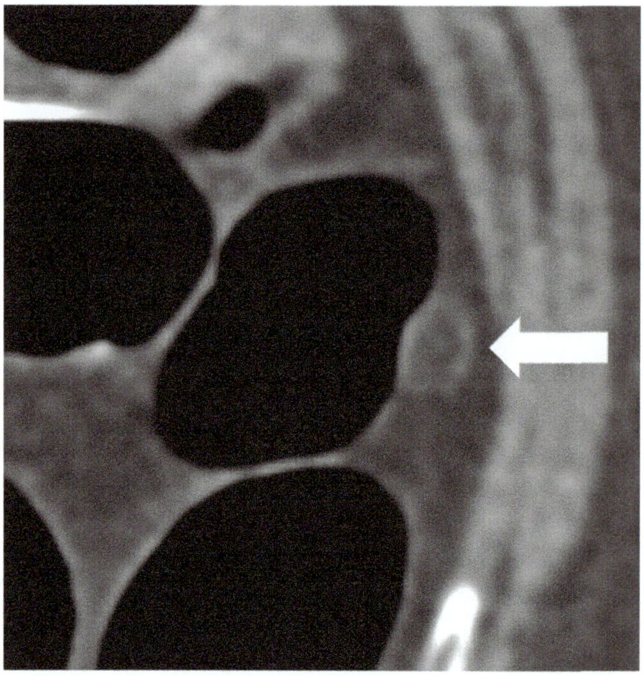

Fig. 12b The corresponding axial image shows a paracolonic ringlike density with fatty centre and central isodense dot consistent with (old) mesenteric appendagitis in this asymptomatic patient (*white arrow*)

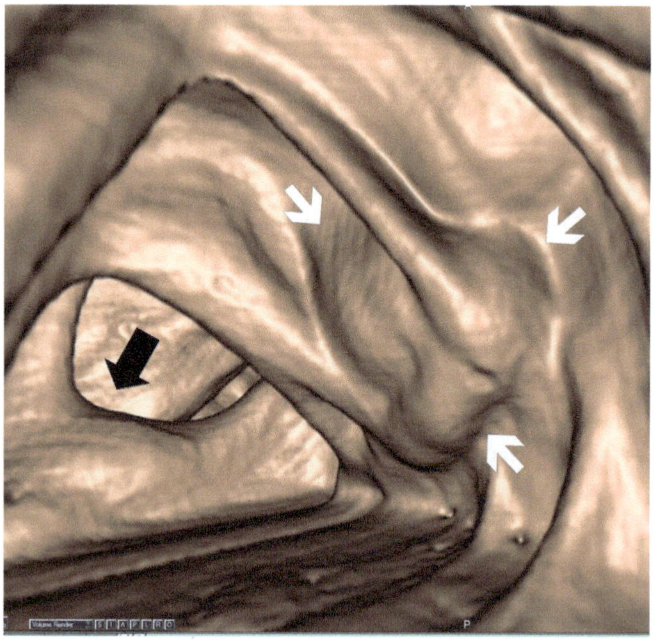

Fig. 13a Antegrade view of the descending colon with the triangular aspect of the colonic lumen. There is a large luminal defect with submucosal characteristics, extending over a semilunar fold (*white arrows*). Broad fold with flattened aspect more distally: ileocecal valve (*black arrow*)

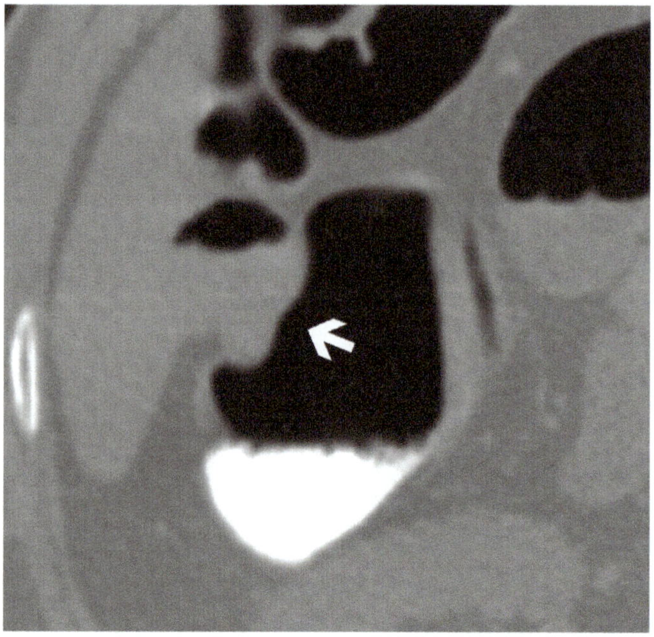

Fig. 13b The corresponding axial image shows a fluid-filled jejunal loop pinched between the liver and the ascending colon, causing an extrinsic impression on the ascending colon (*white arrow*)

Case 8. Polyp Measurement

Problem

There is a consensus that only patients with a polyp ≥6 mm need immediate optical colonoscopy for removal of the polyp. As a consequence, accurate measurement is mandatory to correctly categorise the polypoid lesions. It is necessary to look for the largest dimension of the lesion: for a sessile lesion, take the widest dimension; for a pedunculated polyp, take the widest dimension of the head; and for a flat lesion, take its widest base. Despite these directives, sometimes lesions are incorrectly categorised with underestimation of the lesion size (Fig. 14a–c).

Solution

Always look for the largest dimension of the lesion and do not restrict the measurement of the lesions to the axial images. Use also the sagittal and coronal reformats and 3D images for determining the largest dimension of the lesion.

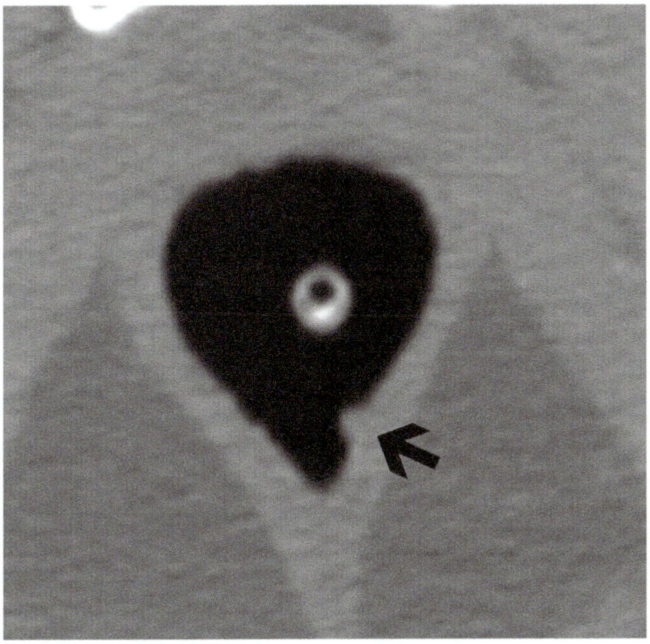

Fig. 14a Axial view of the rectum: sessile polyp measuring 4–5 mm and hence categorised as nonsignificant finding (*black arrow*)

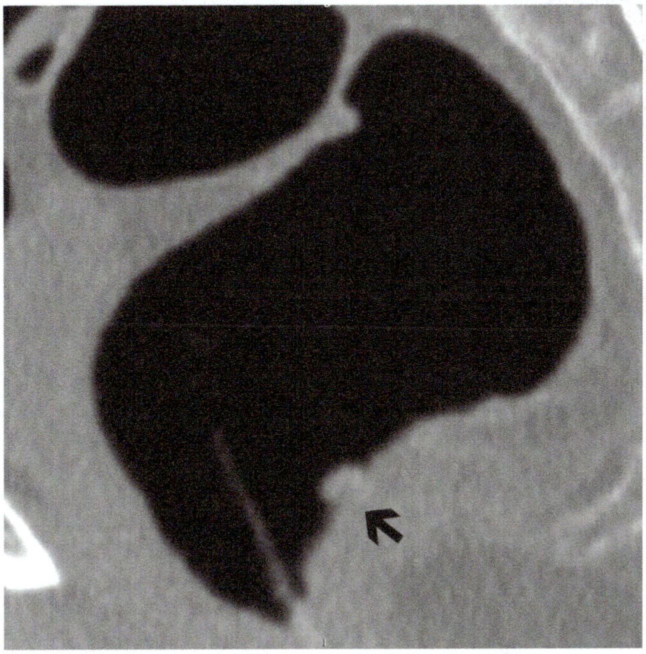

Fig. 14b The sagittal view shows the longest diameter of the polyp. On this view, the polyp has a size of 8 mm, making it a significant lesion prompting optical colonoscopy (*black arrow*)

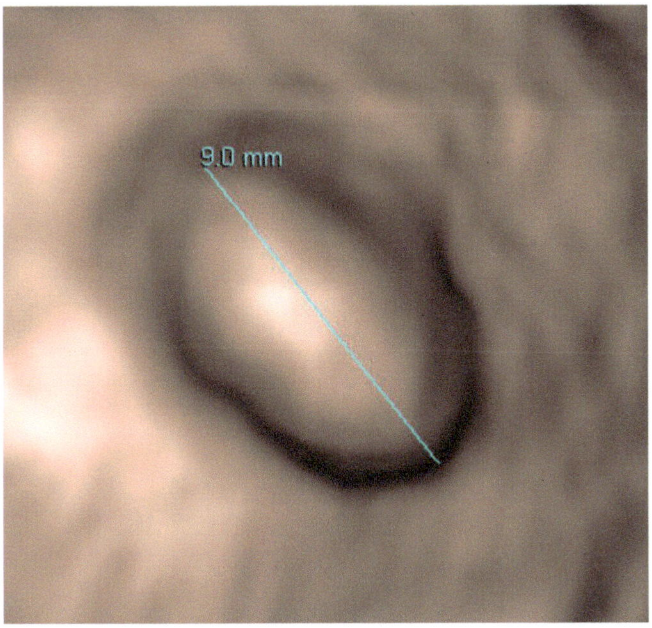

Fig. 14c En face 3D view of the same polyp. Automated measurement shows a size of 9 mm. 3D imaging allows for determining the largest dimension of this lesion

Diverticular Disease

Lorenzo Faggioni, Rossella Scandiffio,
Annalisa Mantarro, and Pietro Bemi

Contents

Abstract

Diverticula are outpouches of the colonic wall formed by the mucosal layer bulging out through the muscular layer, typically at the sites of entry of penetrating vessels. The development of colonic diverticula is thought to be a result of increased intraluminal colonic pressure. Among the various portions of the large bowel, the sigmoid colon is that with the smallest diameter and is therefore expected to withstand the highest intraluminal pressure. As a consequence, diverticula occur more frequently in the left colon (i.e. descending and sigmoid), although they may involve all colonic segments in the most severe cases of diverticular disease. In this chapter the typical CT colonography patterns of diverticula, chronic diverticulosis and diverticulitis are described, and the differential diagnosis between chronic diverticular disease with parietal thickening versus colorectal cancer is discussed. Several 2D and 3D images from CT colonography examinations are provided as examples throughout the text.

Introduction

Diverticula are outpouches of the colonic wall formed by the mucosal layer bulging out through the muscular layer, typically at the sites of entry of penetrating vessels. The development of colonic diverticula is thought to be a result of increased intraluminal colonic pressure. Among the various portions of the large bowel, the sigmoid colon is that with the smallest diameter and is therefore expected to withstand the highest intraluminal pressure. As a consequence, diverticula occur more frequently in the left colon (i.e. descending and sigmoid), although they may involve all colonic segments in the most severe cases of diverticular disease.

L. Faggioni (✉) • R. Scandiffio • A. Mantarro • P. Bemi
Department of Diagnostic and Interventional Radiology,
University of Pisa,
Via Paradisa 2, 56125 Pisa, Italy
e-mail: lfaggioni@sirm.org

E. Neri et al. (eds.), *CT Colonography Atlas*, Medical Radiology,
DOI 10.1007/978-3-642-11149-5_4,

Case 2. Multiple Diverticula of the Descending (Fig. 2a) and Sigmoid Colon (Fig. 2b)

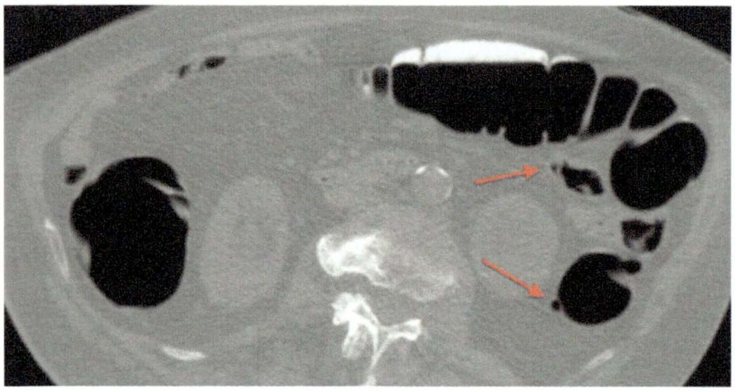

Fig. 2a

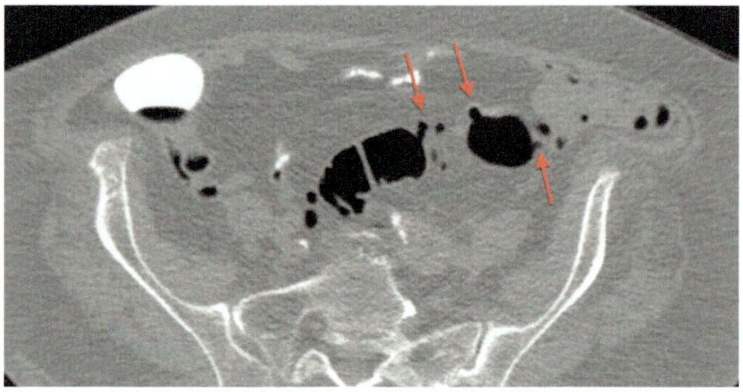

Fig. 2b

Description

Multiple diverticula (*red arrows*) with typical left colonic localisation in an asymptomatic patient. Diverticula without diverticulitis appear as air-filled outpouches of the colonic lining with smooth margins and no significant thickening of the bowel wall or peridiverticular tissues.

Case 3. Chronic Diverticular Disease with Parietal Thickening and Stenosis (Fig. 3a, b)

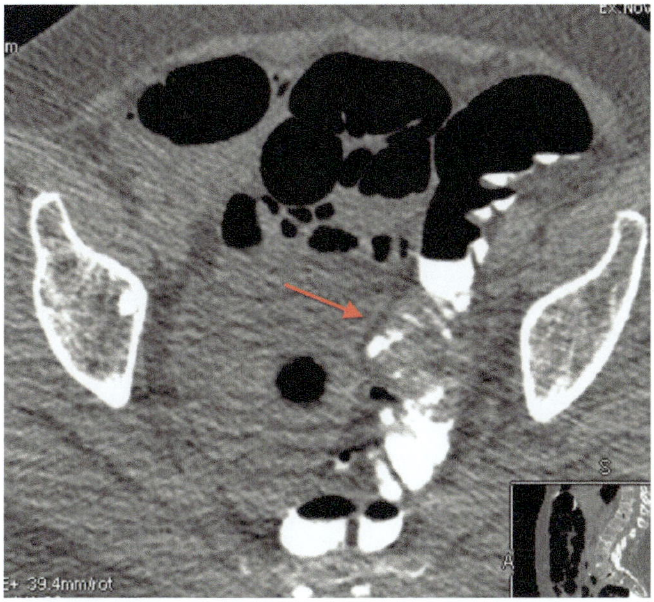

Fig. 3a Axial CT image shows marked thickening of the sigmoid walls (*red arrow*) due to chronic diverticular disease

Description

Marked parietal thickening and stenosis (overestimated as complete luminal obstruction in the double-contrast barium enema-like VR reconstruction) of the sigmoid colon due to chronic diverticular disease.

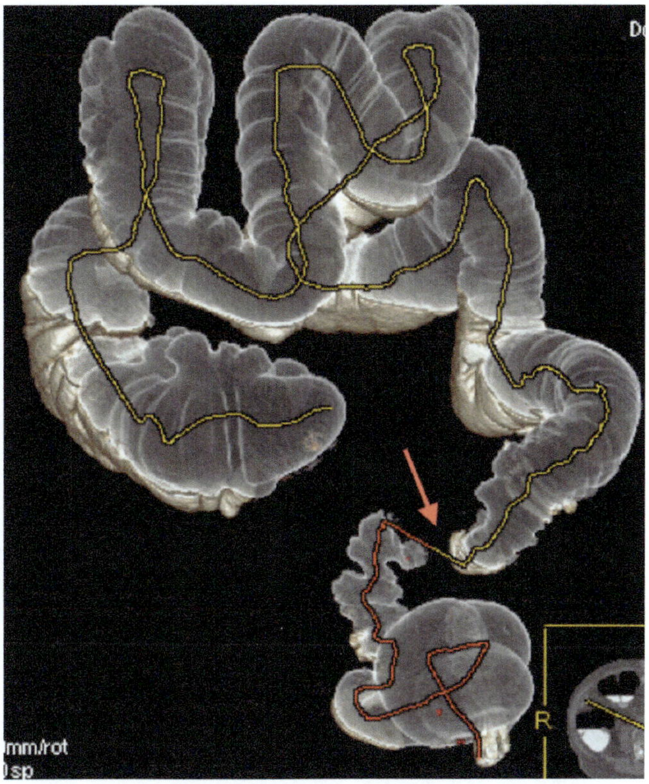

Fig. 3b On VR reconstruction, the marked parietal thickening of the sigmoid colon mimics complete luminal obstruction

Case 4. Chronic Diverticular Disease with Parietal Thickening Versus Colorectal Cancer

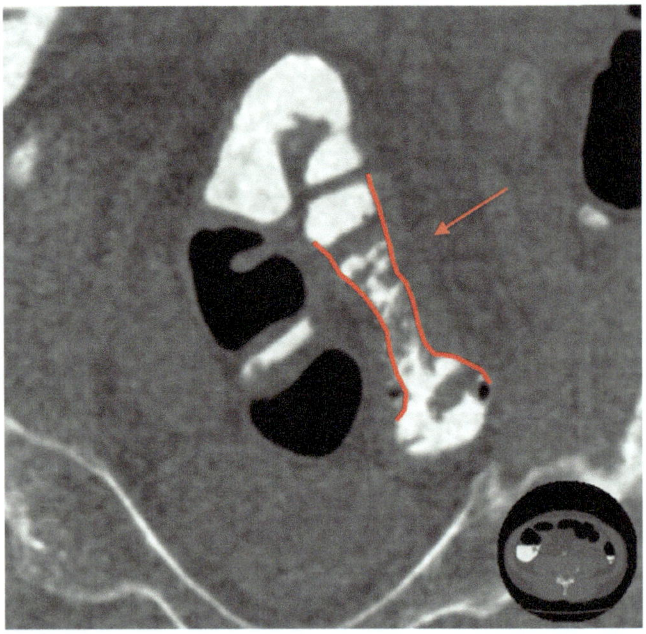

Fig. 4a

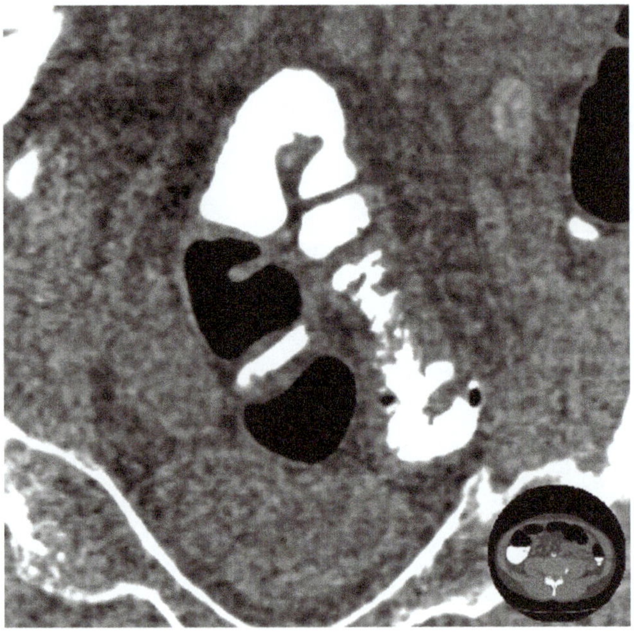

Fig. 4b

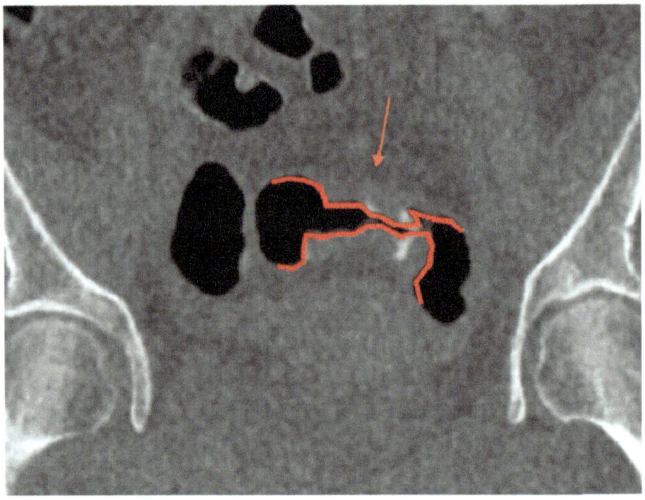

Fig. 4c

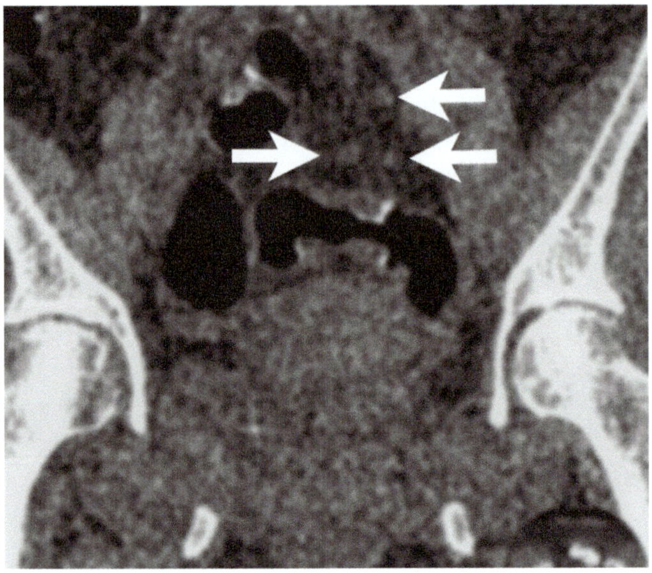

Fig. 4d

Description

In chronic diverticular disease (Fig. 4a, b), there is a smooth transition between regular and thickened colonic wall (*red arrows* in Fig. 4a). Conversely, in annular stenosing colorectal cancer (Fig. 4c, d) an abrupt segmental luminal narrowing usually occurs (*red arrows* in Fig. 4c) and enlarged pericolic lymph nodes may be present (*white arrows* in Fig. 4d).

Case 5. Peridiverticular Thickening (Diverticulitis)

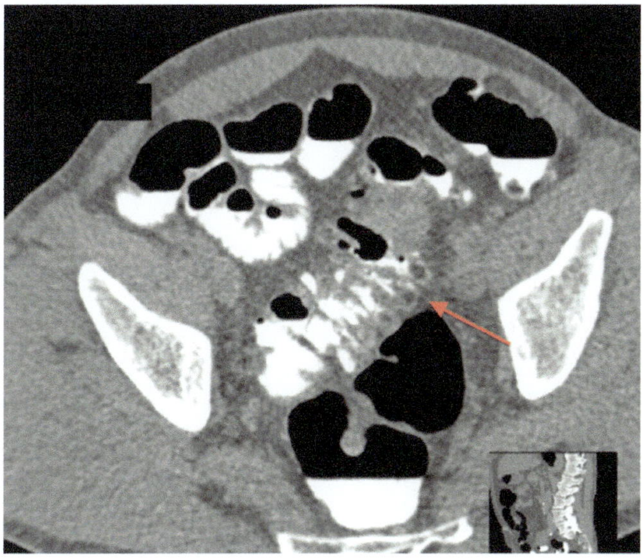

Fig. 5a

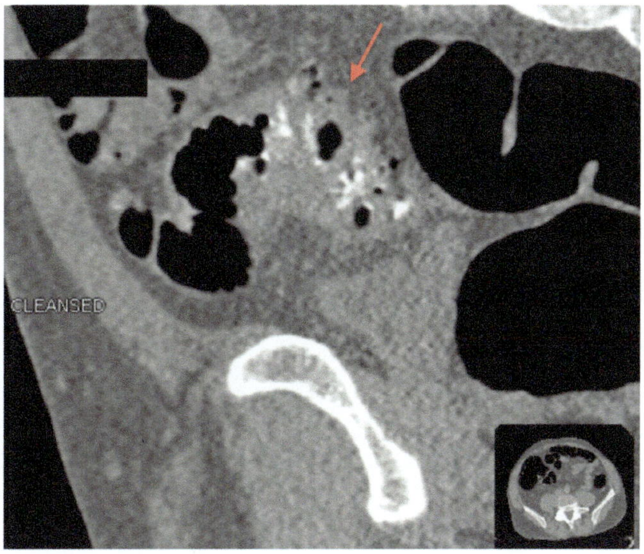

Fig. 5b

Description

Peridiverticular thickening due to peridiverticulitis affecting the sigmoid colon (*red arrows*).

References

1. Stollman N, Raskin JB (2004) Diverticular disease of the colon. Lancet 363:631–639
2. Lefere P, Gryspeerdt S, Baekelandt M, Dewyspelaere J, van Holsbeeck B (2003) Diverticular disease in CT colonography. Eur Radiol 13(S4):L62–L74
3. Mang T, Maier A, Plank C, Mueller-Mang C, Herold C, Schima W (2007) Pitfalls in multi-detector row CT colonography: a systematic approach. Radiographics 27:431–454
4. Chintapalli KN, Chopra S, Ghiatas AA, Esola CC, Fields SF, Dodd GD 3rd (1999) Diverticulitis versus colon cancer: differentiation with helical CT findings. Radiology 210:429–435

Lipomatous Lesions of the Colon

Paola Vagli, Rossella Scandiffio, Eugenia Picano,
and Carlo Bartolozzi

Contents

P. Vagli (✉) • R. Scandiffio • E. Picano • C. Bartolozzi
Department of Diagnostic and Interventional Radiology,
University of Pisa,
Via Paradisa 2, 56127 Pisa, Italy
e-mail: paolavagli@yahoo.it

Abstract

Lipomatous entities of the colon represent a small and definite nosologic group and include lipomatosis of ileocecal valve and lipomas; liposarcomas are extremely rare. CT colonography combines the possibility to measure tissue density to a direct visualization of the bowel wall; this technique allows an increasing sensitivity in the detection of fatty lesions and ensures a definitive diagnosis. This chapter aims to review the colonic lipomatous entities and their clinical features, to present the most important imaging findings, and to describe image interpretation and differential diagnosis.

Lipomatous entities of the colon are restricted to fatty infiltration of ileocecal valve (ICV) or lipomatosis, lipomas and the extremely rare liposarcomas.

As a matter of fact, the detection rate of such lesions seems to be improved by CT colonography, and probably the incidence rates now available and mainly based on autopsy reports underestimate the real frequency. CT colonography in fact providing a direct visualization of the bowel wall and the direct measure of tissue attenuation values allows not only to visualize these lesions with a higher conspicuity but also to rule out any differential diagnosis in one shot.

Lipomatosis of the ICV

It is characterized by fatty submucosal infiltration causing enlargement of the valve lips; streaks of fat could be also contained in most non-lipomatous thin valves while the lack of a distinct capsule differentiates the fat in this condition from true lipoma arising from the valve.

It is difficult to qualify an ICV as being enlarged, but currently, the range of normal for either lip is up to 1.5 cm in thickness; on the other hand, the assessment of the fatty nature of the lips by measuring negative attenuation values (range −40/−120 HU) is very easy by means of CT colonography.

E. Neri et al. (eds.), *CT Colonography Atlas*, Medical Radiology,
DOI 10.1007/978-3-642-11149-5_5, © Springer-Verlag Berlin Heidelberg 2013

Although lipomatosis (or better the related enlargement) of ICV may produce intussusception or obstructive symptoms which can be alleviated by resection of the valve, it is often asymptomatic. Therefore, accurate differentiation between lipomatosis and tumoral lesions of the valve is necessary to avoid unnecessary surgery [1, 2]; in this matter, CT colonography can replace the role of biopsy allowing the structural colon examination and the direct measurement of the density.

When tumours involve the valve, a distinct mass may be identified attached to an otherwise normal valve. Nodularity and irregularity of the valve are suggestive for a tumour. The most common tumour is a lipoma, which differs from lipomatosis of the valve because it is encapsulated. Lipomas of the ICV represent the main differential CT colonography diagnostic challenge based on the presence of a fatty smooth lesion adjacent to the valve.

Features of a lipomatous ICV include thick homogeneous fatty lips with regular margins that appear larger and more bulbous than a normal valve in an otherwise normal ileocecal region (Fig. 1) [3]. Lipomas of the ICV, which true incidence is not actually reported, are more oftenly a protruding and obstructing lipomatous mass with regular margins continuous to the ICV (Fig. 2).

Lipomas

Colonic lipomas are benign tumours and constitute the most common non-epithelial (mesenchymal) neoplasm of the gastrointestinal tract (4.4 % of all and 65 % of gastrointestinal lipomas in autopsy reports) and the second most common benign colonic tumour after adenomatous polyps. The largest percentage (45 %) of lipomas in the colon involve the cecum, which is also the most common location when there are multiple lesions. Lipomas are composed of well-differentiated adipose tissue and may vary greatly in size; they average about 3–4 cm (Fig. 3) but can grow as large as 30 cm. They are usually sessile lesions, and rarely, they are pedunculated [4] (Fig. 4). Lipomas are almost always submucosal covered by smooth mucosa, with only about 10 % being subserosal. Usually this tumour is solitary, but cases of multiple lesions have been reported (20 % of patients).

Colon lipomas usually are incidental findings and tend to become symptomatic when their diameter exceeds 3 cm. When present, symptoms are generally nonspecific and have a long duration.

Abdominal pain, constipation and rectal bleeding are the most common clinical presentation of colon lipomas. The symptoms of larger lipomas are mainly due to mechanical interference with the colonic transit caused by acute or intermittent colo-colonic intussusceptions or to lower gastrointestinal bleeding due to ulceration of the mucosa covering the lipoma. Spontaneous expulsion of a sigmoid lipoma has also been recorded.

Ultrasonographic identification of colonic lipoma may be difficult because lipoma can be represented with the typical multilayered appearance consisting of alternating layer of mucosa, bowel wall and mesenteric fat in cross section, but in the case of a large lipoma, a huge hyperechoic intraluminal mass can be seen [5].

On barium enema examination, colon lipoma may appear as ovoid, well delineated and smooth radiolucent mass. Another characteristic feature is the "squeeze sign" with changes in size and shape of the mass caused by peristaltic bowel movements.

Barium enema can detect lipomas, but it is not specific and the lesion can be mistaken for another type of neoplasm [6].

CT scan is a useful method for demonstration of colon lipoma and can provide a definitive preoperative diagnosis. Typical lipoma appear as parietal, usually protruding, spherical or ovoid mass of variable size, with sharp margins, with or without a stalk, with homogeneous appearance and absorption densities of –40 to –120 HU, typical of fatty compositions. Its soft consistence is responsible of some variations in shape moving from the prone to the supine decubitus and vice versa (Fig. 3). Two-dimensional imaging, owing to the direct measurement of densities, has a distinct advantage over 3D images in classifying lipomas as benign lesions [7], but the direct visualization of the capsule is not achievable. Although malignant transformation has not been described in these lesions, lipomas larger than 3 cm may become symptomatic and endoscopic, (if smaller than 2 cm), or surgical resection is generally recommended for larger lesions.

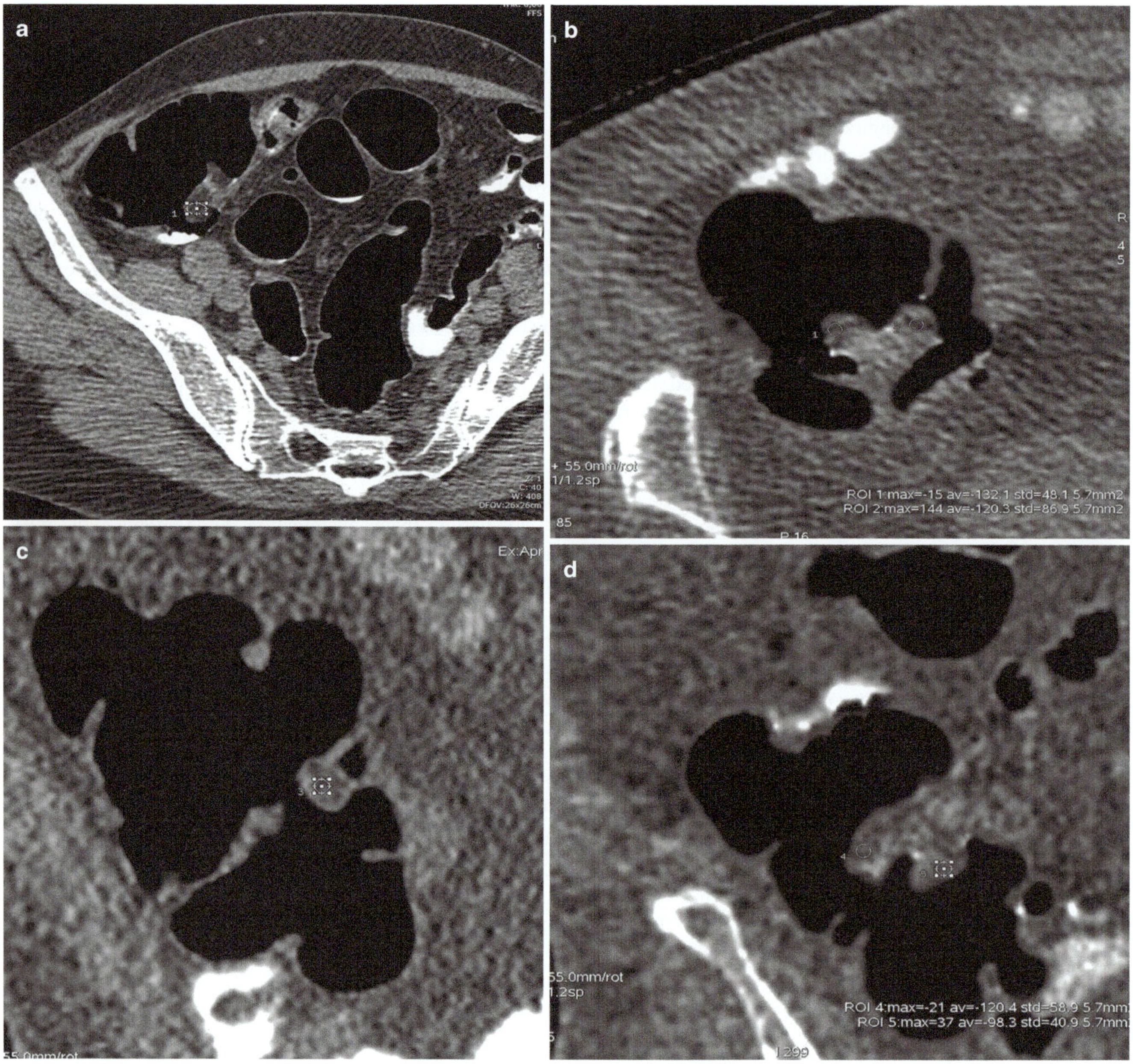

Fig. 1 Lipomatous ICV: three examples (**a**, **b**–**d** and **c**) of prominent ICV as shown by axial (**a**, **b**) and coronal reformatted (**c**, **d**) CT colonography images after electronic cleansing (**b**, **d**). Valvular lips although thickened mantain a normal morphology without signs of obstruction. The attenuation values show homogeneously hypoattenuating values (in **c**, only a valvular lip is mainly involved)

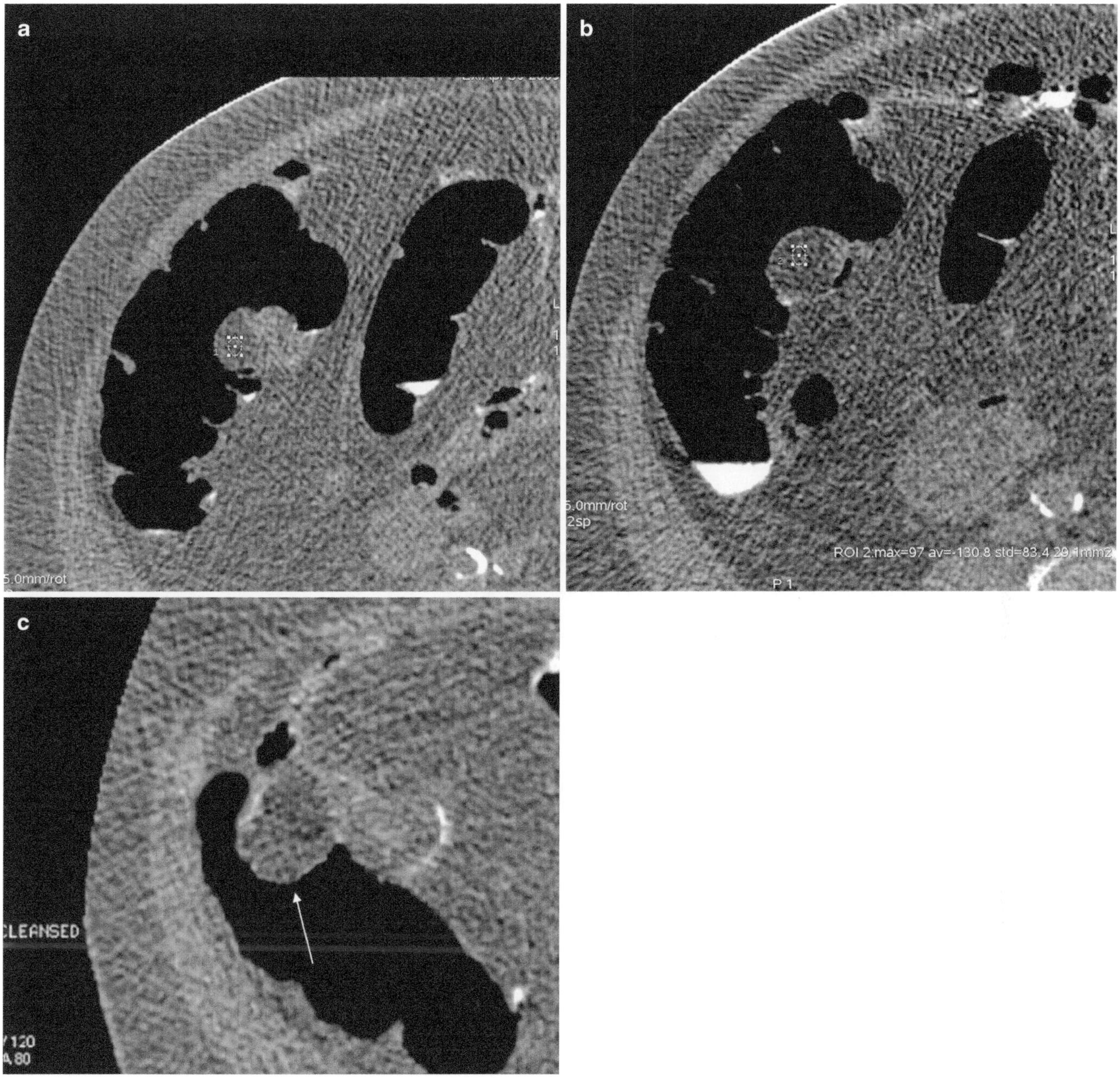

Fig. 2 Lipoma of ICV: nodular homogeneously fatty mass (maximum diameter about 2 cm) adjacent the ICV (**a**–**c**). The mass, close to the distal lip of the valve, preserves the morphology of the cranial lip (**a**). The softness and the mobility of the lipoma are responsible of the mild change in position when moving from supine (**b**) to the prone decubitus (**c**)

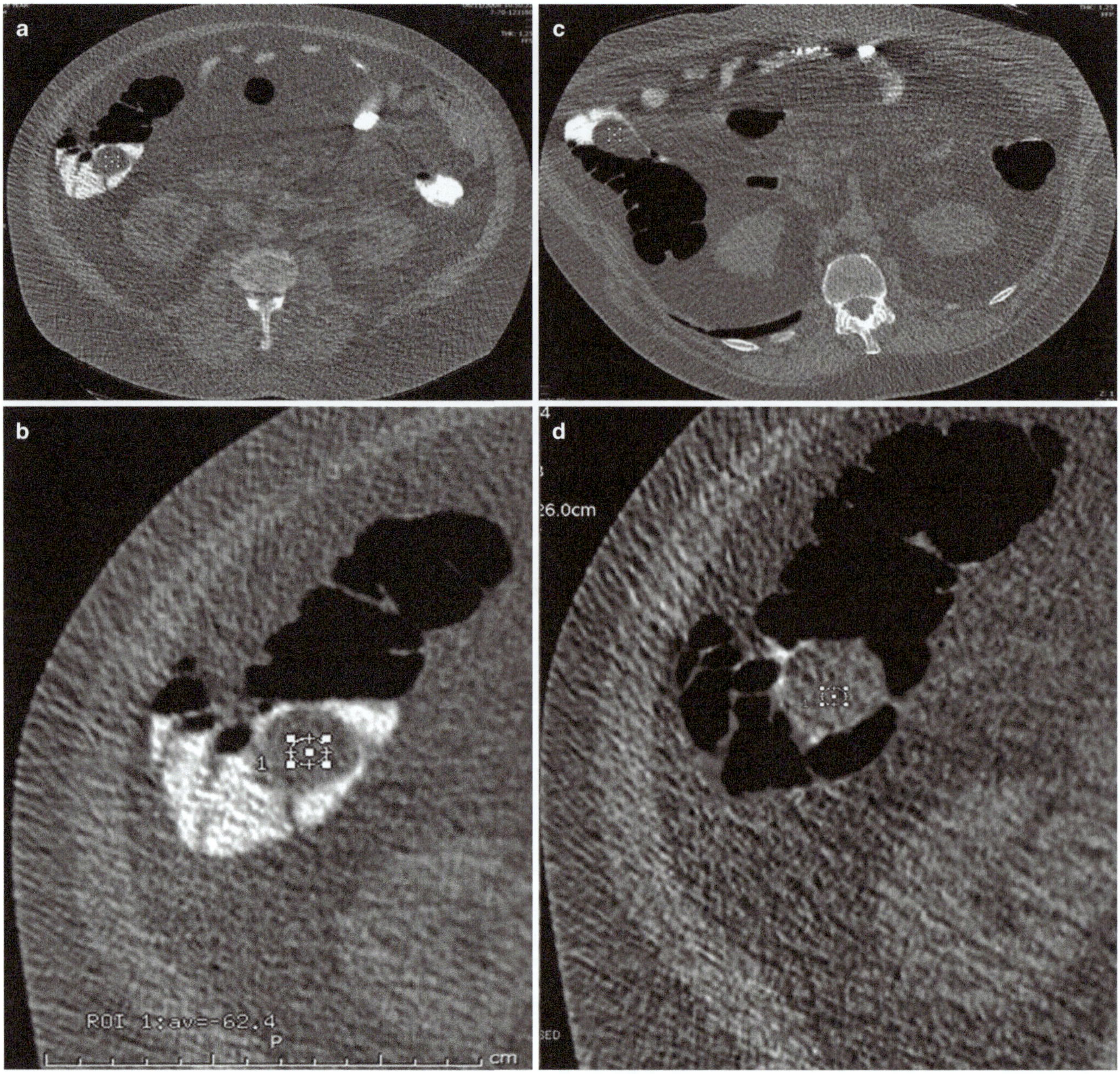

Fig. 3 Lipoma of the right colonic flexure: typical lipoma appearing as an ovoid mass of about 3 cm, with sharp margins, with homogeneous appearance and fat content (–60 HU). Its soft consistence is responsible of some variations in shape and position moving from the prone to the supine decubitus and vice versa (**a**, **b** supine vs. **c** prone). In (**d**) is applied electronic cleansing of the tagging material

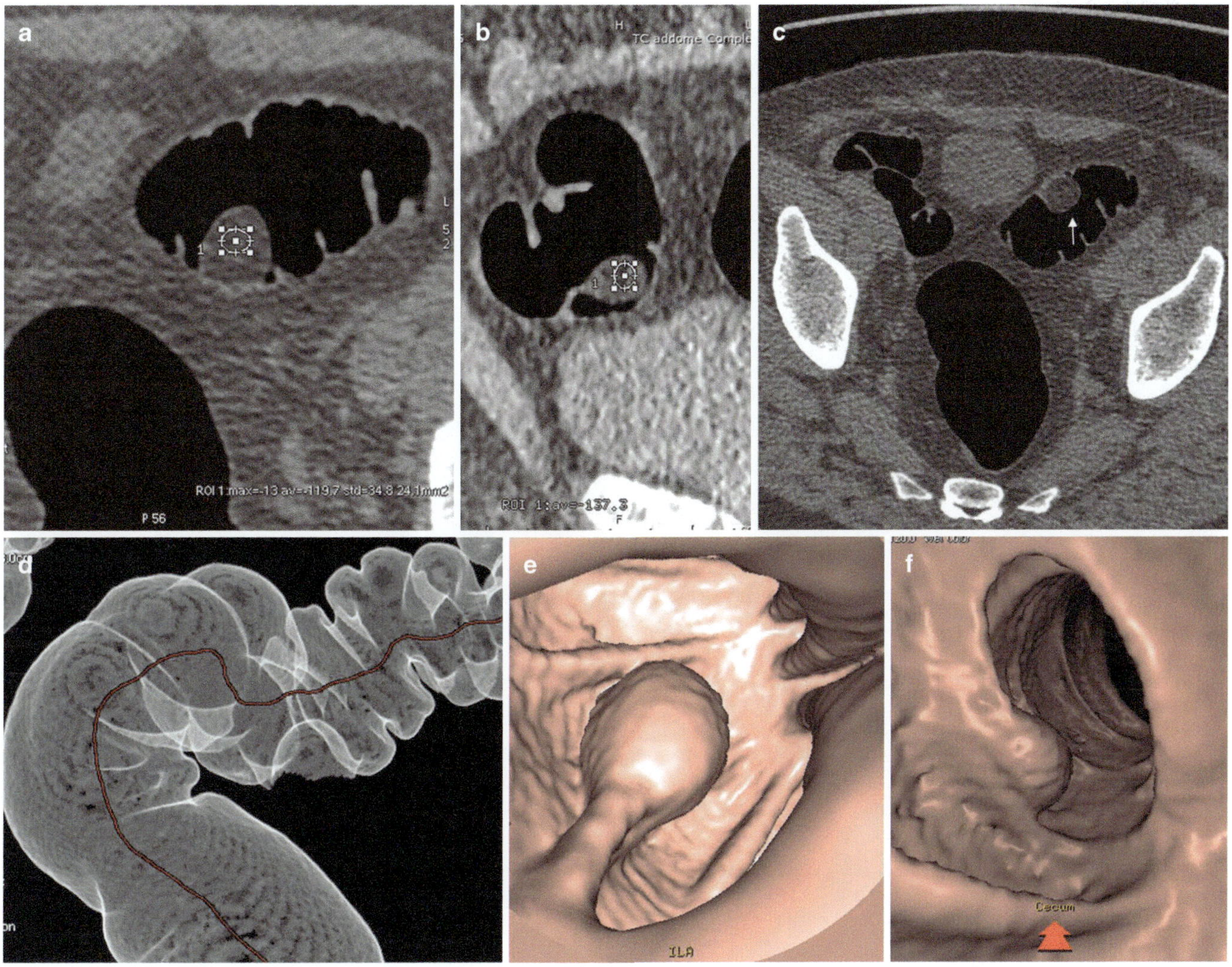

Fig. 4 Pedunculated lipoma of the sigmoid colon: the small (about 2 cm) lipomatous lesion moves from the posterior (supine **a**) to the anterior (prone **c**) colonic surface, thanks to the presence of a stalk that is well displaced in the sagittal reformation (**b**) and at the endoluminal view (**e**). In **d** (volume rendering), and in **e**, **f** (endoluminal view), the lack of tissue densities and of the direct visualization of the wall structure prevents the differentiation with an adenomatous polyp

Liposarcoma

Gastrointestinal tract is an uncommon site for liposarcoma, and primary liposarcoma of the colon is extremely rare. To our knowledge, only eight cases of primary colon liposarcoma have been reported in the world literature to date. Reported lesions are predominantly inhomogeneous parietal massess protruding in the colon with parenchymatous appearance and microscopic fatty components. Lesions present contrast enhancement according to their vascularization and can be accompanied by signs of malignancy as peritoneal nodules or metastases. Clinical features include nonspecific symptoms, such as diarrhoea, abdominal pain, bleeding and obstruction. The prognosis of primary liposarcoma of the colon is not known, and no standardized guidelines have been established for its treatment; however, complete excision can be considered the gold standard [8–10].

References

1. Berk RN, Davis GB, Cholhassey EB (1973) Lipomatosis of the ileocecal valve. AJR Am J Roentgenol 119(2):323–328
2. Silva AC, Beaty SD, Hara AK, Fletcher JG, Fidler JL, Menias CO, Johnson CD (2007) Spectrum of normal and abnormal CT appearances of the ileocecal valve and Cecum with endoscopic and surgical correlation. Radiographics 27(4):1039–1054, Review
3. Regge D, Gallo TM, Nieddu G, Galatola G, Fracchia M, Neri E, Vagli P, Bartolozzi C (2005) Ileocecal valve imaging on computed tomographic colonography. Abdom Imaging 30(1):20–25, Epub 2004 Nov 17

4. Lazaraki G, Tragiaqnnidis D, Xirou P (2009) Endoscopic resection of giant lipoma mimicking colonic neoplasm initially presenting with massive haemorrhage: a case report. Cases J 2:6462
5. Ross GJ, Amilineni V (2000) Case 26: Jejunojejunal Intussusceptions secondary to a lipoma. Radiology 216:727–730
6. Ghidirim G, Mishin I, Gutsu E et al (2005) Giant Sub mucosal lipoma of the cecum: report of a case and review of literature. Rom J Gastroenterol 14(4):393–396
7. Hara AK, Johnson CD, Reed JE (1997) Colorectal lesions: evaluation with CT colography. Radiographics 17(5):1157–1167; discussion 1167–1168
8. Parks RW, Mullan FJ, Kamel HMH, Walsh MY, McKelvey STD (1994) Case report. Liposarcoma of the colon. Ulster Med J 63(1): 111–113
9. D'Annibale M, Cosimelli M, Covello R, Stasi E (2009) Liposarcoma of the colon presenting as an endoluminal mass. World J Surg Oncol 7:78
10. Choi YY, Kim YJ, Jin SY (2010) Primary liposarcoma of the ascending colon: a rare case of mixed type presenting as hemoperitoneum combined with other type of retroperitoneal liposarcoma. BMC Cancer 10:239

Case 1. Ulcerative Colitis of the Rectum

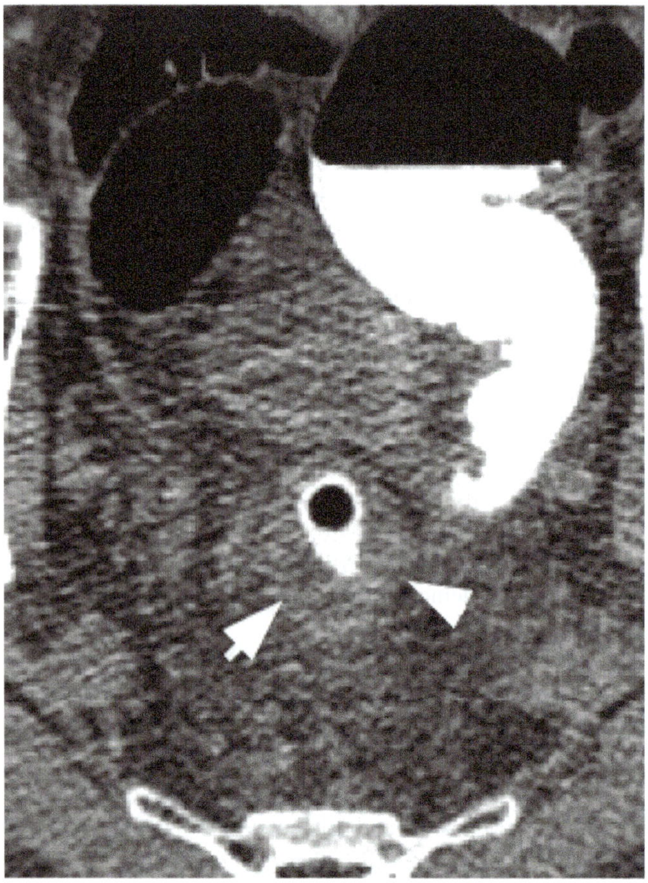

Fig. 1a Axial view. Circumferential thickening of the rectum (*arrow heads*)

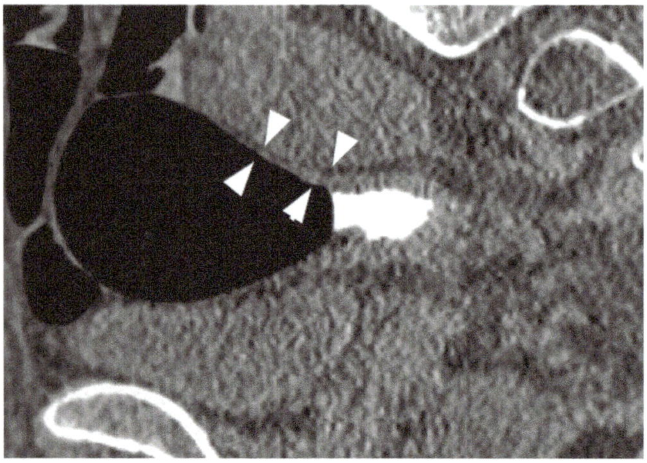

Fig. 1b Sagittal MPR. Circumferential thickening of the rectum (*arrow heads*) with partial luminal stenosis and dilatation of the sigmoid colon. Note the smooth surface and progressive reduction of thickening between rectum and the normal sigmoid colon, which is typical of inflammation

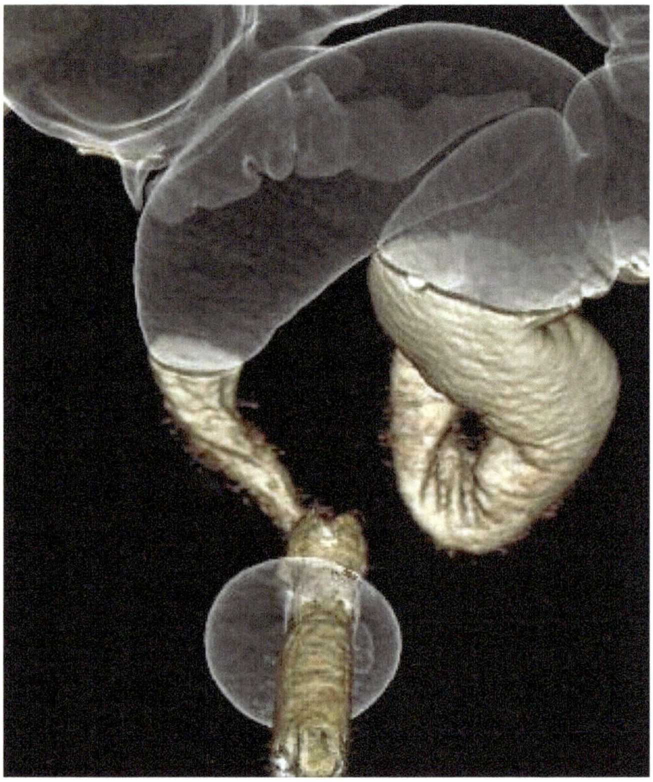

Fig. 1c 3D Volume rendering of the rectum and sigmoid colon

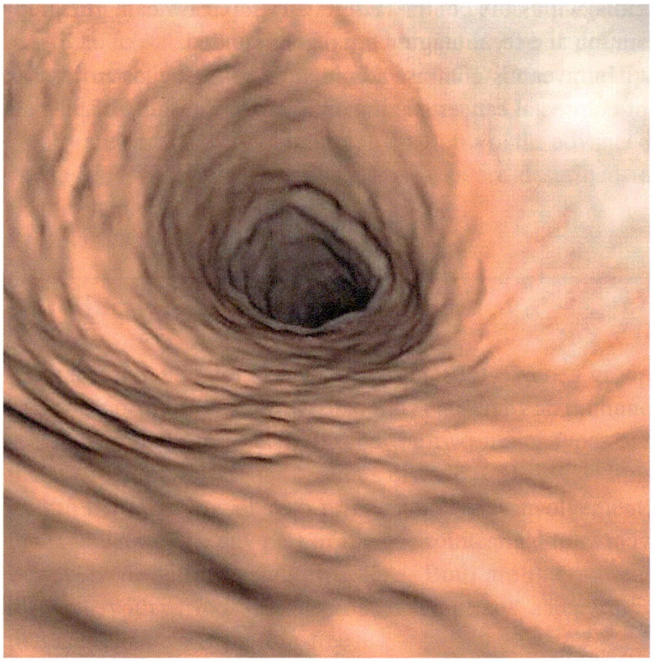

Fig. 1d Endoluminal view that demonstrate the stenosis and the complete loss of the Houston valves

Case 2. Ulcerative Colitis of the Rectum and Sigmoid Colon

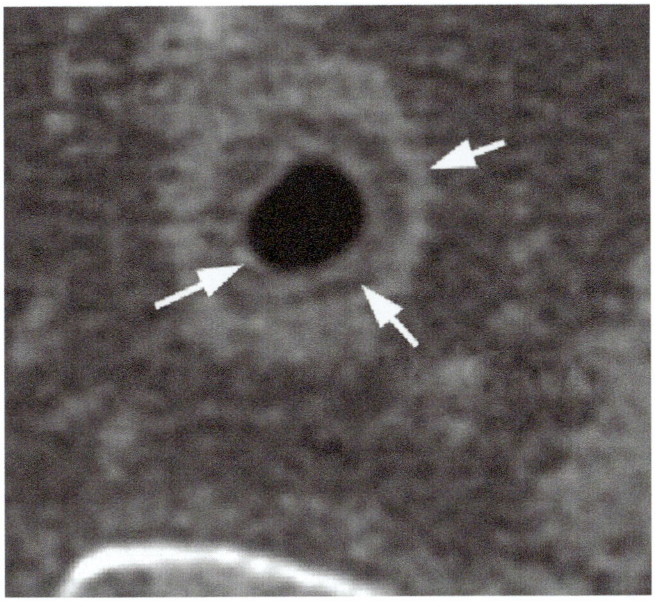

Fig. 2a Axial view. Halo sign in the rectum with clear evidence of the three wall layers (*arrows*) from the lumen, mucosa. submucosa and sierosa

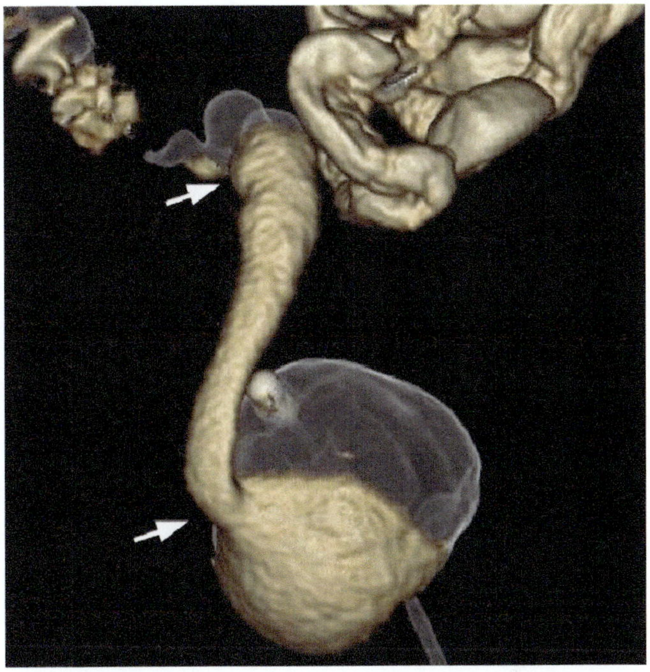

Fig. 2c 3D panoramic view demonstrates the luminal stenosis and extension (*arrows*)

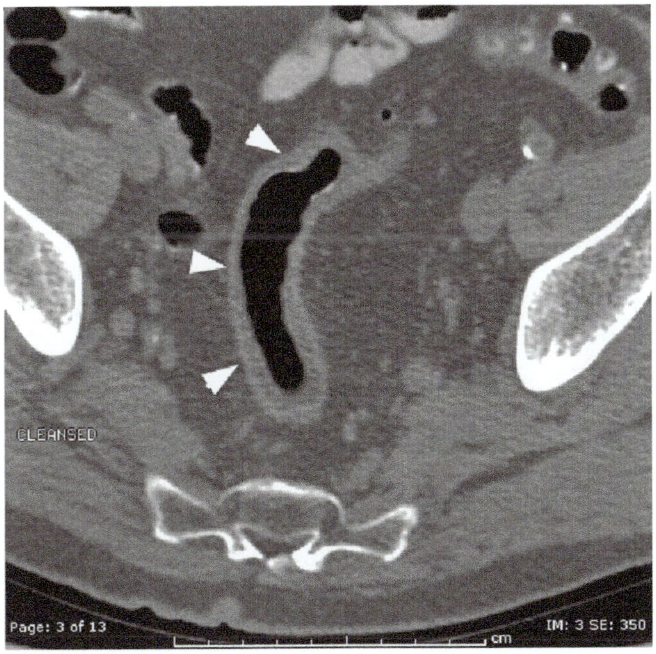

Fig. 2b Axial view. Progressive extension of the circumferential thickening from the rectum to the sigmoid colon (*arrow heads*)

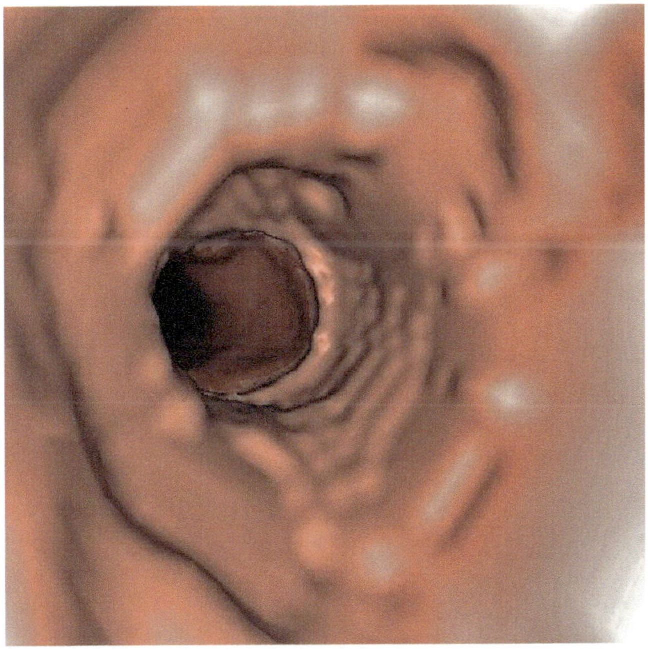

Fig. 2d 3D endoluminal view through the rectum shows the stenosis and the absence of Houston Valves

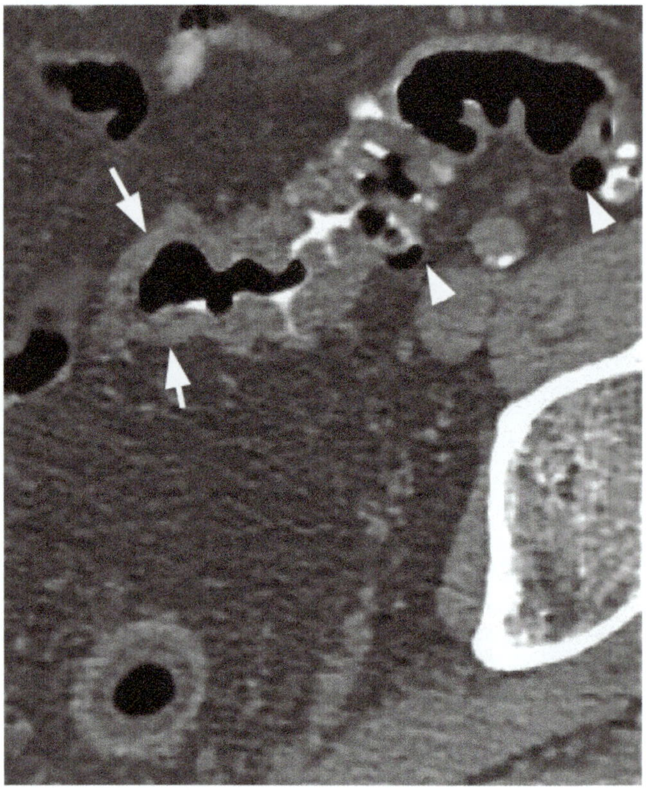

Fig. 2e Axial view. The rectal thickening extends to the sigmoid colon (*arrows*) where multiple diverticula are present (*arrow heads*)

Case 3. Crohn's Disease of the Transverse Colon

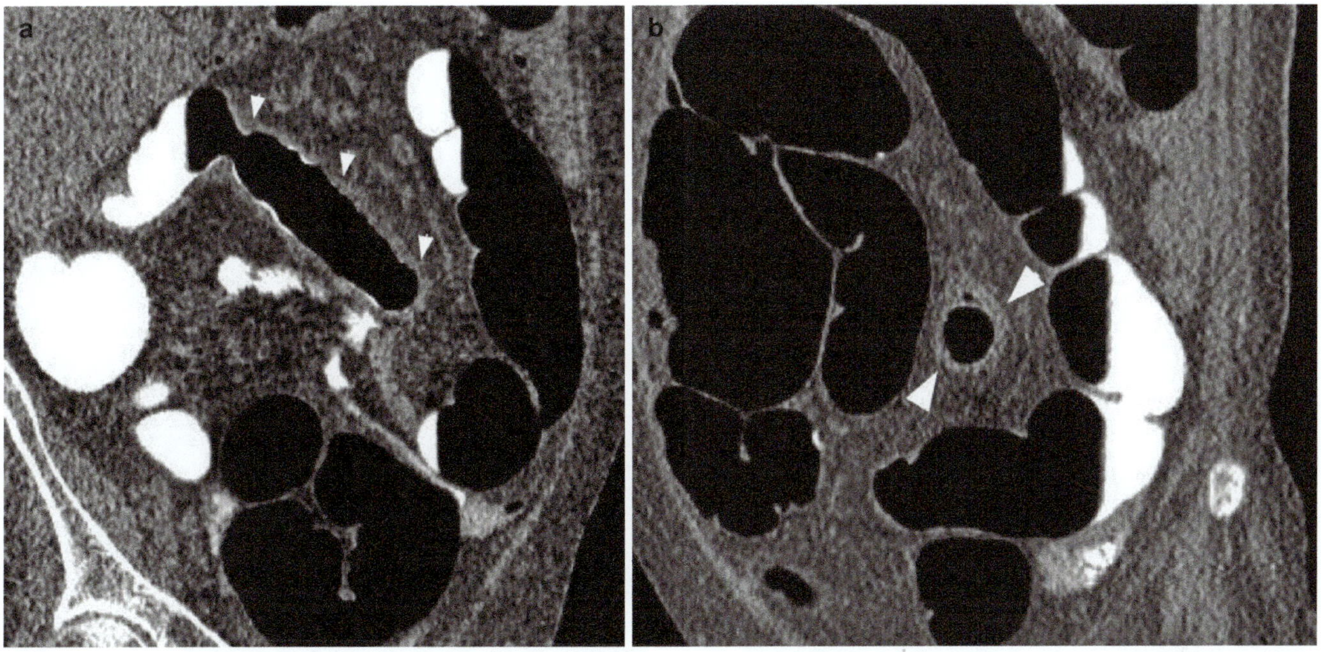

Fig. 3a and b Coronal (**a**) and Sagittal (**b**) MPR views. Annular thickening and stenosis of a large portion of the transverse colon (*arrow heads*)

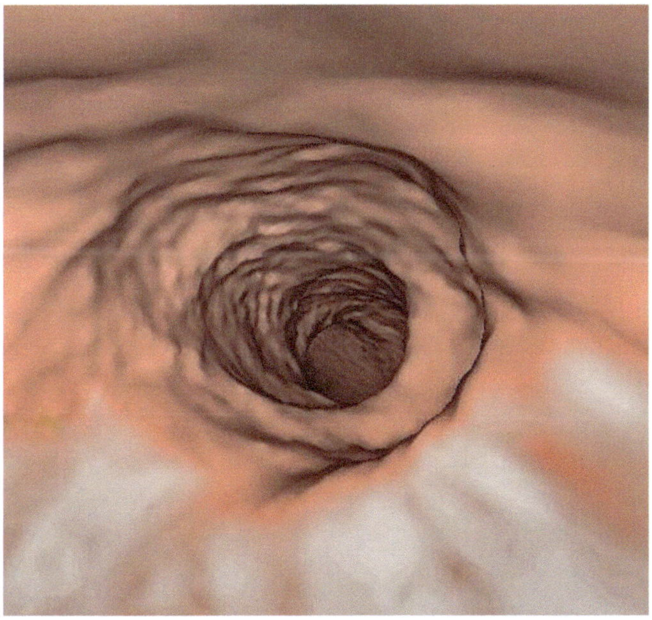

Fig. 3c Endoluminal view. Demonstrates the loss of haustral folds

Case 4. Crohn's Disease of the Rectum

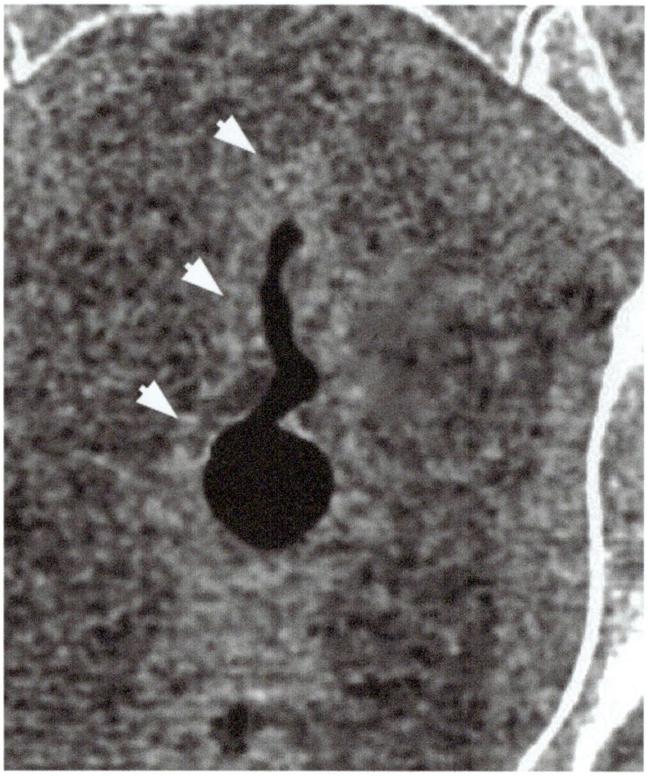

Fig. 4a Axial view demonstrates the annular thickeking of the rectum with luminal stenosis (*arrow heads*)

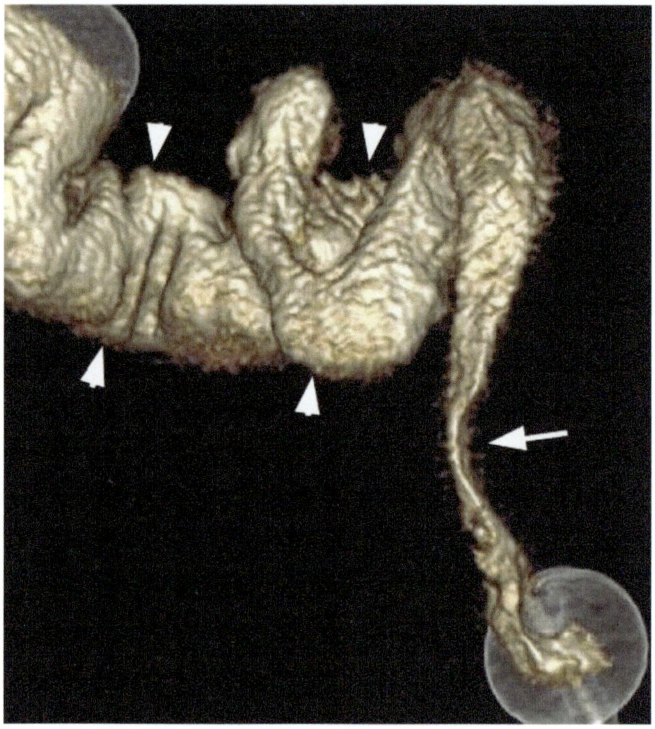

Fig. 4b The 3D panoramic view shows the luminal stenosis (*arrow*) and the dilatation of the sigmoid colon (*arrow heads*)

Case 5. Crohn's Disease of the Terminal Ileum

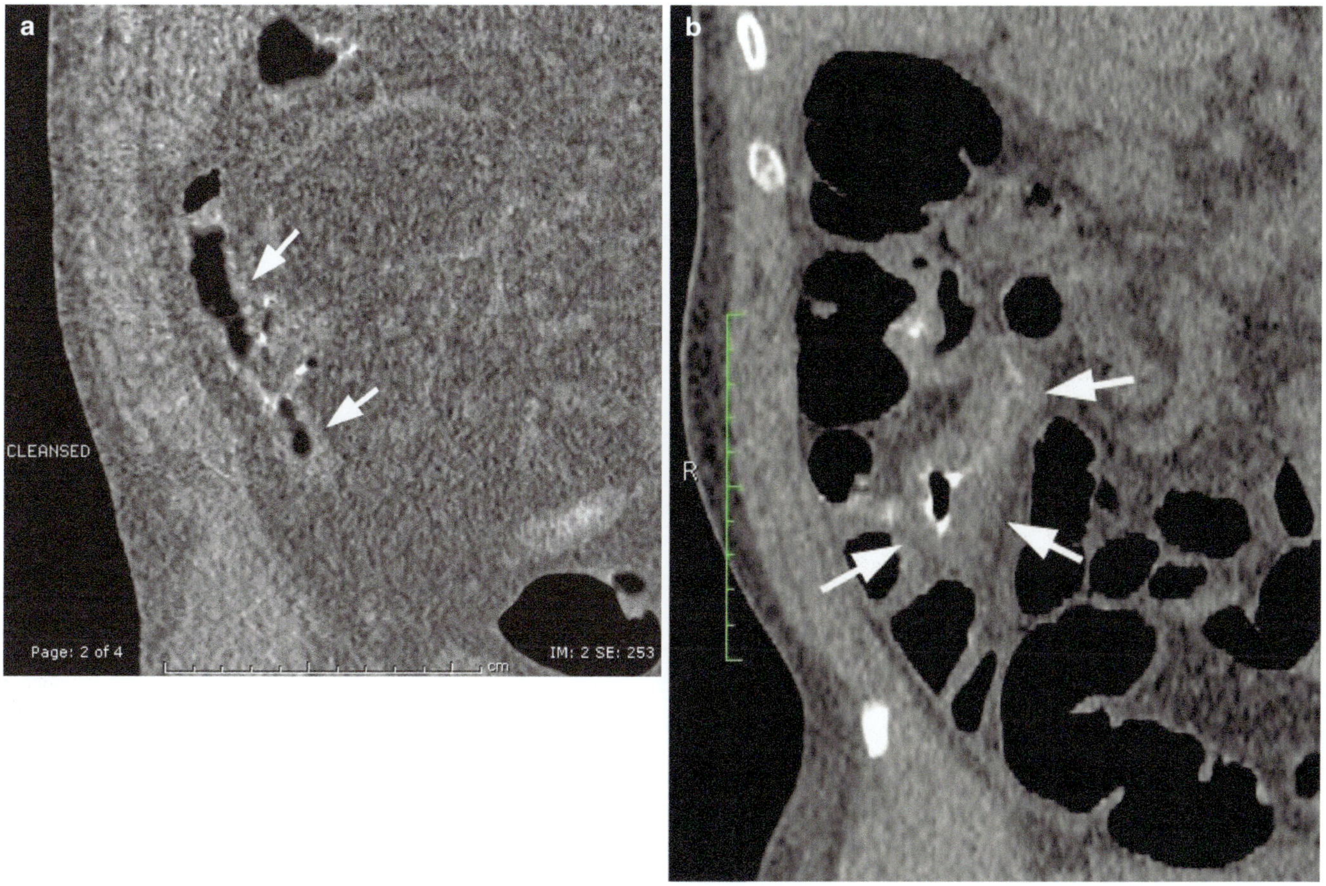

Fig. 5a and b Coronal MPR views demonstrates the annular thickening of the terminal ileum (*arrows*) in two different cases

References

1. Regge D, Neri E, Turini F, Chiara G (2009) Role of CT colonography in inflammatory bowel disease. Eur J Radiol 69(3):404–408
2. Carrascosa P, Castiglioni R, Capuñay C, López EM, Carrascosa J (2007) CT colonoscopy in inflammatory bowel disease. Abdom Imaging 32(5):596–601
3. Andersen K, Vogt C, Blondin D et al (2006) Multi-detector CT-colonography in inflammatory bowel disease: prospective analysis of CT-findings to high resolution video colonoscopy. Eur J Radiol 58(1):140–146
4. Tarján Z, Zágoni T, Györke T, Mester Á, Karlinger K, Makó EK (2000) Spiral CT colonography in inflammatory bowel disease. Eur J Radiol 35(3):193–198

Polyps: Pedunculated

Andrea Laghi, Franco Iafrate, and Maria Ciolina

Contents

A. Laghi (✉) • F. Iafrate • M. Ciolina
Department of Radiological Sciences, Oncology and Pathology,
Sapienza – University of Rome,
Rome, Italy
e-mail: andlaghi@gmail.com

Abstract

In this chapter will be discussed the morphological features of pedunculated polyps giving the readers some few imaging pearls to recognize them and differentiate them from other entities like sessile polyp or stool residues.

Introduction

A polyp is defined as a protrusion or as a projecting mass of overgrown tissue arising from colonic wall. Polyp's morphology can be sessile, pedunculated, or flat. Pedunculated lesion is defined as a polyp with a stalk attaching the polyp head to the colonic wall. Although most colonic pedunculated polyps are asymptomatic, the symptoms and their severity depend upon the size (2 cm or more in diameter) of the polyp and the length of its stalk. Commonly, symptomatic pedunculated polyps also present with a lower gastrointestinal bleeding which may range from occult bleeding, as detected by fecal occult testing to frank blood per rectum. Lower gastrointestinal bleeding associated with acute abdominal pain may be caused by torsion of stalk. Large pedunculated polyps may also cause profuse watery diarrhea or constipation.

Pathology

Pedunculated polyps have a connecting stalk between mucosal surface and polyp head. Pedunculated polyps are more common than sessile ones, but the risk of cancer is much higher in sessile villous adenomas than in pedunculated tubular adenomas. According to histology, as for sessile ones, even pedunculated polyps are classified as neoplastic (or adenomatous), hyperplastic, juvenile, hamartomatous, inflammatory, and other subtype including submucosal polyps (carcinoid tumors, hematogenous metastases, GIST, and serosal endometriomas). Removal of the benign precursor lesion, represented by adenomatous polyp, is the

E. Neri et al. (eds.), *CT Colonography Atlas*, Medical Radiology,
DOI 10.1007/978-3-642-11149-5_7, © Springer-Verlag Berlin Heidelberg 2013

aim of colorectal cancer screening [1]. The World Health Organization (WHO) classifies adenomas into tubular (less than 20 % villous architecture), tubulovillous, and villous, with approximately 87 % of adenomas being tubular, 8 % tubulovillous, and 5 % villous [2]. The probability of high-grade dysplasia and of carcinomatous transformation increases with polyp size, especially when they are larger than 1 cm and with presence of villous component [3].

CT colonography Pattern

At 2D CT colonography images, pedunculated polyp appears like a homogenous soft-tissue filling defect with a nodular part, the head, suspended in the colonic lumen through a stalk. Positional change of polyp head according to gravity can be found comparing axial supine and prone images. 3D images allow virtual visualization of head surface, smooth or lobulated, of stalk length and its relationship with haustral folds [4]. An important issue concerning pedunculated polypoid lesion is that they can move, sometime dramatically when the stalk is long, during changing of decubitus due to gravity and they represent so-called mobile polyps. They may move not only from the anterior to posterior surface (or vice versa) but axially along the length of the colon as well. The automatic supine to prone linking done by the workstation software will need to be "unlinked" to show the comparison properly. Pedunculated polypoid lesion at CT colonography must be measured only considering the diameter of the head.

Case 1. Pedunculated Polyp with a Long Thin Stalk

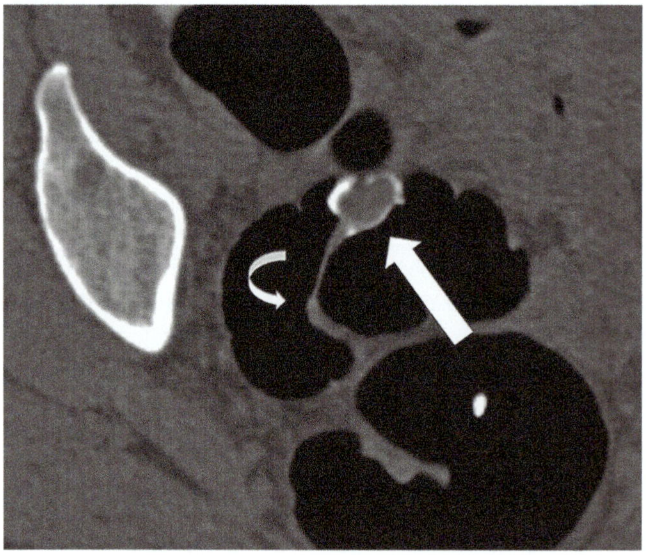

Fig. 1a Prone axial CT scan of sigmoid colon

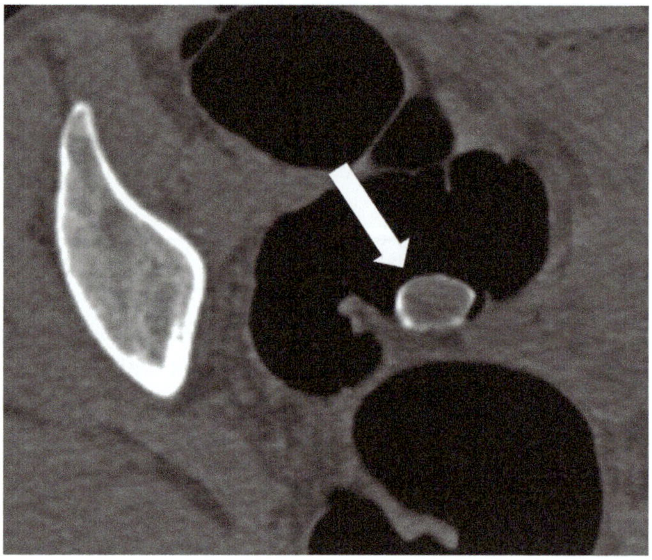

Fig. 1b Supine axial CT colonography image

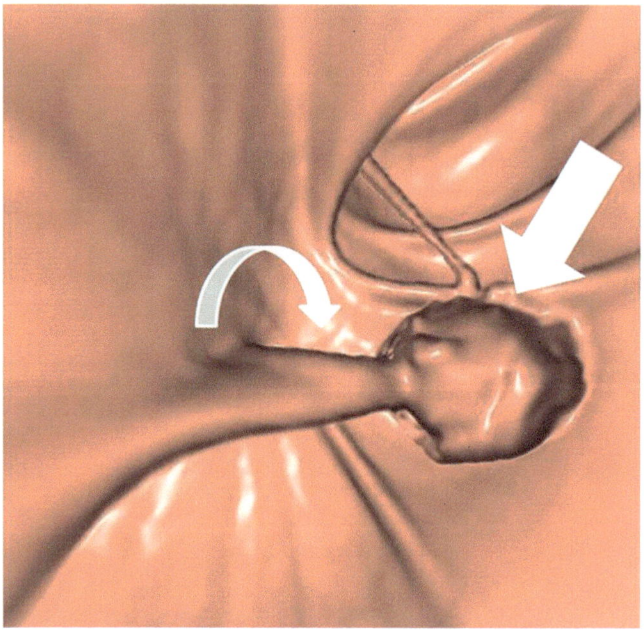

Fig. 1c Endoluminal 3D CT colonography image

Description

CT colonography 2D prone image of sigmoid colon (a) shows polyp's head as a soft-tissue nodular filling defect (arrow) connected to colonic wall through a long and thin stalk (curved arrow).

Changing patient's position from prone to supine (b), polyp's head (arrow) falls down on the posterior colonic wall according to gravity with consequent disappearing of the stalk.

3D endoluminal CT colonography image (c) shows an endoscopic view of the polyp's head (arrow) and its stalk (curved arrow).

Case 2. Pedunculated Polyp with Lobulated Contours

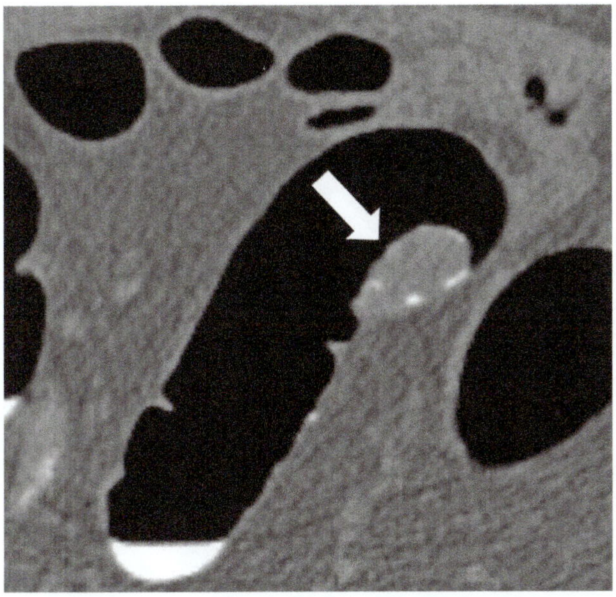

Fig. 2a Supine axial CT scan of sigmoid colon

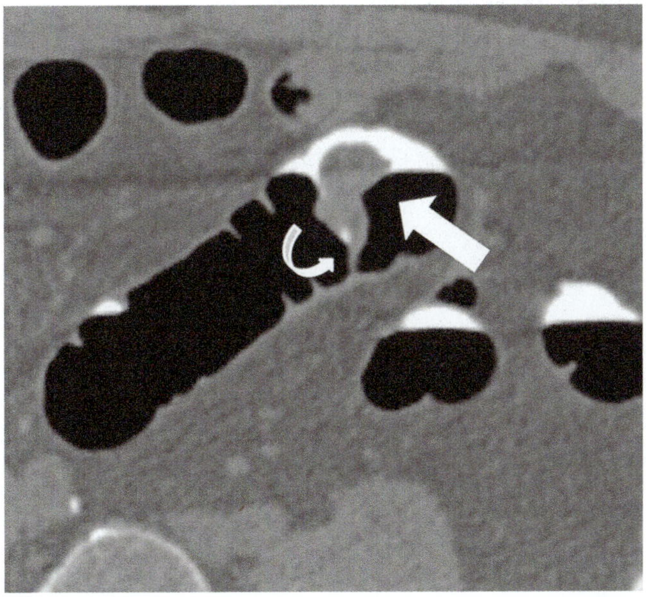

Fig. 2b Prone axial CT scan

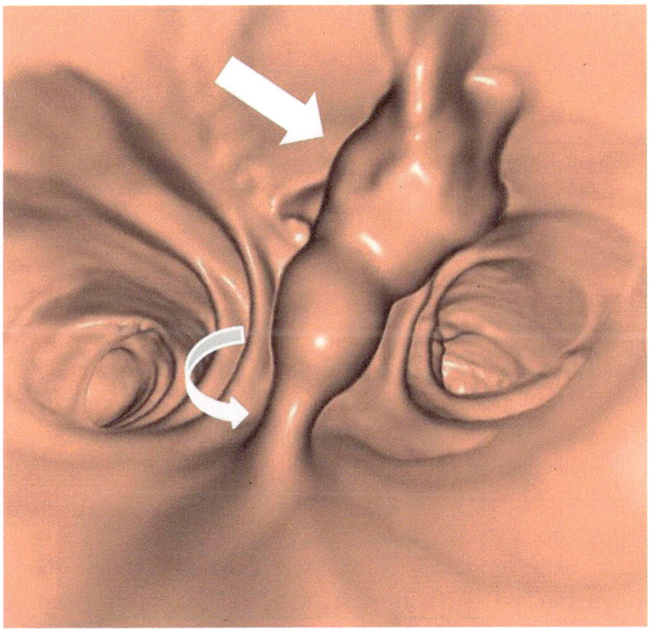

Fig. 2c Endoluminal 3D CT colonography image

Description

2D CT colonography axial supine image (a) shows a soft-tissue filling defect (arrow) with homogenous mucosal density and contours marked by oral iodinated contrast thus providing an easier differentiation from stool.

2D CT colonography axial prone image (b) reveals soft-tissue filling defect is due to the presence of a pedunculated polyp with its lobulated head (arrow) and its short stalk (curved arrow).

3D CT colonography image (c) showing the bulbous aspect of polypoid lesion's head (arrow) and depicting the short stalk (curved arrow).

Case 3. Pedunculated Polyp with a Short Stalk

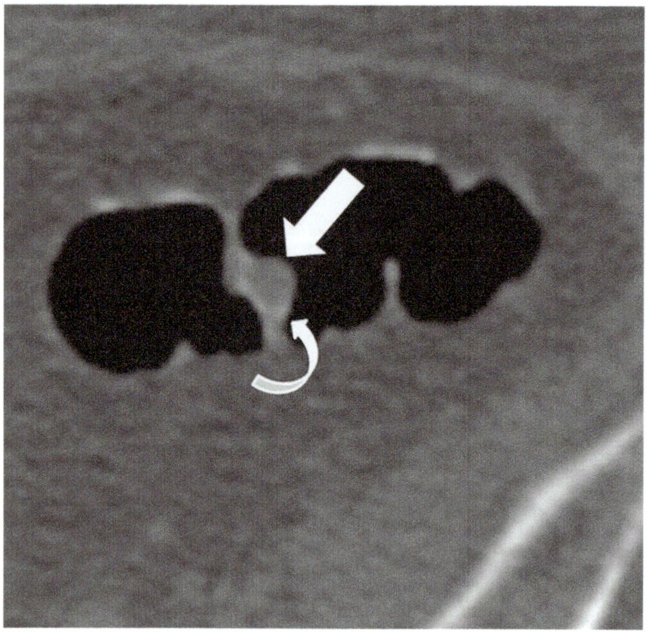

Fig. 3a Prone axial CT colonography image

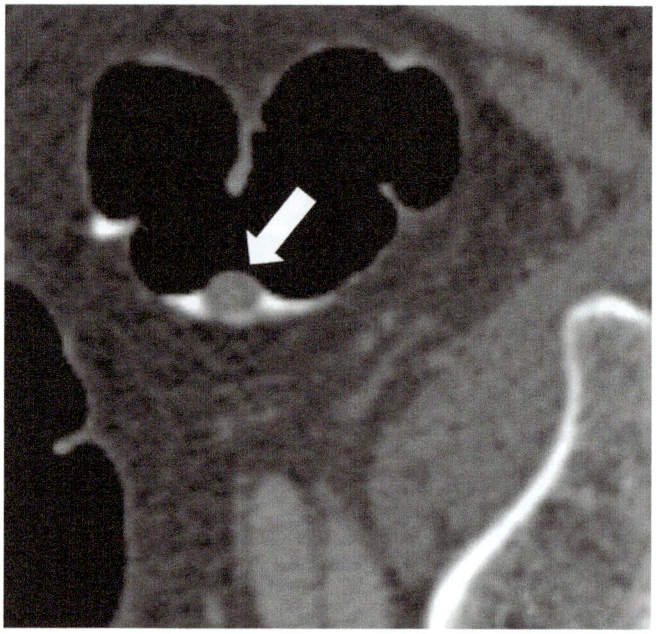

Fig. 3b Supine axial CT colonography image

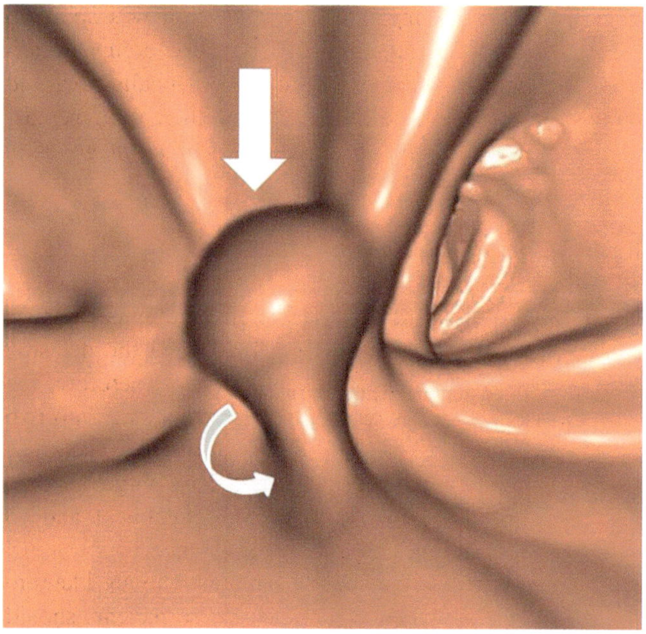

Fig. 3c Endoluminal 3D CT colonography image

Description

Axial prone CT colonography images shows a 10-mm pedunculated polypoid lesion at sigmoid colon with the head (arrow) suspended within colonic lumen by a short stalk linked to colonic posterior wall (curved arrow). From the anterior colonic wall, a haustral fold reaches polyp's head mimicking a stalk.

On axial supine CT colonography scan (b), pedunculated polyp (arrow) is easily detectable, thanks to surrounding iodinated positive contrast agent.

3D endoluminal CT colonography image (c) of polyp's head (arrow) and its stalk (curved arrow).

Case 4. Small Pedunculated Polyp Mimicking a Sessile Polyp

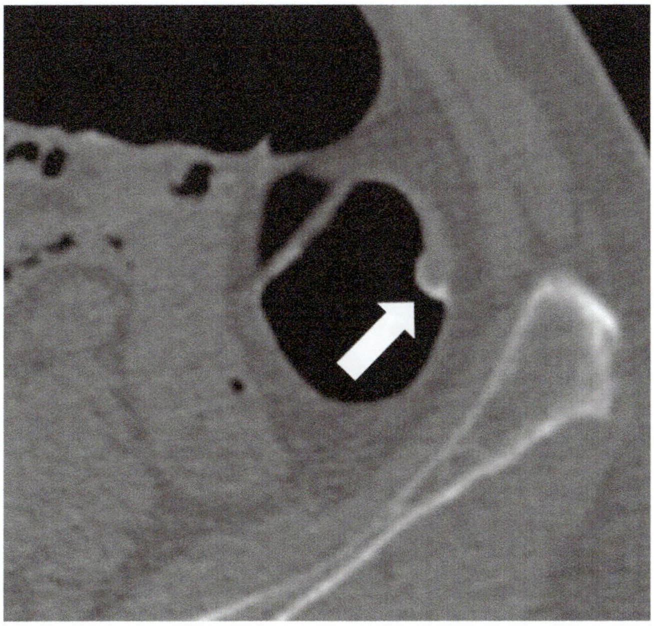

Fig. 4a Supine axial CT colonography image

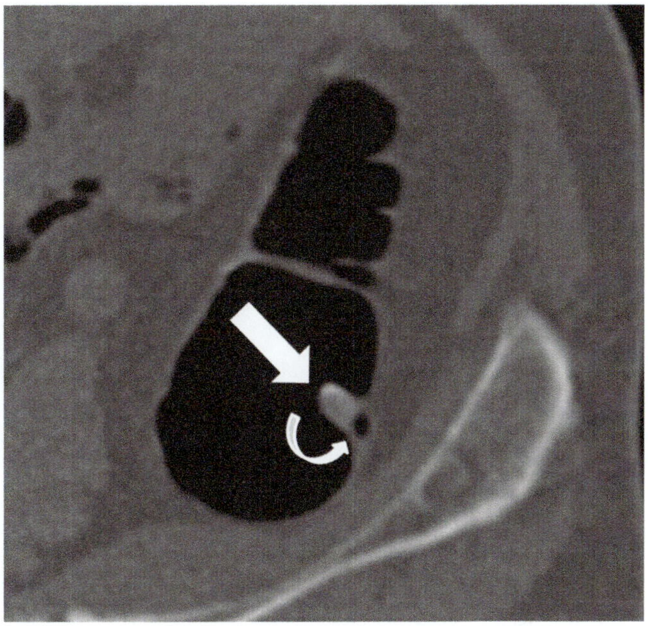

Fig. 4b Supine axial CT colonography image

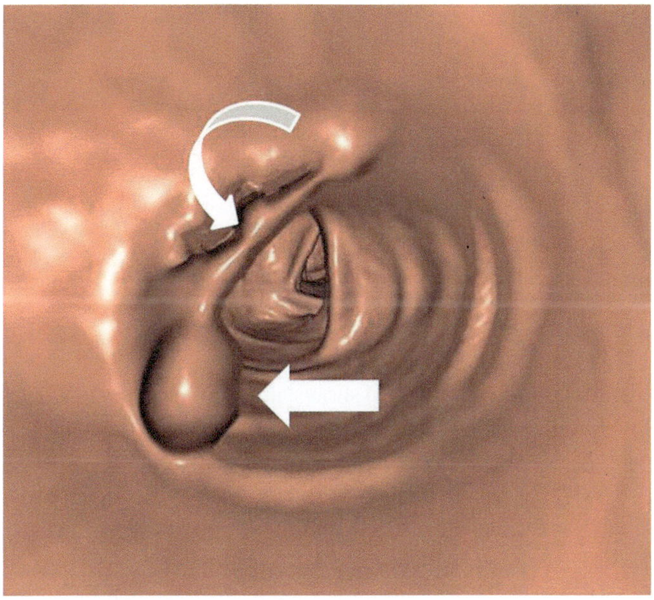

Fig. 4c Endoluminal 3D CT colonography image

Description

2D axial prone CT colonography image (a) showing a small nodular homogenous filling defect (arrow) that seemed to be directly attached to colonic wall as a polypoid sessile lesion, partially submerged by tagging agent.

2D axial supine (b) CT colonography image clarifies polypoid lesion has a head (arrow) and a tiny stalk (curved arrow).

3D image (c) confirms the presence of a pedunculated lesion with a head (arrow) and a stalk (curved arrow).

Case 5. Pedunculated Polyp with Curved Stalk

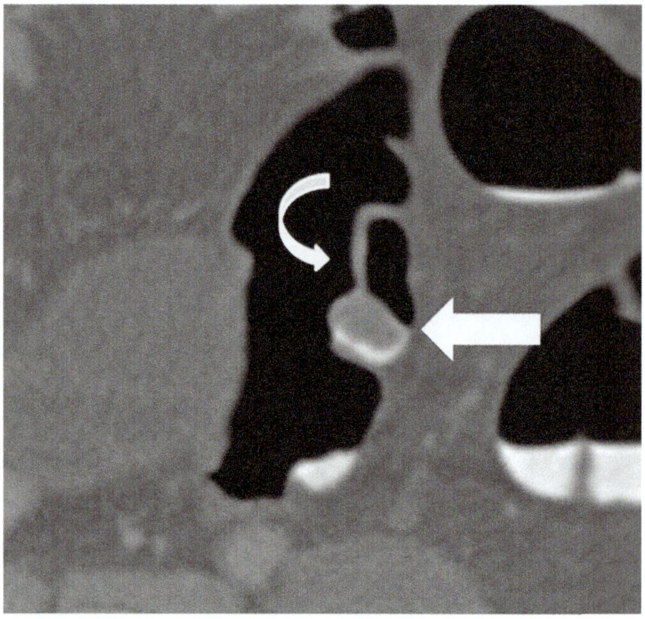

Fig. 5a Supine axial CT colonography image

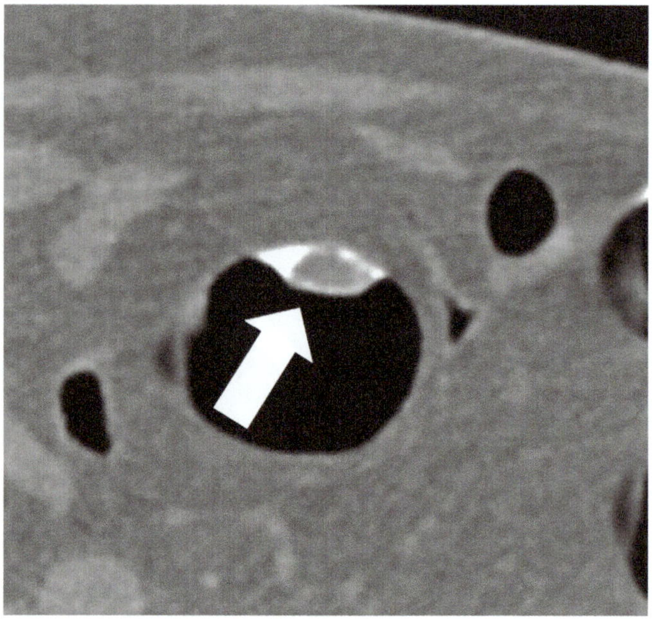

Fig. 5b Prone axial CT colonography image

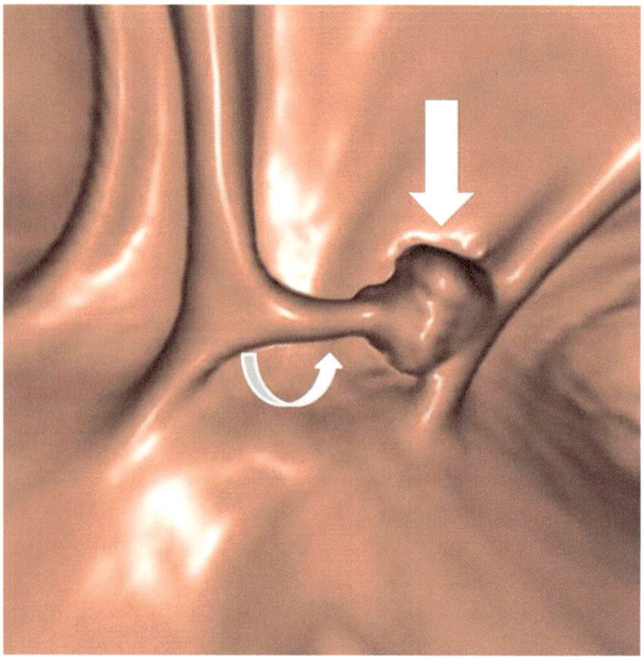

Fig. 5c Endoluminal 3D CT colonography image

Description

Axial CT supine image (a) shows, at sigmoid colon, a 20-mm polypoid lesion with a head (arrow) connected to colonic wall by a long and curved stalk (curved arrow).

Axial CT prone image (b) showing the typical positional change of the head (arrow) that moves according to gravity falling on the anterior wall of sigma.

At 3D CT colonography image (c), the pedunculated polyp with its head (arrow) and its long stalk (curved arrow) are clearly visible.

References

1. Winawer SJ, Zauber AG (2002) The advanced adenoma as the primary target of screening. Gastrointest Endosc Clin N Am 12:1–9
2. Bujanda L, Cosme A, Gil I et al (2010) Malignant colorectal polyps. World J Gastroenterol 16(25):3103–3111
3. Regula J, Rupinski M, Kraszewska E et al (2006) Colonoscopy in colorectal-cancer screening for detection of advanced neoplasia. N Engl J Med 355:1863–1872
4. Laghi A, Iannaccone R, Carbone I et al (2002) Detection of colorectal lesions with virtual computed tomographic colonography. Am J Surg 183(2):124–131

Sessile Polyps

Daniele Regge and Gabriella Iussich

Contents

D. Regge (✉) • G. Iussich
Division of Radiology Unit,
Institute for Cancer Research and Treatment,
Candiolo-Torino, Italy
e-mail: daniele.regge@ircc.it; gabriella.iussich@ircc.it

Abstract

Sessile polyps are broad based lesions usually arising from the colon mucosa. Most sessile polyps are either adenomas or hyperplastic in nature. Occasionally sessile lesions may arise from the bowel wall or may represent extraparietal lesions. Fecal residues and other foreign objects may occasionally be misinterpreted as sessile lesions. This chapter will provide the reader with a detailed description of how sessile lesions appear at CT colonography and on how to discriminate true lesions from false findings

Introduction

Prevalence, Distribution, and Pathology

Sessile polyps are broad-based lesions arising from the mucosa, less than 3 cm in largest diameter. Their height should be more than 3 mm; otherwise, they are defined as flat. These definitions are used for reporting CT colonography, and they are largely unrelated to the histological and endoscopic classifications. Most commonly sessile appearing lesions are either hyperplastic or adenomatous polyps (i.e., adenomas). Almost all hyperplastic polyps are sessile, and they represent the vast majority of polyps sized 5 mm or less, approximately 30 % of the intermediate-size lesions (6–9 mm) and less than 10 % of the 10-mm or larger lesions. Therefore, the larger sessile polyps are usually advanced adenomas (i.e., >20 % villous component and/or high-grade dysplasia); occasionally, even the smaller polyps may be advanced or malignant. Malignant polyps are defined as cancerized. Rarely, sessile lesions may originate within the bowel wall and appear at CT colonography as a mucosal lesion. Intramural lesions include lipomas, leiomyomas, hamartomas, carcinoids, and juvenile polyps. Occasionally, extraparietal lesions may also protrude within the bowel lumen and have a polyp-like structure.

Sessile polyps are usually asymptomatic. Occasionally, they may ulcerate and bleed, and their presence may be detected by

E. Neri et al. (eds.), *CT Colonography Atlas*, Medical Radiology,
DOI 10.1007/978-3-642-11149-5_8, © Springer-Verlag Berlin Heidelberg 2013

the fecal occult blood test. However, sessile polyps bleed less commonly than pedunculated lesions. Sessile polyps are found in all colon segments. They are more common in the rectum and sigmoid colon, and their frequency decreases moving toward the cecum. However, even in the cecum, the prevalence of sessile polyps is still higher than that of pedunculated polyps.

CT colonography Findings

At CT colonography, sessile polyps are endoluminal formations with a broad base, a soft tissue, and homogeneous density. They do not modify their location when patient decubitus is changed from prone to supine. Therefore, in most cases, they are easy to distinguish from fecal residues. Feces have irregular margins and are inhomogeneous as they trap air bubbles within their texture. Air has a distinctive low density and may be readily identified within fecal residues. Furthermore, feces usually, but not always, change their position with gravity. Sticky residues are occasionally observed in subjects undergoing a low-regimen preparation. Occasionally, foreign objects such as seeds or pills may appear as sessile polyps, homogeneous and with regular margins. However, they are mobile and contrast material can sometimes seep within these objects and between the objects and the bowel wall on CT colonography, allowing a differential diagnosis. Occasionally, volume averaging may occur between the soft tissue density of polyps and the contrast material coating, making diagnosis more difficult.

Case 1. Sessile Polyp < 6 mm (Hyperplastic Polyp)

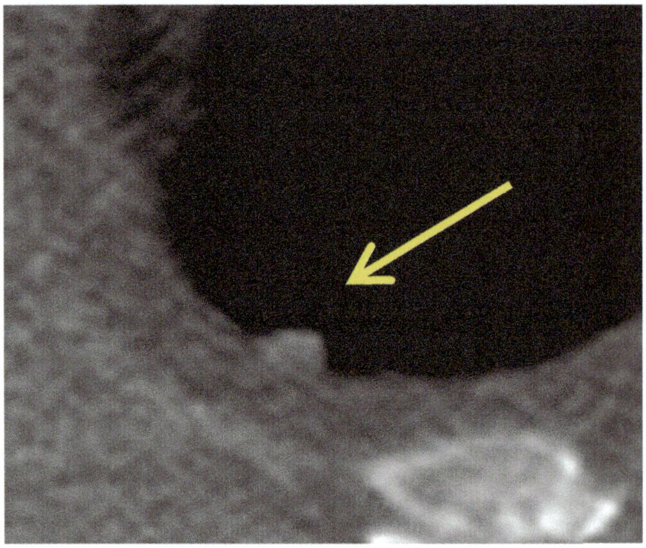

Fig. 1a

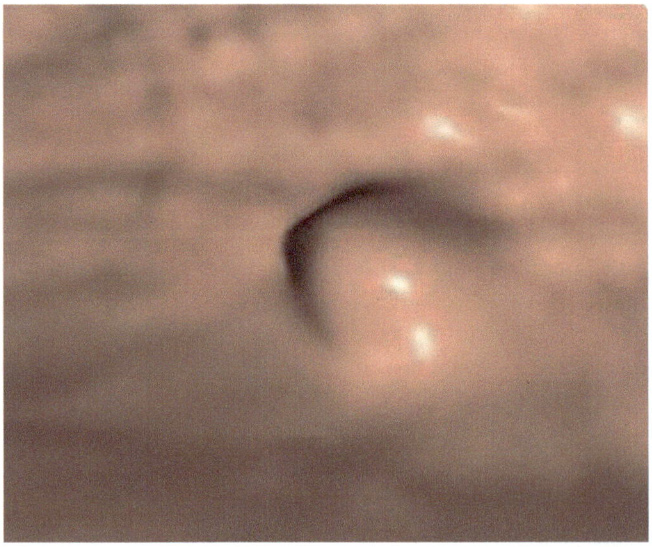

Fig. 1b

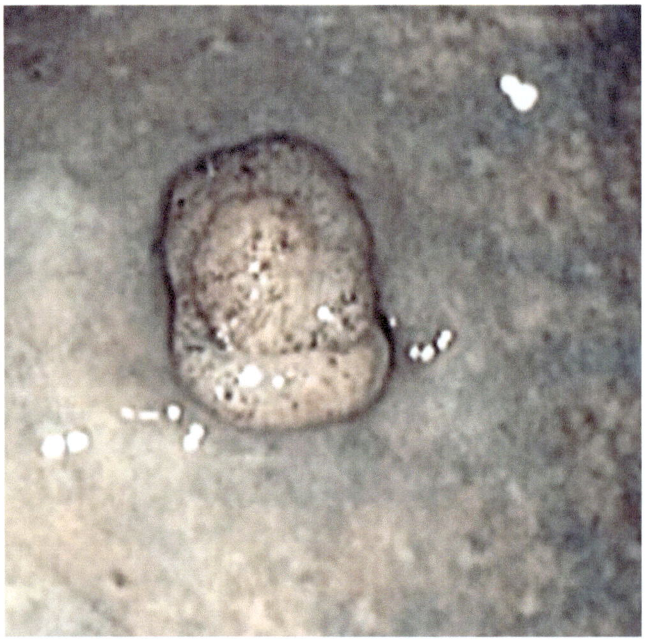

Fig. 1c

Description

A 5-mm polyp of the posterior wall of the rectum can be observed in the axial (yellow arrow) and 3D endoluminal views (a–b). Endoscopy (c) was performed using narrow band imaging, which enhances the vascular network. At histology, the lesion was a hyperplastic polyp

Case 2. Sessile Polyp 6–9 mm (Tubular Adenoma)

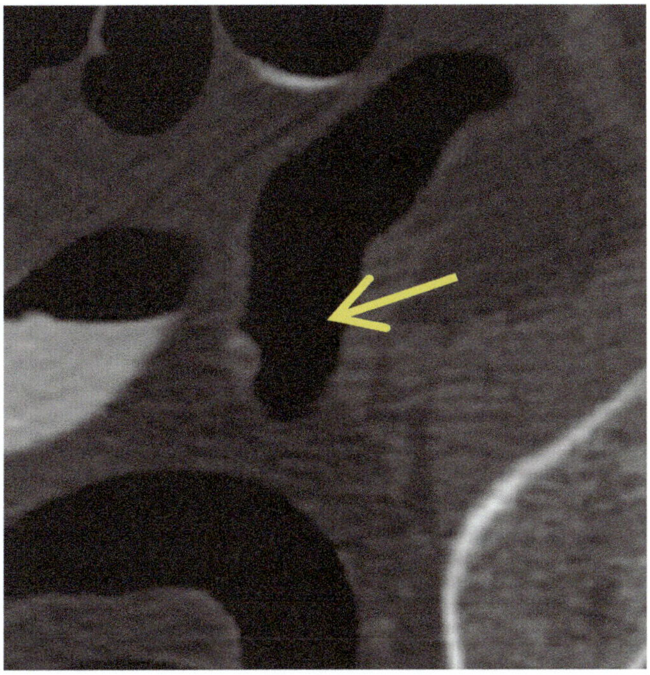

Fig. 2a

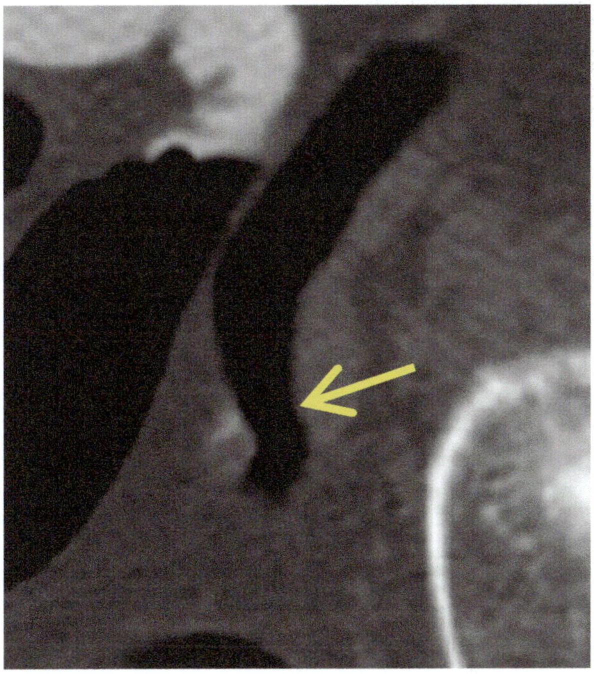

Fig. 2b

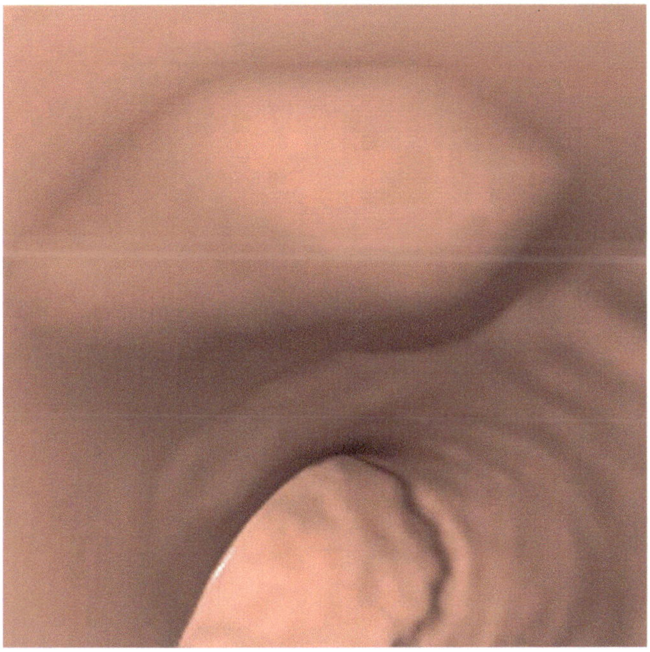

Fig. 2c

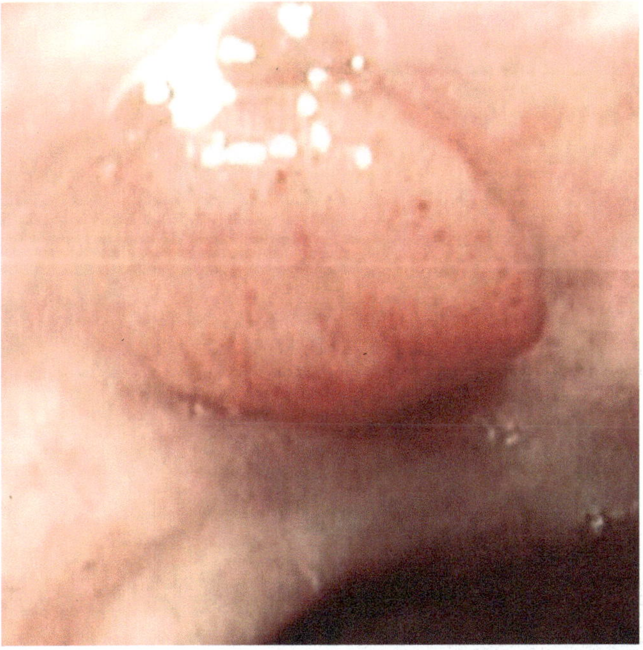

Fig. 2d

Description

The axial prone and supine images (a–b, yellow arrows) and the 3D endoluminal (c) view show a 6-mm sessile polyp of the sigmoid colon. The polyp lies adjacent to a fold (d). Lesion histology was tubular adenoma with low-grade dysplasia

Case 3. Sessile Polyp ≥ 10 mm (Adenoma, Regular Margins)

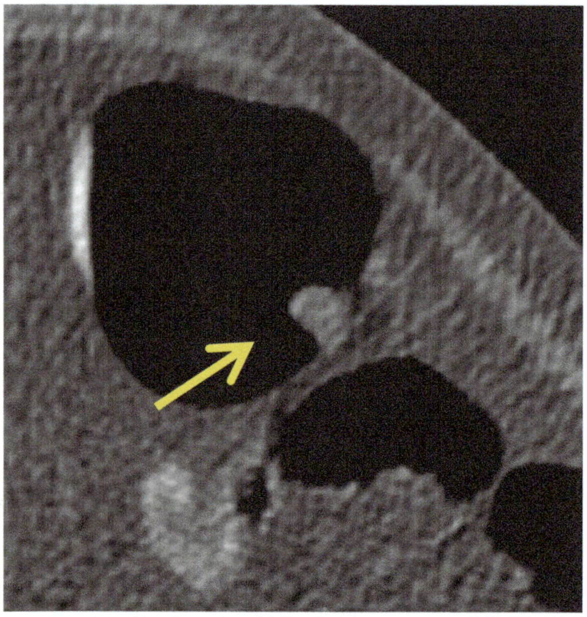

Fig. 3a

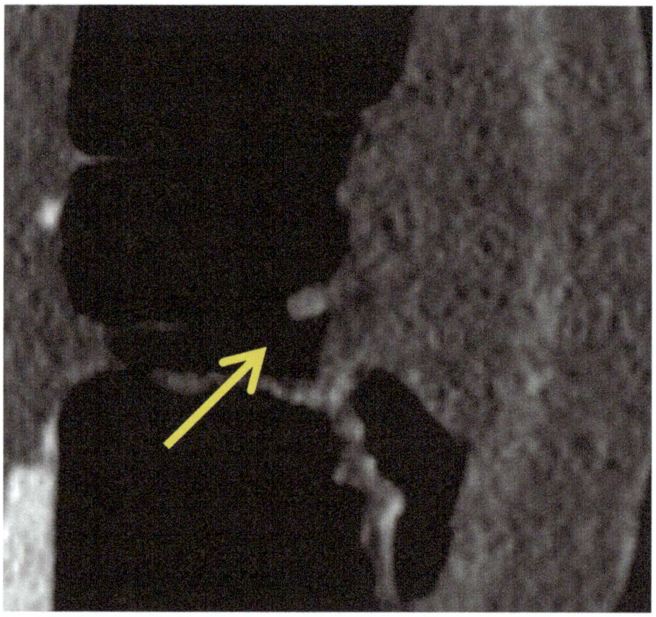

Fig. 3b

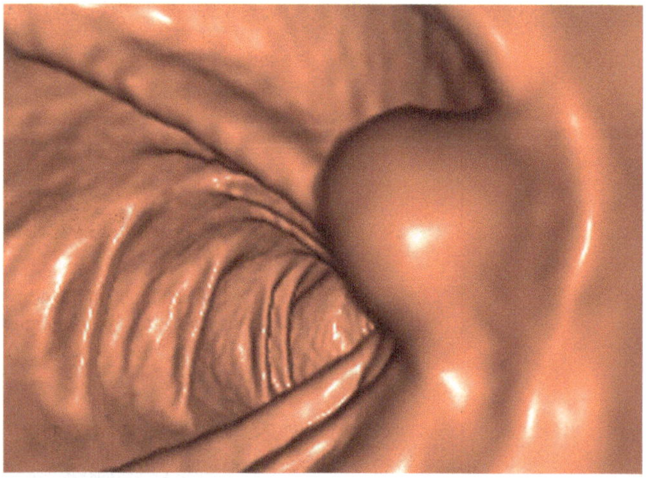

Fig. 3c

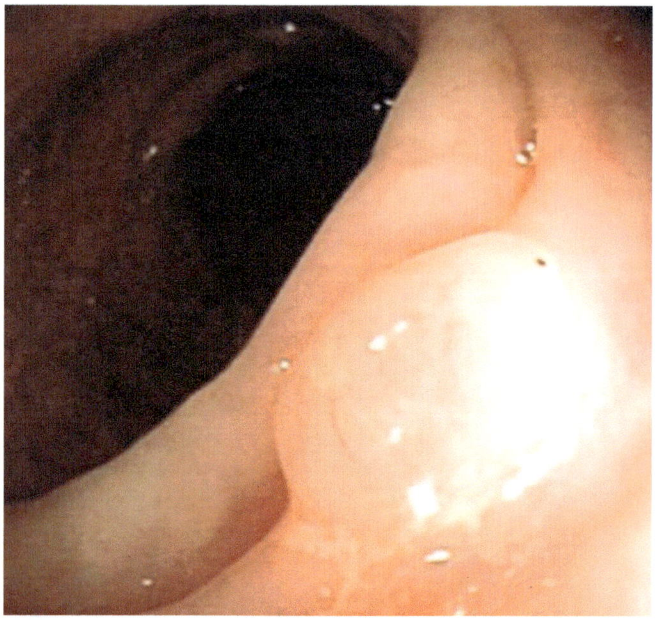

Fig. 3d

Description

The axial (a, yellow arrow) coronal (b, yellow arrow) reformats and 3D endoluminal view (c) show a 10-mm sessile polyp of the ascending colon. The polyp has regular margins and is located on top of a fold. The finding is confirmed by endoscopy (d). At histology, the lesion was a tubular adenoma with low-grade dysplasia

Case 4. Sessile Polyp ≥ 10 mm (Adenoma, Irregular Margins)

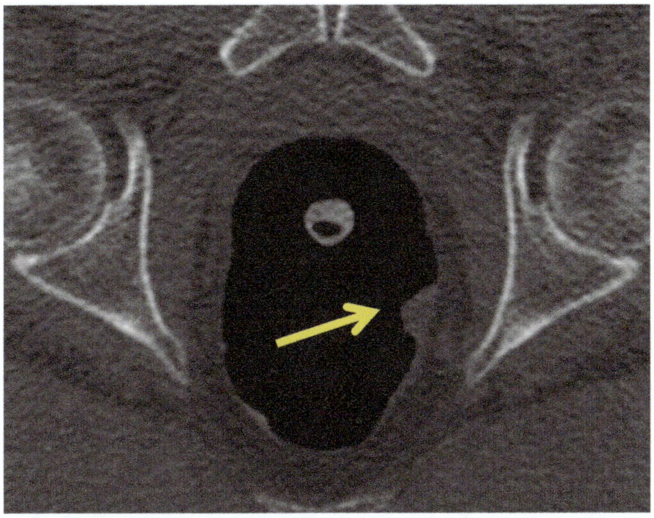

Fig. 4a

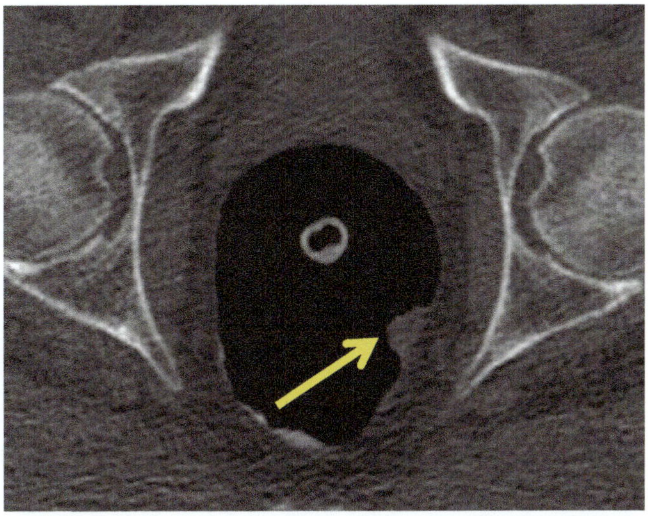

Fig. 4b

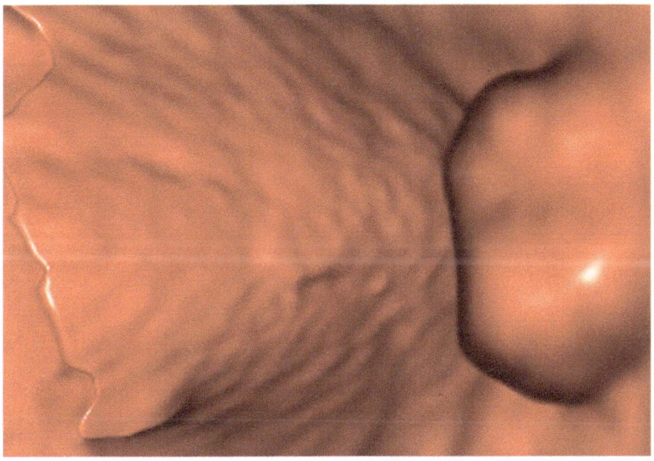

Fig. 4c

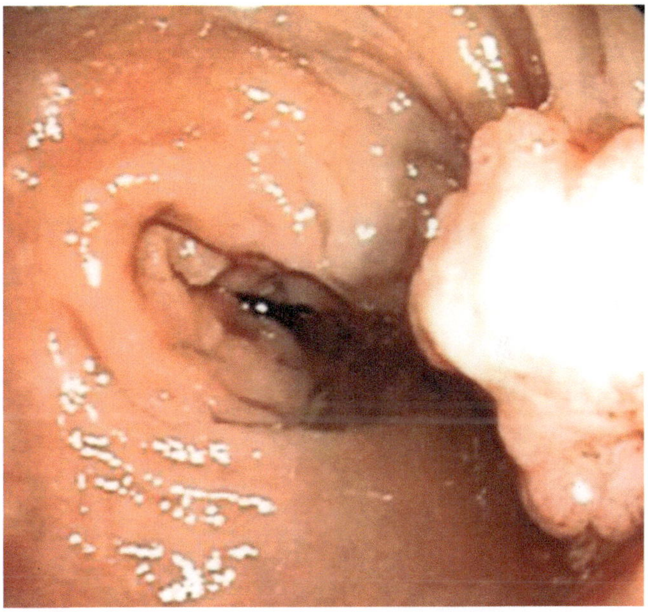

Fig. 4d

Description

The axial scan in the prone (a, yellow arrow) and supine positions (b, yellow arrow), and the 3D endoluminal view (c) shows a 15-mm broad-based lesion of left lateral wall of the rectum. The lesion hass irregular margins and homogeneous attenuation. The polyp was removed during endoscopy (d). At histology, the lesion was a tubulo-villous adenoma with high-grade dysplasia

Case 5. Multiple Polyposis

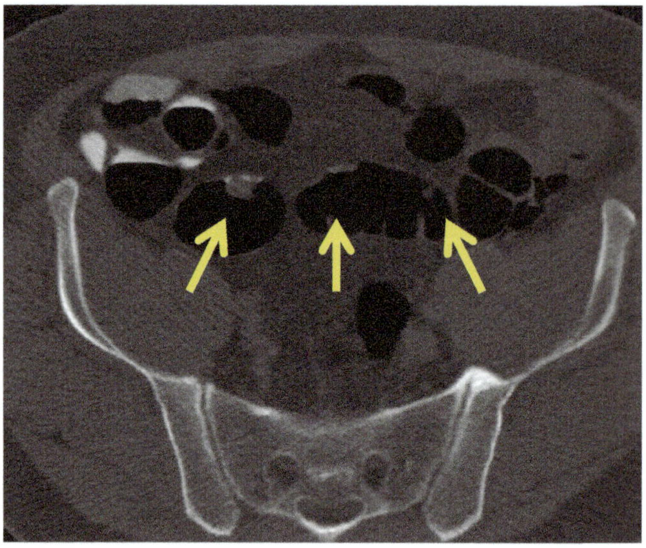

Fig. 5a

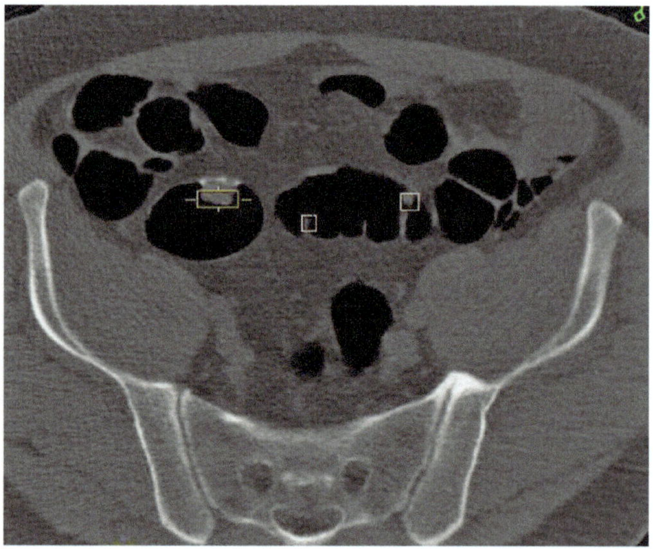

Fig. 5b

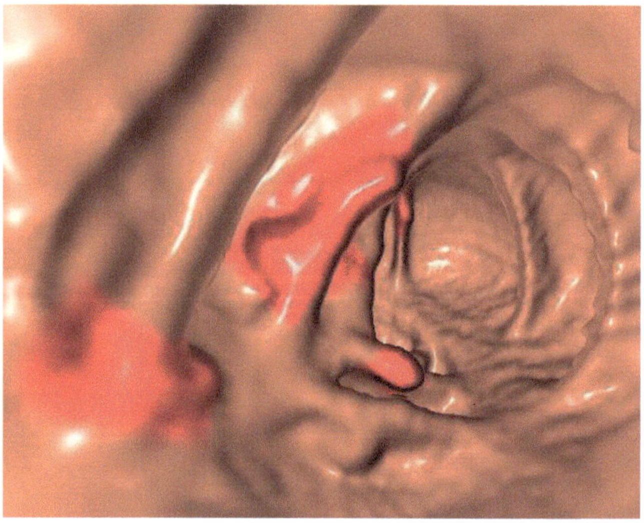

Fig. 5c

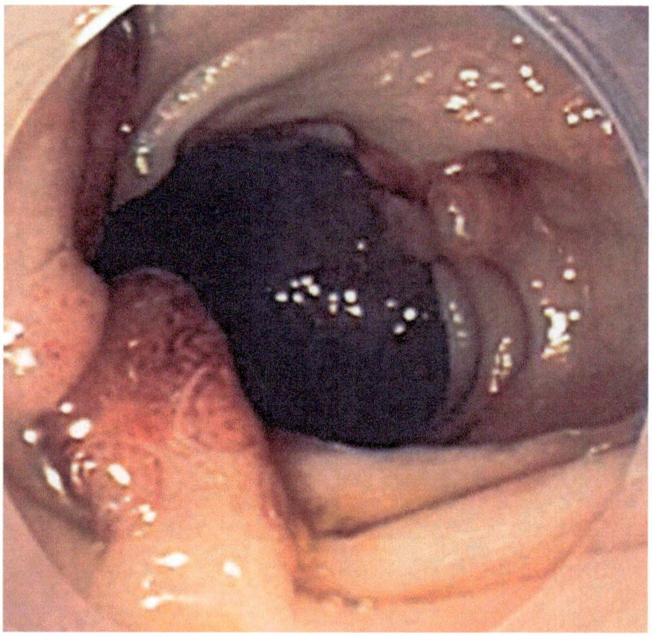

Fig. 5d

Description

The axial 2D image (a, three yellow arrows) shows three sessile polyps of the sigmoid colon. In these cases, CAD can be useful to highlight most significant lesions on both the 2D axial images (b, yellow boxes) and on the 3D endoluminal view (c, red coloring of the air-mucosal interface). The patient was diagnosed with familial adenomatous polyposis (FAP) (d) (Courtesy of Dr. Nicola Flor)

Case 6. Cancerized Polyp (8 mm)

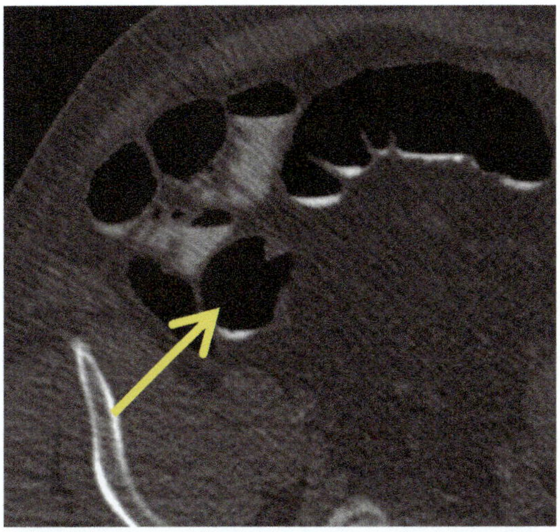

Fig. 6a

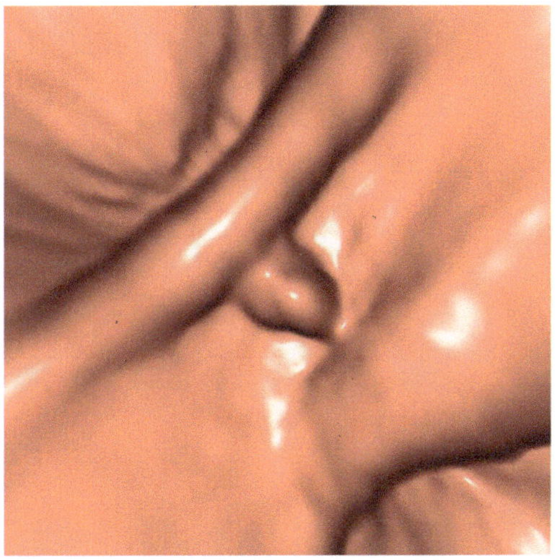

Fig. 6b

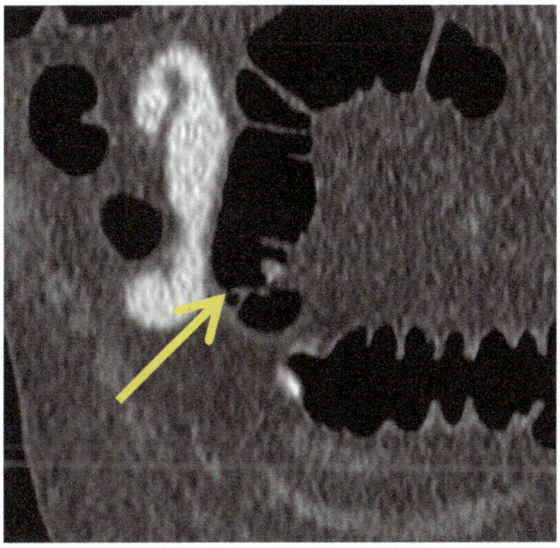

Fig. 6c

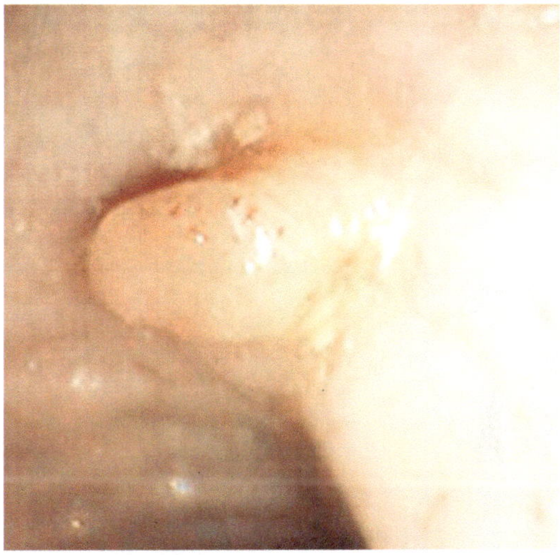

Fig. 6d

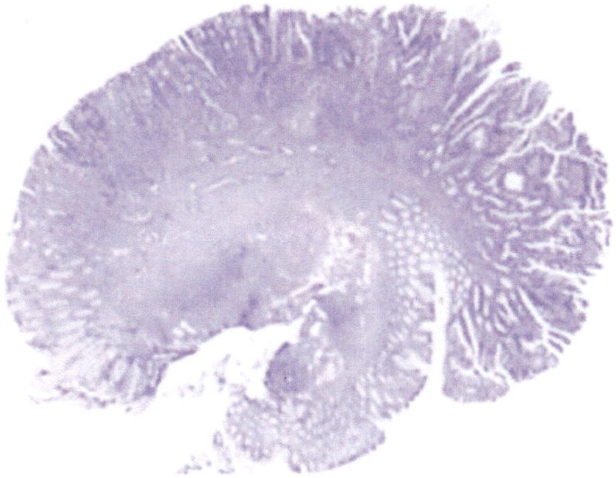

Fig. 6e

Description

An 8-mm sessile polyp of the sigmoid is shown in the axial 2D scan (a, yellow arrow) and in the 3D endoluminal view (b, yellow arrow). The polyp was confirmed at endoscopy (c) and removed by polypectomy. Histology (d) revealed a serrated polypoid lesion with adenocarcinoma infiltrating the submucosa (stage pT1) (Courtesy of Dr. Mauro Risio)

Case 7. Small Sessile Cancer

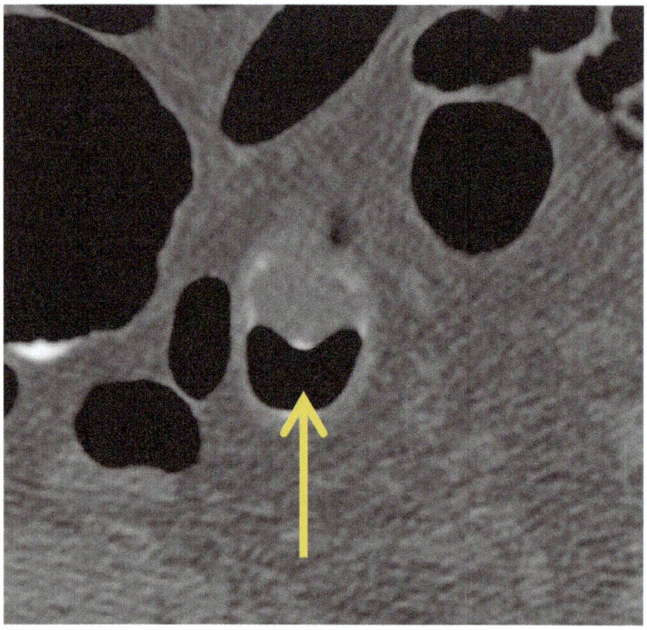

Fig. 7a

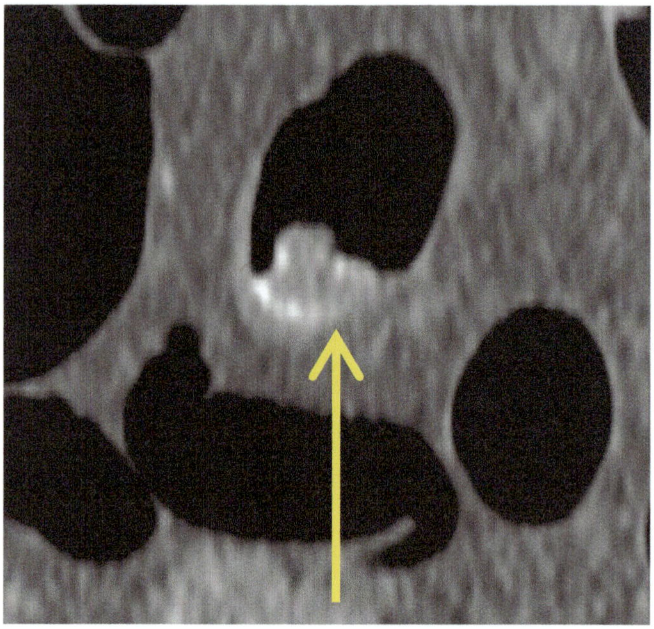

Fig. 7b

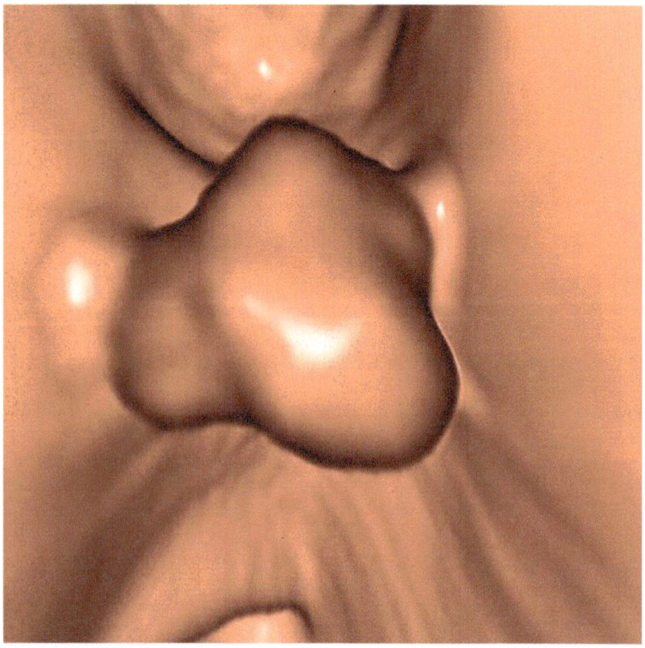

Fig. 7c

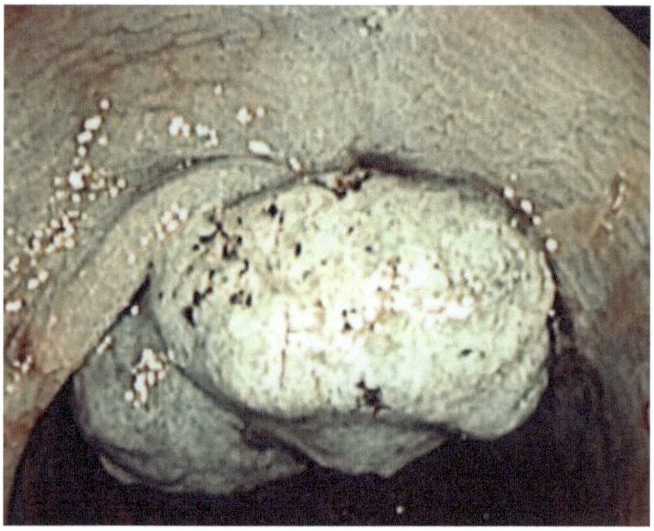

Fig. 7d

Description

A 12-mm sessile lesion of the sigmoid is shown in the axial and coronal 2D scan (a–b, yellow arrows) and in the 3D endoluminal view (c). The polyp was confirmed at endoscopy (d) and removed by polypectomy. Histology revealed an adenocarcinoma infiltrating the submucosa

Case 8. Sessile Polyp Coated by Tagged Fluid

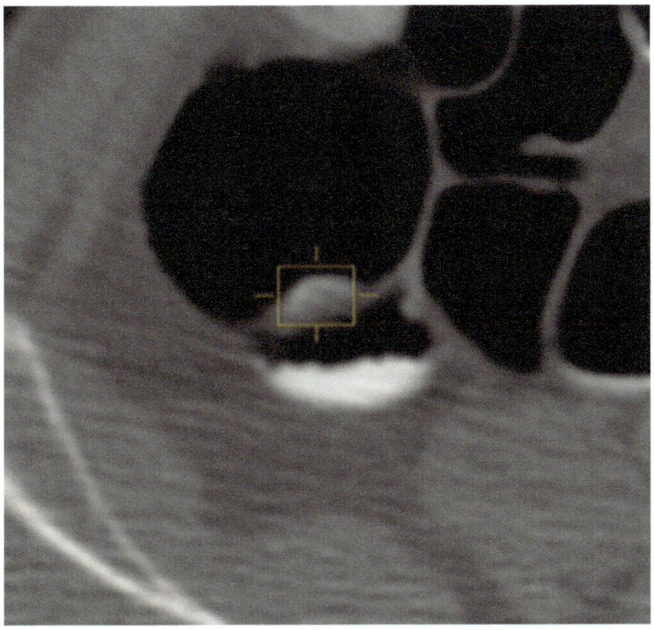

Fig. 8a

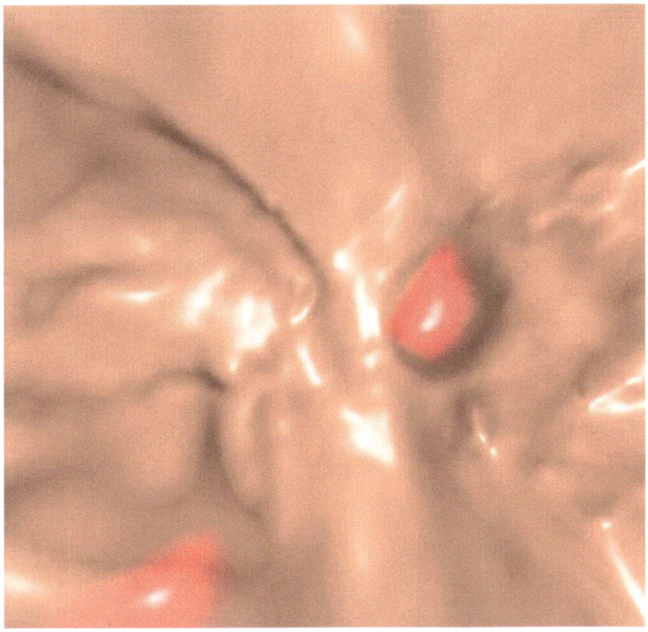

Fig. 8b

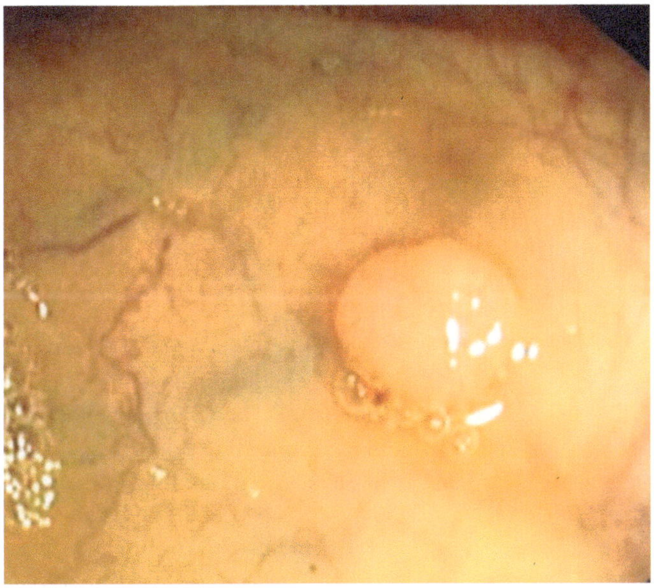

Fig. 8c

Description

This polyp was highlighted by CAD (a, yellow box) but was rejected by the reader that considered the finding a marked fecal residue. Volume averaging between the soft tissue density and the thin layer of tagged fluid may have deceived the radiologist. In these cases, careful observation of the 3D endoluminal view (b) may facilitate the diagnosis. The polyp was confirmed by endoscopy (c) and histology revealed low-grade dysplasia

Case 9. Sessile Polyp on Top of a Fold

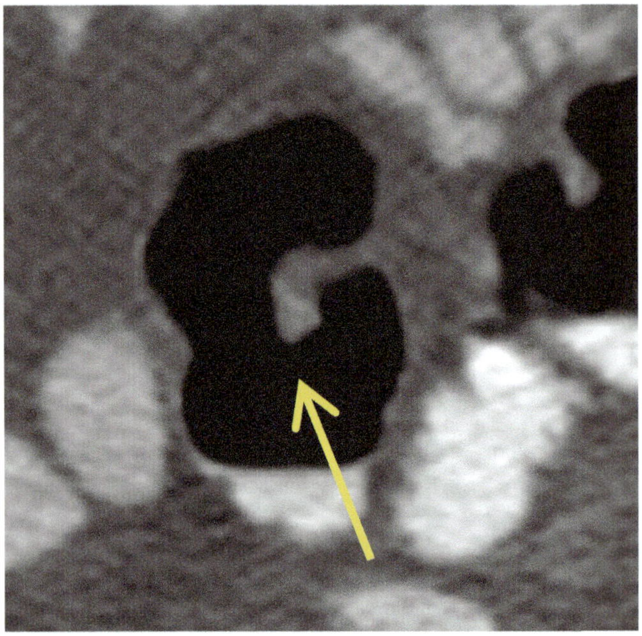

Fig. 9a

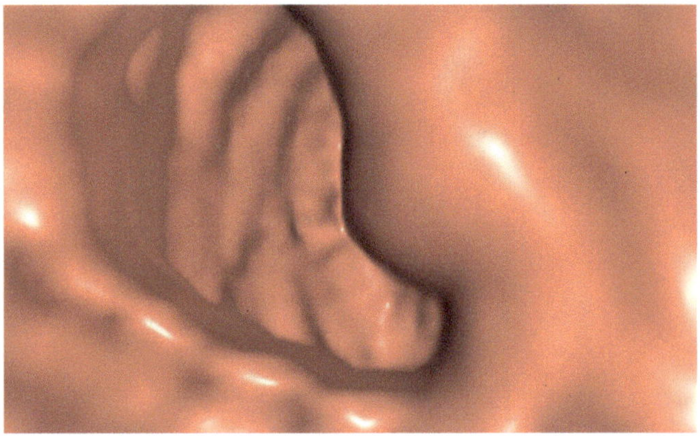

Fig. 9b

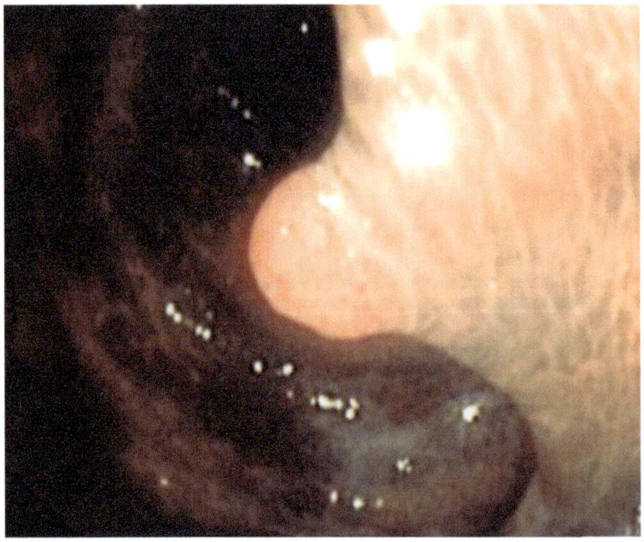

Fig. 9c

Description

Small polyps located on fold crests may be difficult to detect. In these cases, careful review of both the axial 2D reformats (a, yellow arrow) and the 3D endoluminal views (b) may facilitate diagnosis. Detection may be even more difficult when, as in this case, polyps are located in a poorly distended segment of the sigmoid colon or if folds are thicker than normal as may occur in a prediverticular condition. Endoscopy (c) confirms CT colonography findings of a 6-mm hyperplastic polyp

Case 10. Sessile Polyp on ICV

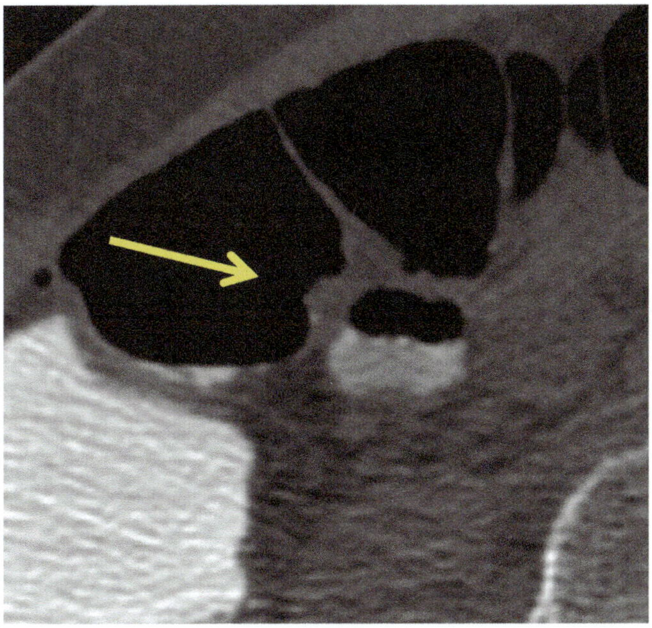

Fig. 10a

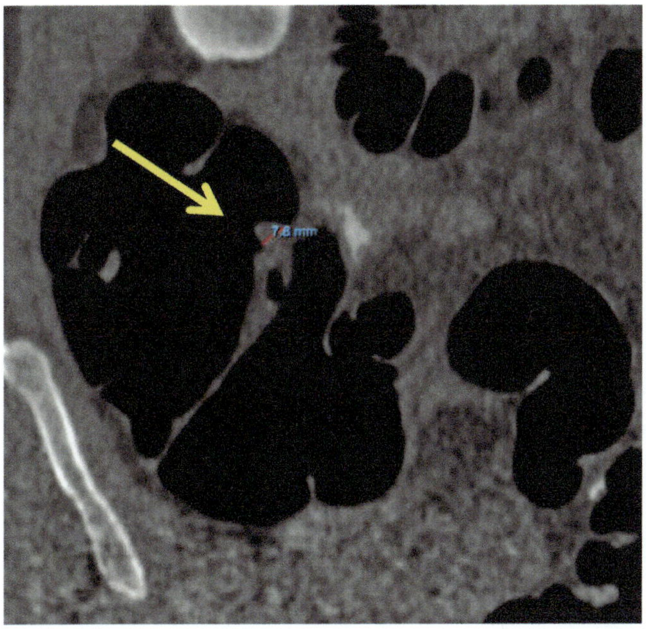

Fig. 10b

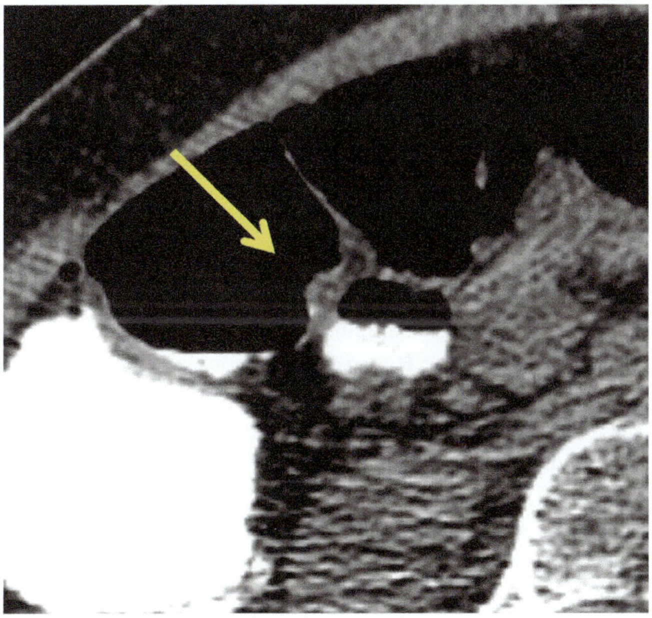

Fig. 10c

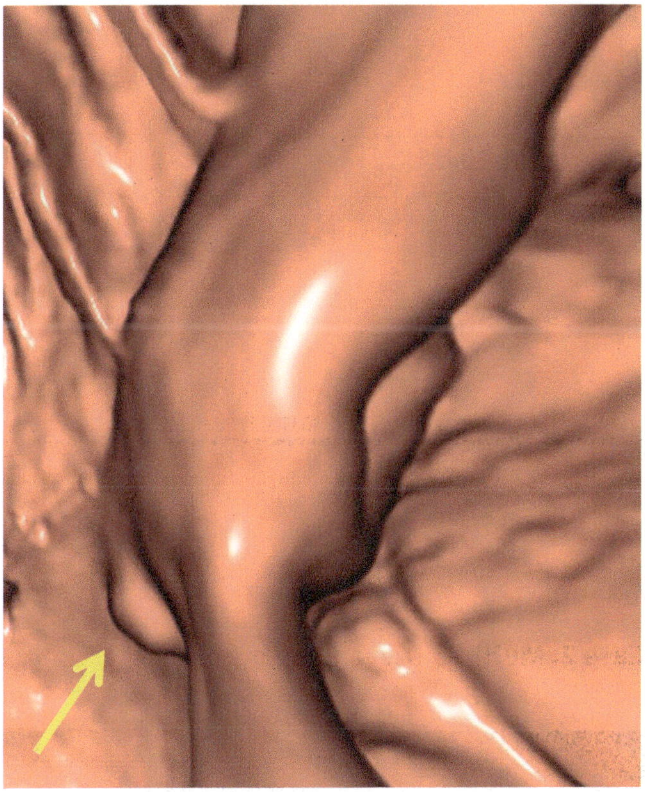

Fig. 10d

Description

Polyps growing on the ileocecal valve are difficult to diagnose as they may be considered as part of the valve, which has a polyp-like structure and a variable morphology. In this case, a 7-mm sessile polyp, located on the lower lip of the ileocecal valve (ICV), is shown on both the axial (a, yellow arrow) and coronal (b, yellow arrow) 2D reformats and on the 3D endoluminal view (c). Visualizing the valve with an abdominal window setting may facilitate diagnosis (d). As in this case, polyps have a soft tissue density (yellow arrow), while the ICV has a prevalent fatty density. At histology, the polyp was a tubulo-villous lesion with low-grade dysplasia

Case 11. Pills

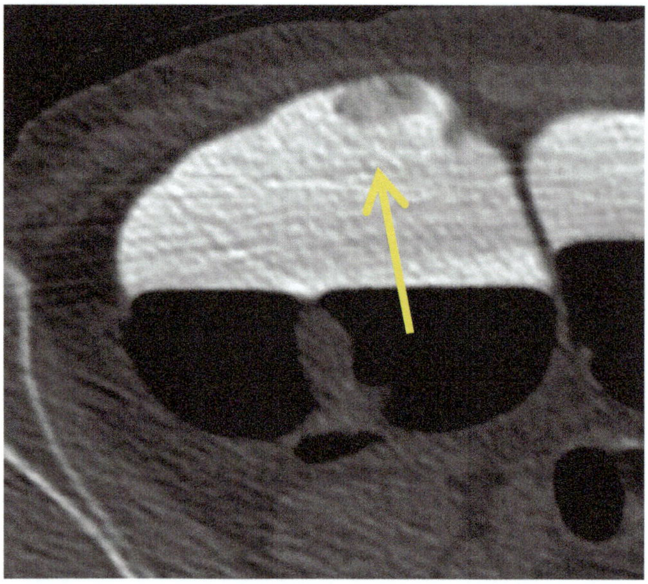

Fig. 11a

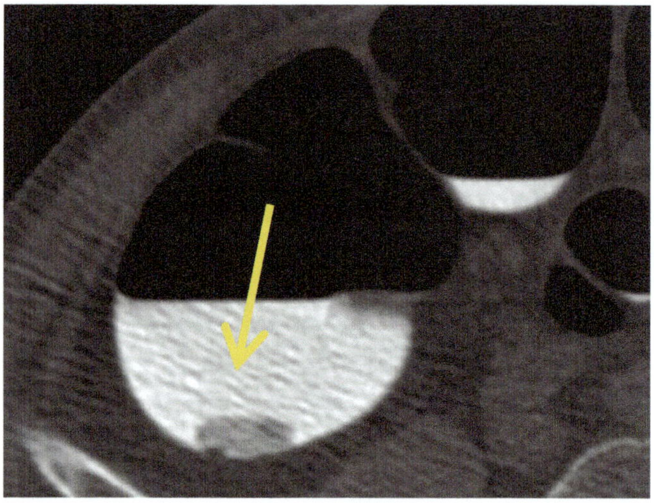

Fig. 11b

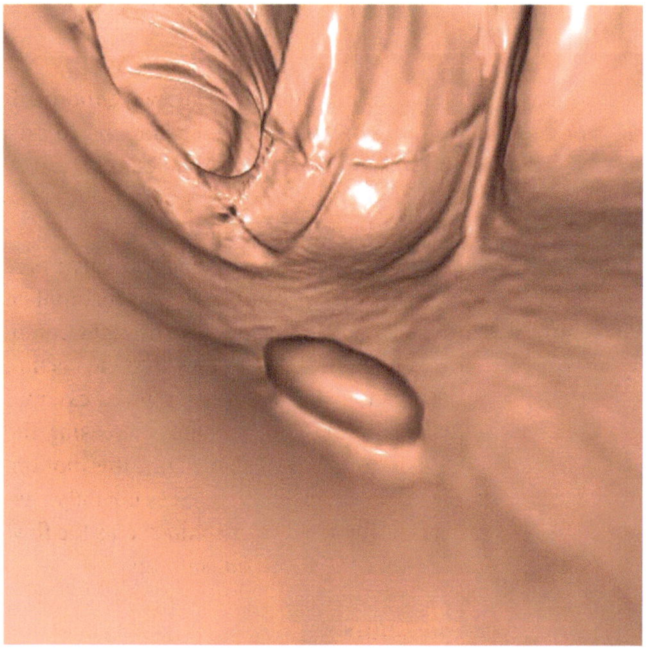

Fig. 11c

Description

False-positive findings are uncommon when using the fecal-tagging preparation. However, occasionally filling defects within the tagged fluid may mimic a sessile polyp. In this case, the prone axial 2D scan (a, yellow arrow) shows an ovoid-shaped filling defect lying adjacent to the posterior cecal wall, with a relatively high density. The finding is confirmed at the 3D endoluminal view (c). However, the position of the object changed dramatically on the supine 2D axial scan (b, yellow arrow). Patient questioned after the CT colonography exam revealed intake of antihypertensive pills a few hours before the test

Case 12. Hypertrophic Anal Papilla

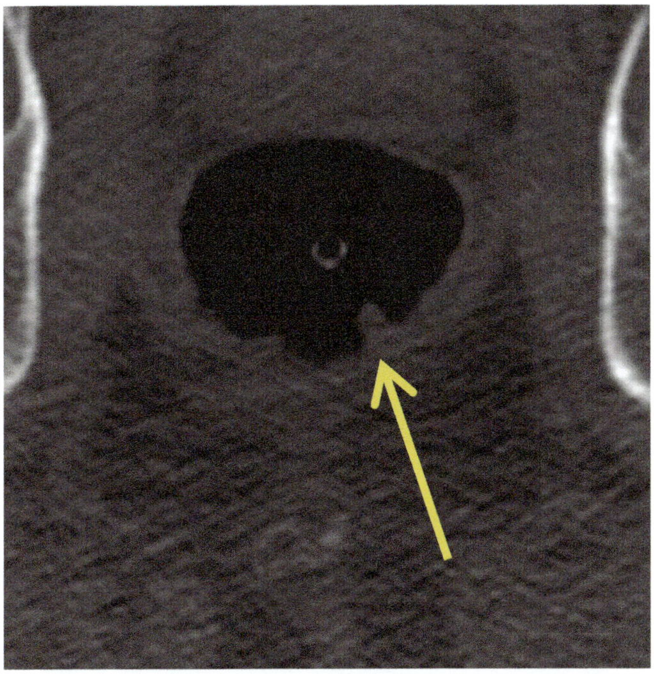

Fig. 12a

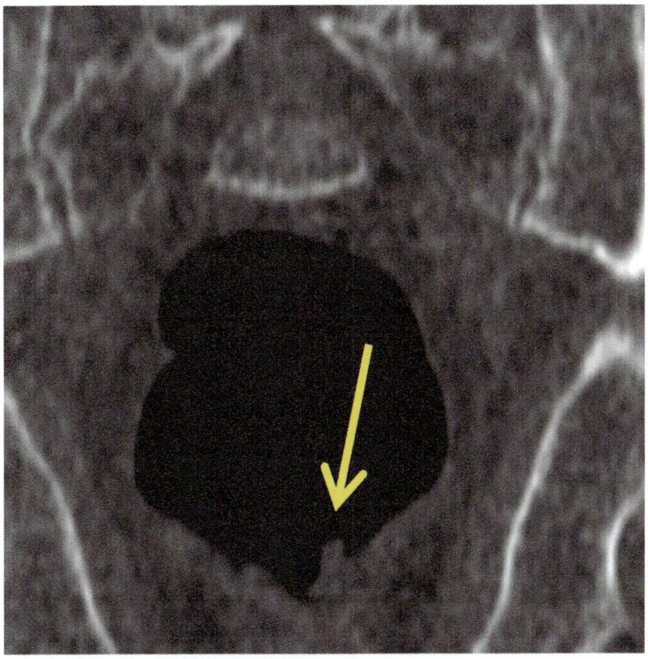

Fig. 12b

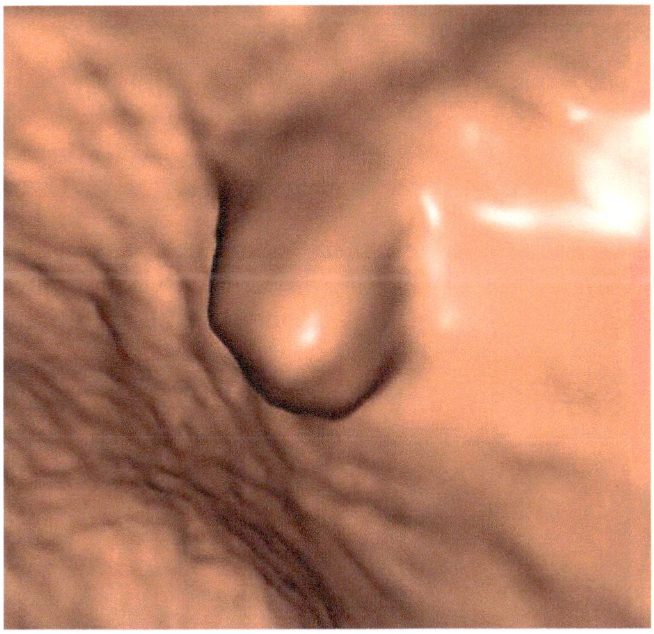

Fig. 12c

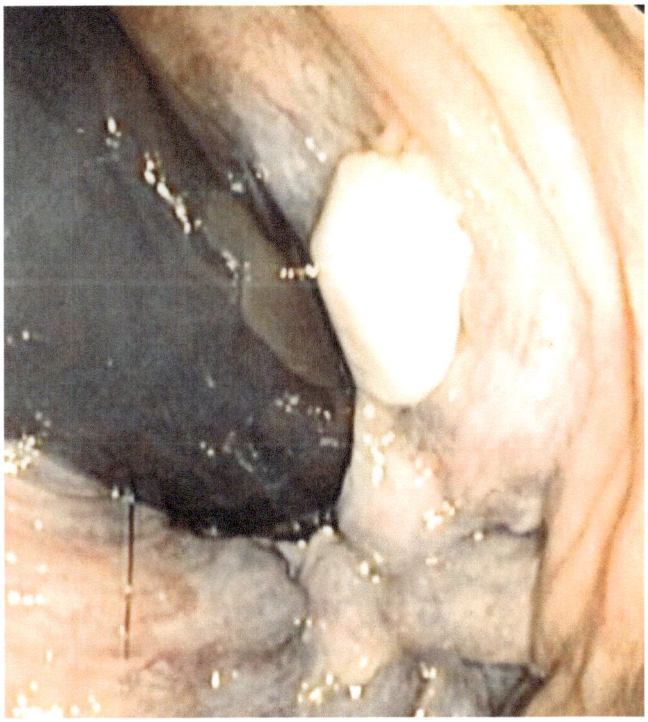

Fig. 12d

Description

The lower rectum is a difficult segment to examine with CT colonography. The inflated balloon catheter, commonly used to assure adequate colon distension, could flatten the smaller and unconspicuous polyps that may be missed by readers. In addition, small hemorrhoidal varices may be diagnosed as polyps or vice versa. Digital exploration of the distal rectum should be recommended in patients undergoing CT colonography.

In this case, the axial (a, yellow arrow) and coronal (b, yellow arrow) 2D reformats show an endoluminal filling defect of the distal rectum that is confirmed by the 3D endoluminal view (c) that was diagnosed as a subcentimeter polyp. Endoscopy (d) shows the whitish aspect of the sessile lesion, a typical finding in hypertrophic anal papillae

Flat Lesion

Franco Iafrate, Maria Ciolina, and Andrea Laghi

Contents

F. Iafrate (✉) • M. Ciolina • A. Laghi
Department of Radiological Sciences, Oncology and Pathology, Sapienza – University of Rome, Rome, Italy
e-mail: francoiafrate@gmail.com

Abstract
In this chapter will be underlined the importance of a correct definition and categorization of flat or non polypoid lesion according to Paris Classification. CT colonography morphological features of flat lesions are then reported giving the readers some few imaging pearls to recognize them.

Introduction

Flat lesions represent a subset of sessile polyps that, as the name implies, have a "nonpolypoid" plaque-like morphology and are usually endoscopically diagnosed as <3-mm-height neoplasms. Both the prevalence and the clinical significance of flat lesions have been the source of recent debate. Flat lesions represent a major problem in the US and European screening population. However, a single-center Veterans Administration (VA) study suggested that nonpolypoid lesions may be more common in the US than in other parts of the world and more histologically ominous, than previously thought [1].

Pathology

Advanced adenomas may be morphologically classified in two broad categories, polypoid colorectal neoplasm (P-CRN) and nonpolypoid or flat colorectal neoplasm (NP-CRN) [2]. It is widely accepted that the majority of colorectal cancers develop slowly through polypoid growth. However, recent studies have shown that nonpolypoid colorectal lesions also contribute to the development of colorectal cancers [3]. Following Paris classification, flat lesions are categorized according to the level of the underlying mucosa into slightly elevated (IIa), completely flat (IIb), slightly depressed (IIc), ulcerated lesions (III), and other mixed variants such as "slight elevation with depression" (IIc + IIa) and "depressed with slightly elevated border" (IIa + IIc) [4, 5]. Large (1 cm) superficially elevated

E. Neri et al. (eds.), *CT Colonography Atlas*, Medical Radiology,
DOI 10.1007/978-3-642-11149-5_9,

NP-CRN are often labeled as "carpet lesions" in the United States and "laterally spreading tumors" in Japan. Flat lesions have been extensively reported in Japanese literature but when applying dedicated endoscopic techniques, such as chromoendoscopy and magnifying endoscopy, have been consistently reported even in Western countries [6]. Several studies have shown that flat lesions have an increased risk of harboring high-grade dysplasia and of rapidly progressing to invasive carcinoma than polypoid lesions. It has been postulated that nonpolypoid lesions may account for 20–30 % of colorectal cancer. In particular, depressed nonpolypoid lesions, which have been described as the most difficult lesions to detect, have the highest risk to be cancerous at the time of diagnosis.

CT colonography Pattern

At CT colonography, flat lesion can appear as plaque-shaped mucosal elevation, with or without a central depression, as a thickened haustral fold with typical "cigar-like" morphology, or as several nodular mucosal surfaces [3, 7]. From a morphological point of view, flat lesions have been classified as lesions less than 3 mm in elevation, as very broad lesions 5-mm high, or as lesions three times larger than higher. There is controversy regarding the prevalence, clinical importance, and appropriate screening methods for nonpolypoid (flat and depressed) polyps in the colon. Because flat lesions are generally less conspicuous than polypoid lesions, they tend to be more challenging to initially detect at CT colonography, as with optical colonoscopy. The importance of nonpolypoid (also colloquially referred to as "flat") colorectal adenomas as precursors of colorectal cancer is increasingly recognized [2, 3]. Some studies suggested a greater risk for malignancy of nonpolypoid adenomas compared with that of polypoid lesions [3, 4], although there are also contradicting results [5].

Case 1. Slightly Elevated Flat Lesion (IIa)

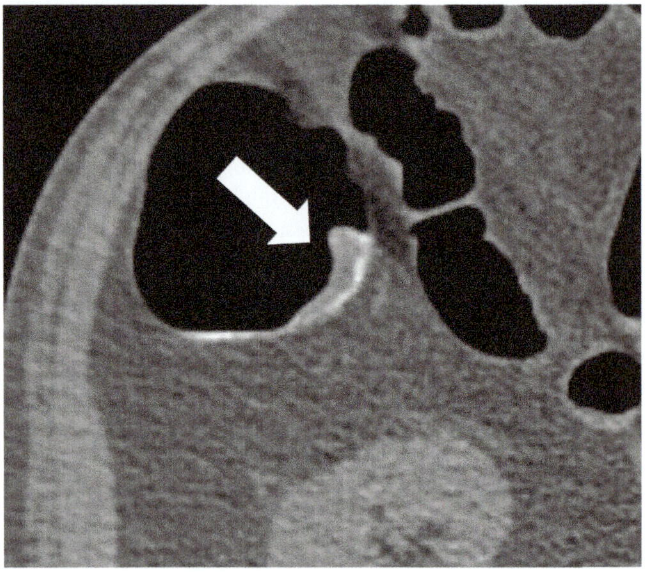

Fig. 1a Supine axial CT scan of ascending colon

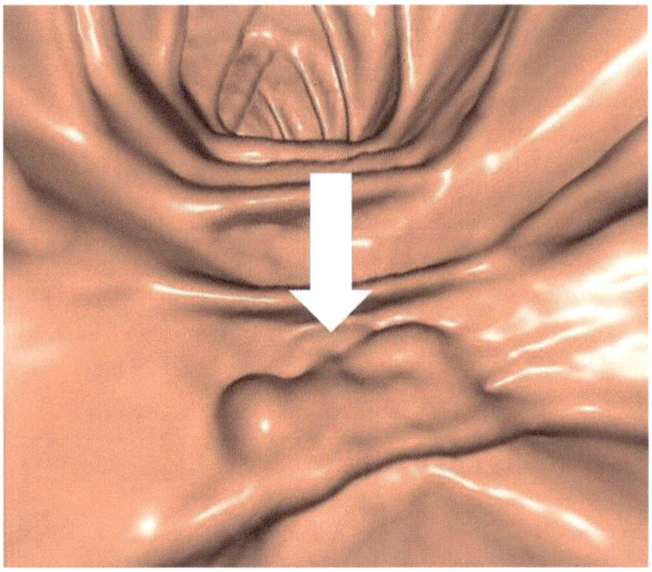

Fig. 1b Endoluminal 3D CT image

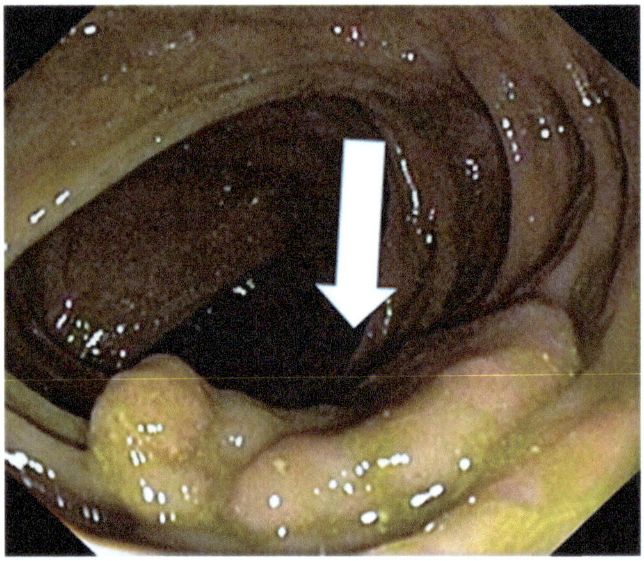

Fig. 1c Endoscopic image

Description

2D CT colonography axial supine image (a) using CT colonography window-level setting showing a flat lesion (arrow) arising between two haustral folds.

3D endoluminal CT colonography image (b) showing flat lesion (arrow) and better depicting its relationship with adjacent haustral folds within ascending colon.

Endoscopic image (c) showing precise correlation with 3D endoluminal CT colonography image

Case 2. Flat Lesion with "Carpet-Like" Appearance or Laterally Spreading Tumor

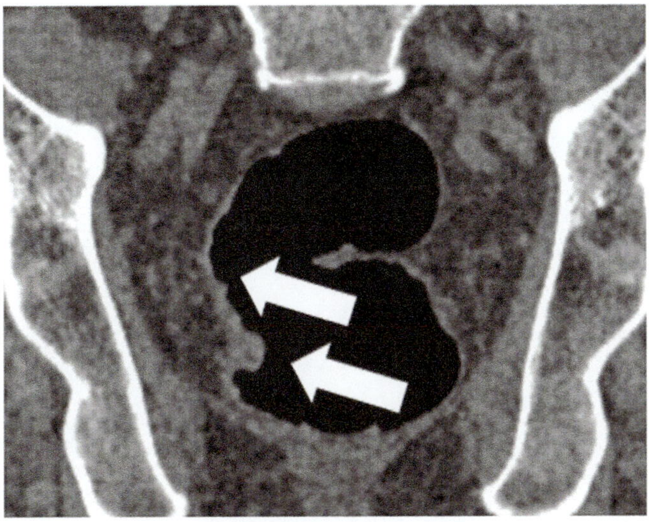

Fig. 2a Coronal 2D reformatted image

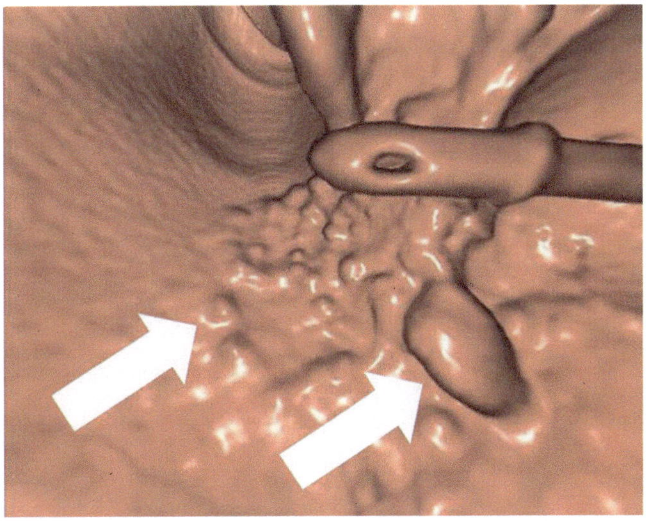

Fig. 2b 3D CT colonography endoluminal image

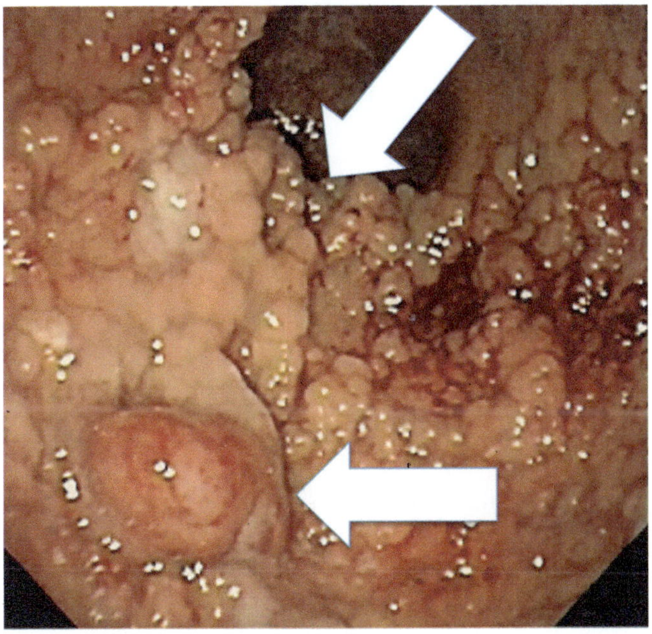

Fig. 2c Endoscopic image

Description

2D coronal prone image (a) showing flat elevation with nodular surfaces (arrows) involving the entire rectal circumference. 3D endoluminal CT colonography image (b) shows diffuse and irregular mucosal nodularities (arrows) surrounding Foley catheter. Colonoscopy (c) shows typical carpet-like appearance of the flat lesion (arrows)

Case 3. Flat Lesion with "Cigar-Like Shape" Appearance (IIa)

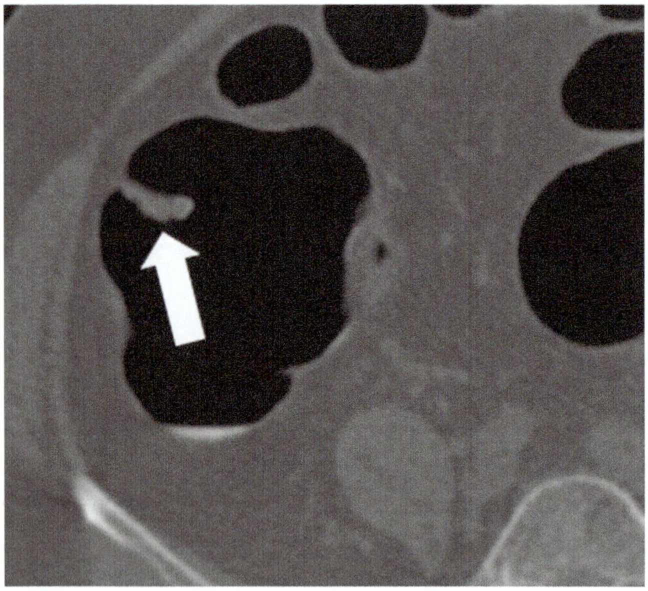

Fig. 3a Supine axial CT scan of ascending colon

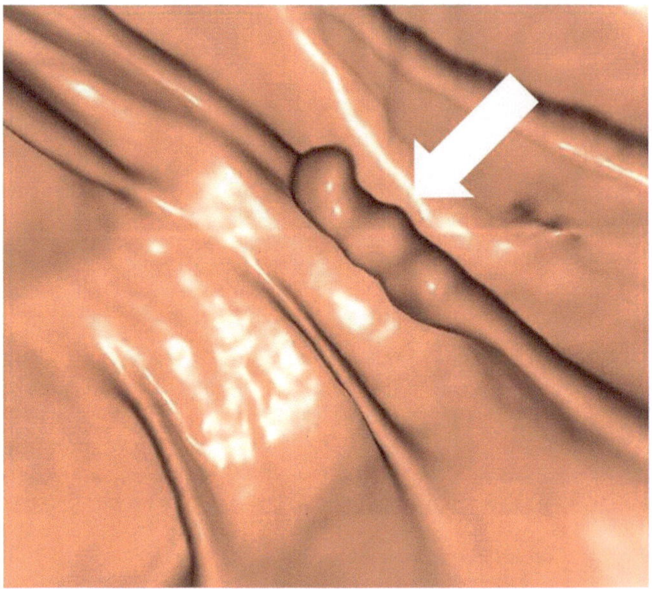

Fig. 3b Endoluminal 3D CT image

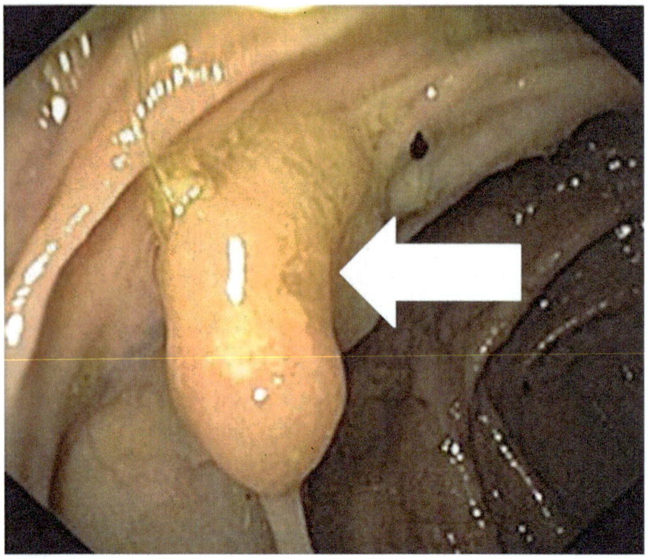

Fig. 3c Endoscopic image

Description

Occasionally, flat lesion has a small focal attachment to the colonic fold with the majority of the lesion protruding within bowel lumen. When this occurs, flat lesion acquires a "cigar-shaped" appearance. Note this appearance of flat lesion (arrow) in the right colon at CT colonography axial supine (a), at 3D endoluminal view (b), and at colonoscopy (c)

Case 4. Ulcerated Flat Lesion (III) with Central Depression

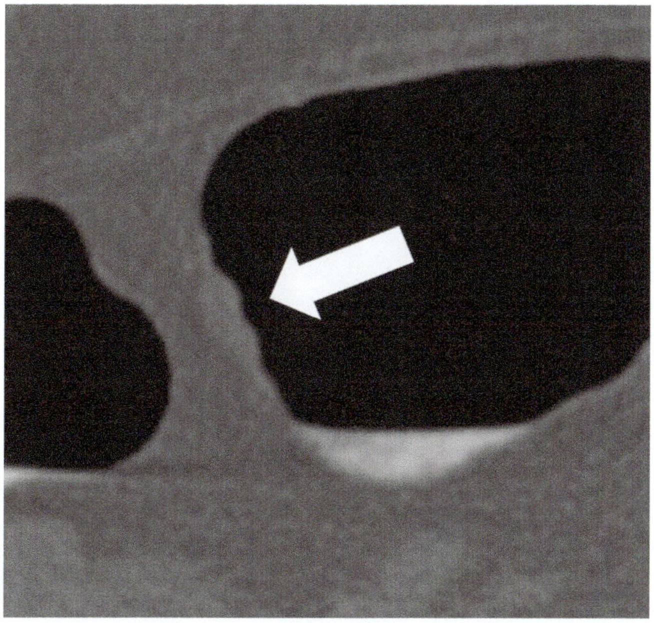

Fig. 4a Axial supine CT image

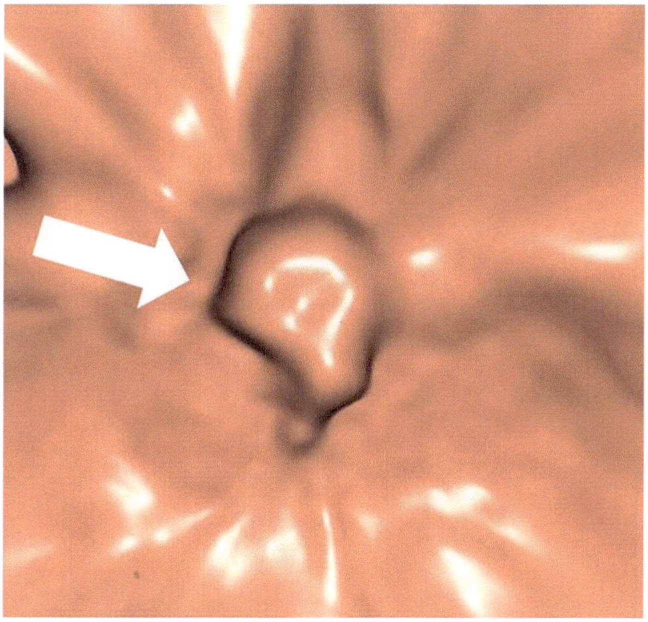

Fig. 4b 3D CT colonography endoluminal image

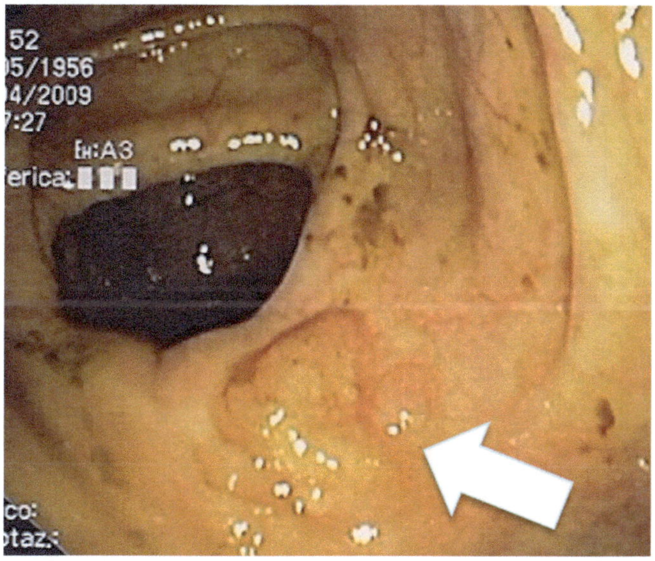

Fig. 4c Endoscopic image

Description

Axial 2D CT colonography supine image (a) showing an ulcerated flat lesion at the apex of the caecum, easily appreciable using 2D CT colonography window-level setting and fecal-tagging technique. 3D CT colonography endoluminal (b) image shows the typical flat morphology of the lesion (arrow), depicting tiny central ulceration confirmed by colonoscopy (c)

Case 5. Slightly Elevated Flat Lesion with Depression (IIc + IIa)

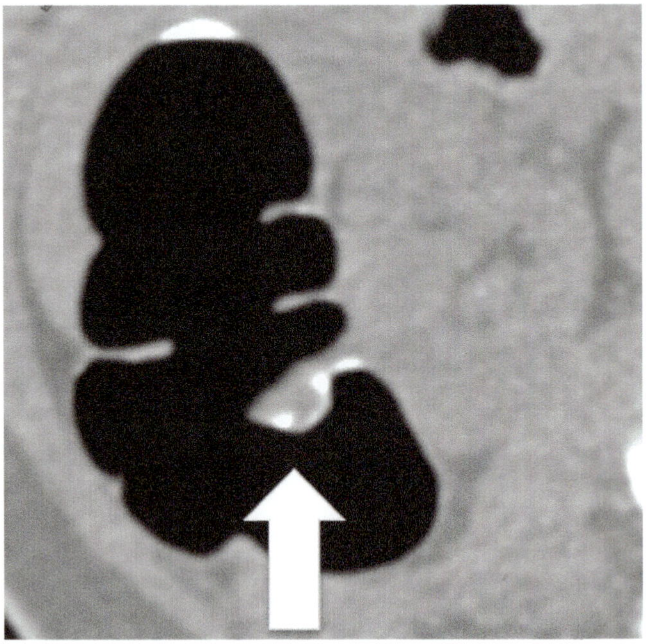

Fig. 5a 2D CT colonography axial prone image

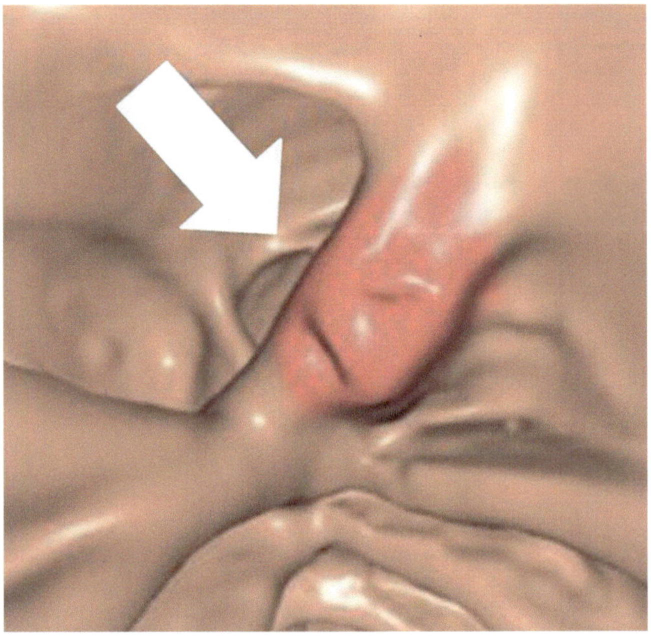

Fig. 5b 3D CT colonography endoluminal image

Description

3D endoluminal CT colonography image (b) shows focal thickening of a fold (arrow) within the ascending colon; this appears to be just adherent tagged stool, but 2D correlation, with axial (a), shows that this is a true soft tissue lesion (arrow) with contrast coating of its surface. Note how the contrast clings only to the polyp and not the normal mucosa. Endoluminal 3D reconstruction after applying CAD software (b) that automatically detected the lesion (arrow) and marked in red

References

1. Soetikno RM, Kaltenbach T, Rouse RV et al (2008) Prevalence of nonpolypoid (flat and depressed) colorectal neoplasms in asymptomatic and symptomatic adults. JAMA 299(9):1027–1035
2. Soetikno R, Friedland S, Kaltenbach T et al (2006) Nonpolypoid (flat and depressed) colorectal neoplasms. Veterans Affairs Palo Alto Health Care System and Stanford University School of Medicine, Palo Alto, California; and Hiroshima University School of Medicine, Hiroshima, Japan. Gastroenterology 130:566–576
3. Kaltenbach T, Friedland S, Maheshwari A et al (2007) Short- and long-term outcomes of standardized EMR of nonpolypoid (flat and depressed) colorectal lesions > or = 1 cm (with video). Gastrointest Endosc 65(6):857–865
4. No Authors listed (2003) The Paris endoscopic classification of superficial neoplastic lesions: esophagus, stomach, and colon. Gastrointest Endosc 58(Suppl 6):S3–S43
5. Park SH, Lee SS, Choi EK et al (2007) Flat colorectal neoplasms: definition, importance, and visualization on CT colonography. AJR Am J Roentgenol 188:953–959
6. Hurlstone DP, Cross SS, Drew K et al (2004) An evaluation of colorectal endoscopic mucosal resection using high-magnification chromoscopic colonoscopy: a prospective study of 1000 colonoscopies. Endoscopy 36:491–498
7. Pickhardt PJ, Nugent PA, Choi JR et al (2004) Flat colorectal lesions in asymptomatic adults: implications for screening with CT virtual colonoscopy. AJR Am J Roentgenol 183(5):1343–1347

Colon Cancer

Marjolein H. Liedenbaum and Jaap Stoker

Contents

Abstract

Vegetating masses are colorectal carcinomas or large colorectal polyps that protrude into the colonic lumen. A colorectal mass is defined as a lesion with a maximum diameter of at least 30 mm. Although most of these vegetating masses are clearly visible at CT colonography, some might be more difficult to detect or may be missed because of reader fatigue or superficial reading. It is crucial to keep the sensitivity high for detection of these lesions.

Introduction

The lifetime risk of colorectal carcinoma in average-risk individuals in the Western world is about 6 % [4]. Only 10 % of the patients with advanced stage colorectal carcinoma with distant metastasis are still alive 5 years after the diagnosis has been made [7]. This compares to 90 % of patients, with colorectal carcinomas with the least advanced stage, where disease is confined to the bowel only. Timely detection of colorectal cancer is thus important for prognosis.

Little information is available on the prevalence of colorectal masses in different populations. In colorectal carcinoma, screening studies the prevalence of colorectal carcinomas (≥10 mm) varied from 0.3 to 0.8 % [1, 5, 6]. In a CT colonography meta-analysis of studies with symptomatic and surveillance patients, the prevalence of colorectal carcinomas was 4.8 % [3]. To our knowledge, there is no information on the prevalence of vegetating masses and the test accuracy of CT colonography (which is presumably (almost) 100 %)

Pathology

All colorectal carcinomas are thought to develop from adenomas or from flat dysplasia [2, 9]. The gross appearance of these carcinomas can vary from a flat lesion to a large vegetating mass. A mass is a protruding structure with soft-tissue

M.H. Liedenbaum, M.D., Ph.D. (✉) • J. Stoker, M.D., Ph.D.
Department of Radiology,
Academic Medical Center, University of Amsterdam,
Meibergdreef 9, 1105 AZ Amsterdam, The Netherlands
e-mail: m.h.liedenbaum@amc.uva.nl; j.stoker@amc.uva.nl

E. Neri et al. (eds.), *CT Colonography Atlas*, Medical Radiology,
DOI 10.1007/978-3-642-11149-5_10,

attenuation at CT. The largest diameter of a mass has been defined as at least 30 mm [10]. A large vegetating mass at CT colonography will almost always concern adenocarcinoma, although other diagnoses (e.g. lipoma, endometriosis, hemorrhoids, benign polyp, thickened bowel wall after inflammation, GIST, lymphoma, anal abscess) should be considered. Ninety-six percent of the colorectal carcinomas are adenocarcinomas [8].

CT colonography Pattern

At CT colonography, most colorectal carcinomas are clearly visible because they protrude in the colonic lumen or obstruct the lumen. Viewing a suspected lesion at an abdominal window (e.g. W450, L40) helps in evaluating the soft-tissue density. This is important to differentiate between vegetating masses and large untagged stool parts and to identify lipomas (Fig. 8). Further, the extension of the mass outside the colonic wall should be included in the report as well, especially when this includes invasion of surrounding organs and structures. Some masses nearly obstruct the lumen and can appear as so-called apple core lesions based on the appearance at surface-rendered images and formerly contrast enema (for an example, see Fig. 2). It is also possible that the lumen is totally obstructed. Then the mass can mimic a collapsed bowel loop at CT colonography direct distal to dilated large bowel. It is important to differentiate between a mass and a collapsed bowel segment; sufficient distension is therefore mandatory (see Fig. 4 for a colorectal lesion in the rectosigmoid where sufficient distension is needed).

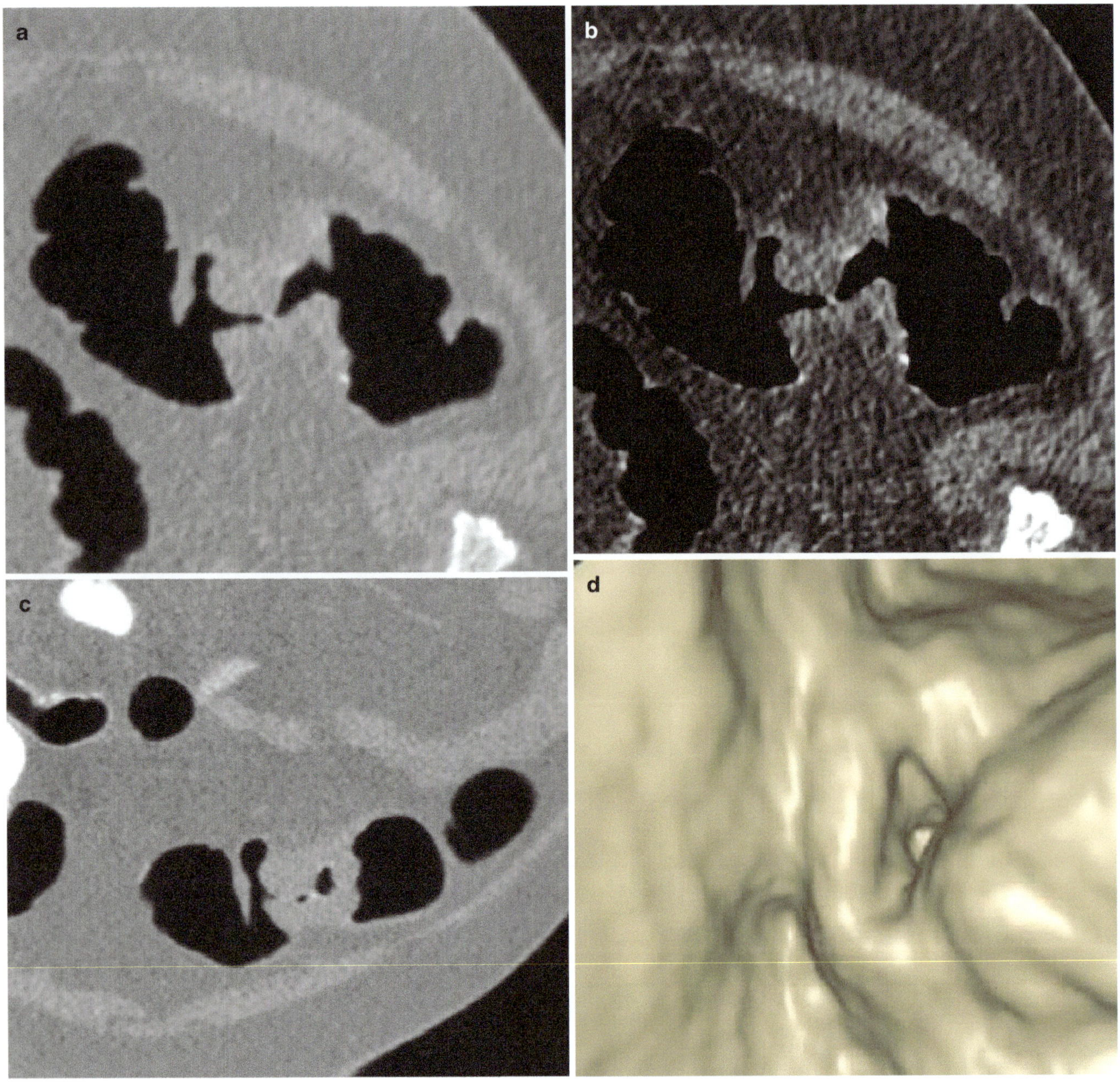

Fig. 1 A 72-year-old man with bowel pain and changing bowel habits. A vegetating mass in the sigmoid colon was found (adenocarcinoma). (**a**) Supine image, axial view. (**b**) Supine image, soft-tissue window setting, axial view. (**c**) Supine, MPR coronal direction. (**d**) Three-dimensional image of the mass

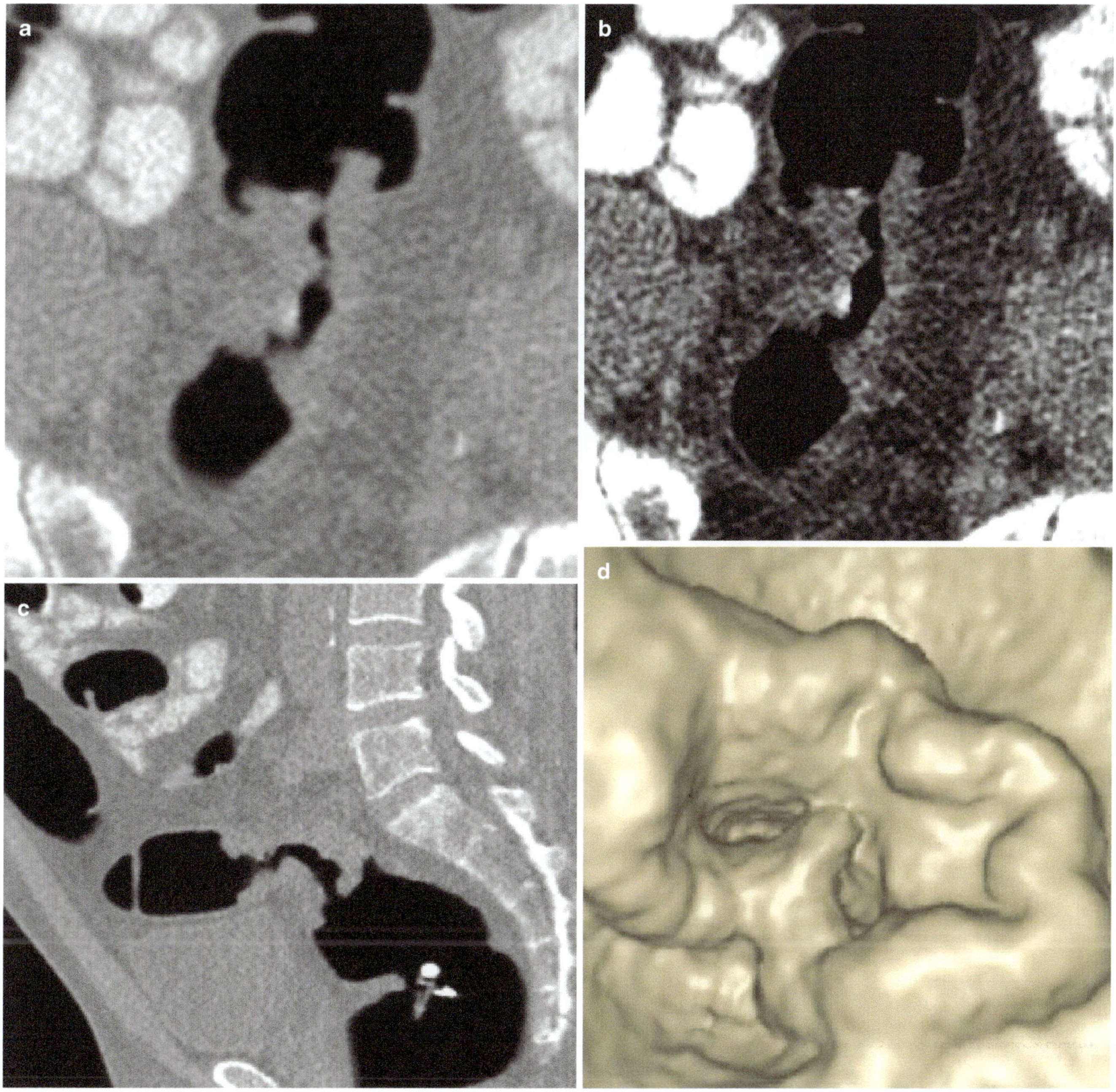

Fig. 2 A 56-year-old man with weight loss and changed bowel habits. A vegetating mass in the sigmoid colon, typical apple core lesion, was found (adenocarcinoma). (**a**) Supine image, axial view. (**b**) Soft-tissue window setting. (**c**) Supine image, MPR sagittal view. (**d**) Three-dimensional image. (**e**) Colonoscopy image

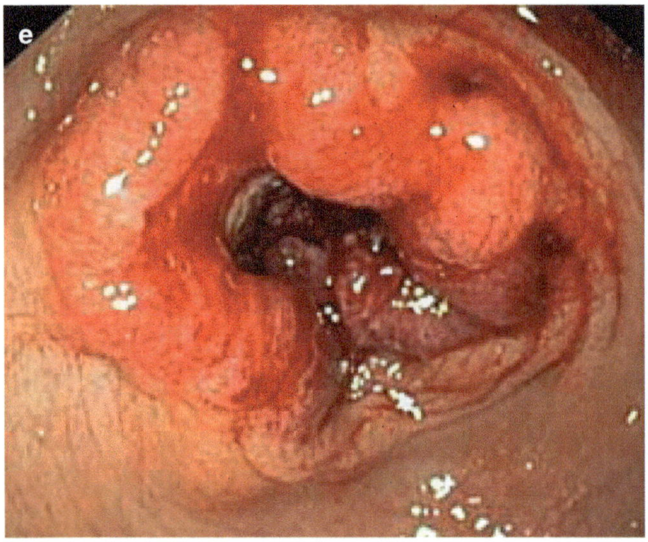

Fig. 2 (continued)

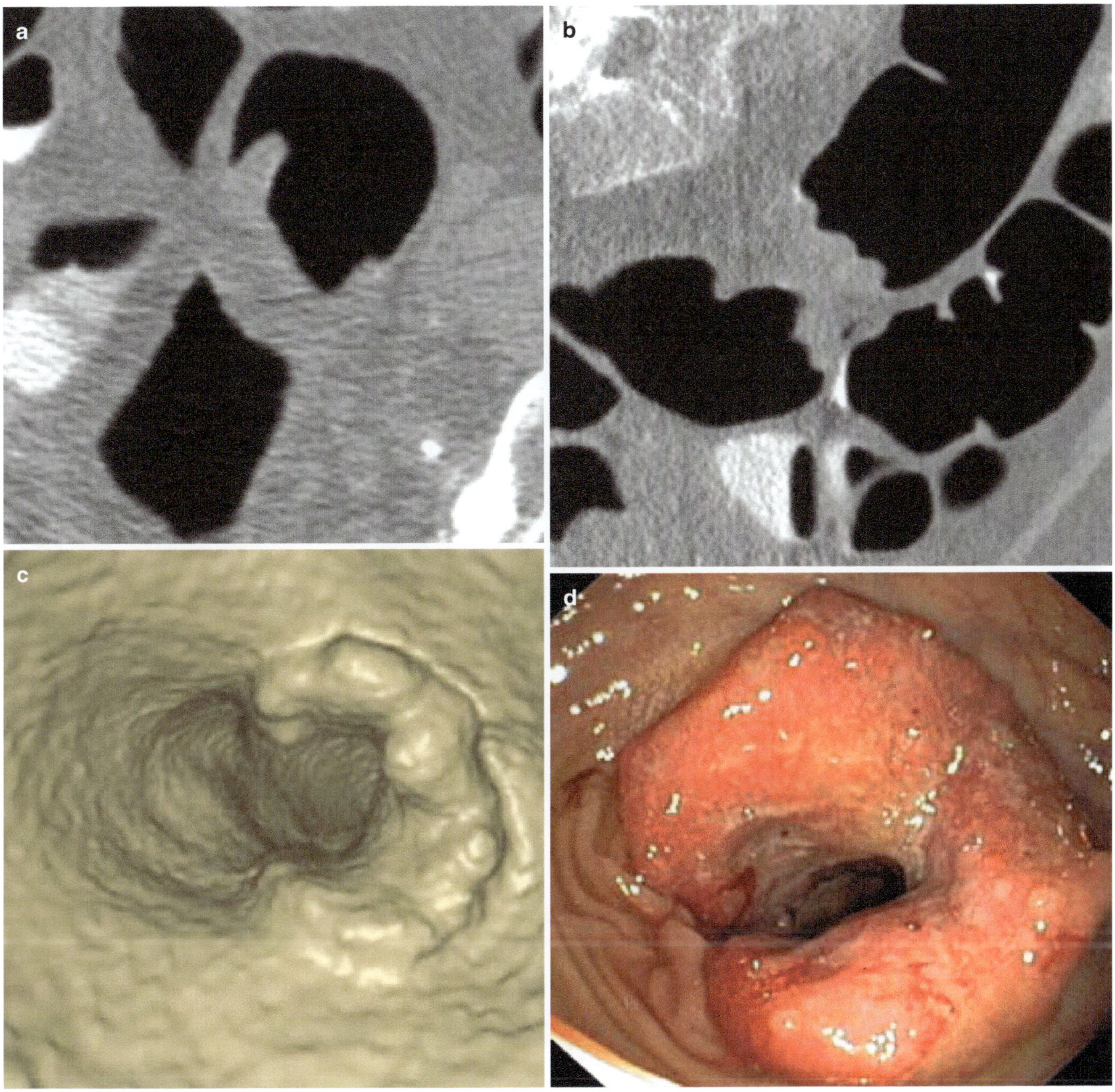

Fig. 3 A 64-year-old woman tested positive in an FOBT screening program. A vegetating mass in the sigmoid colon was found (adenocarcinoma). (**a**) Supine image, axial view. (**b**) Supine image, MPR sagittal view. (**c**) Three-dimensional image. (**d**) Colonoscopy image

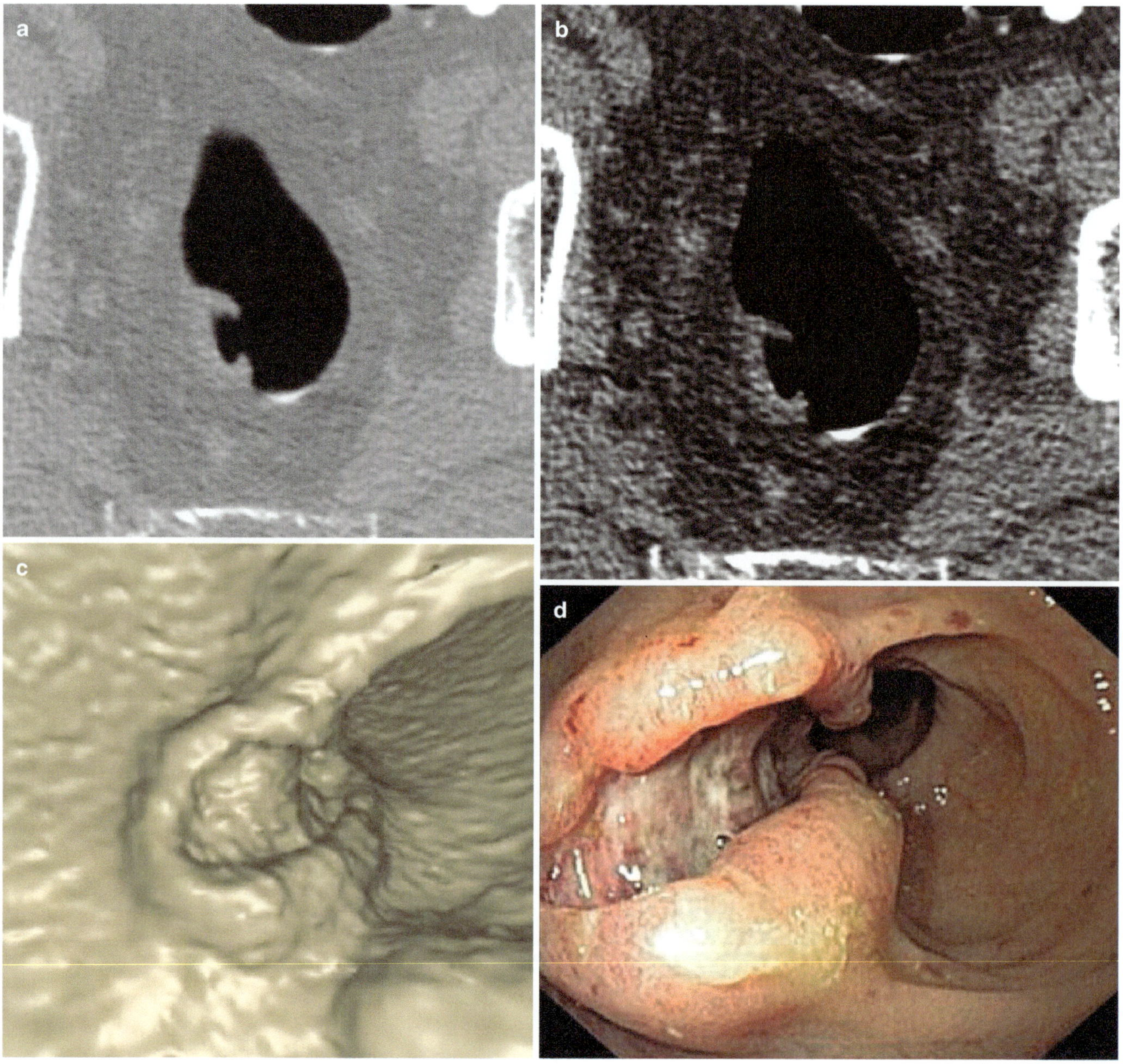

Fig. 4 A 71-year-old man tested positive in an FOBT screening program. A vegetating mass in the rectosigmoid was found (adenocarcinoma). (**a**) Supine image, axial view. (**b**) Soft-tissue window setting. (**c**) Three-dimensional image. (**d**) Colonoscopy image

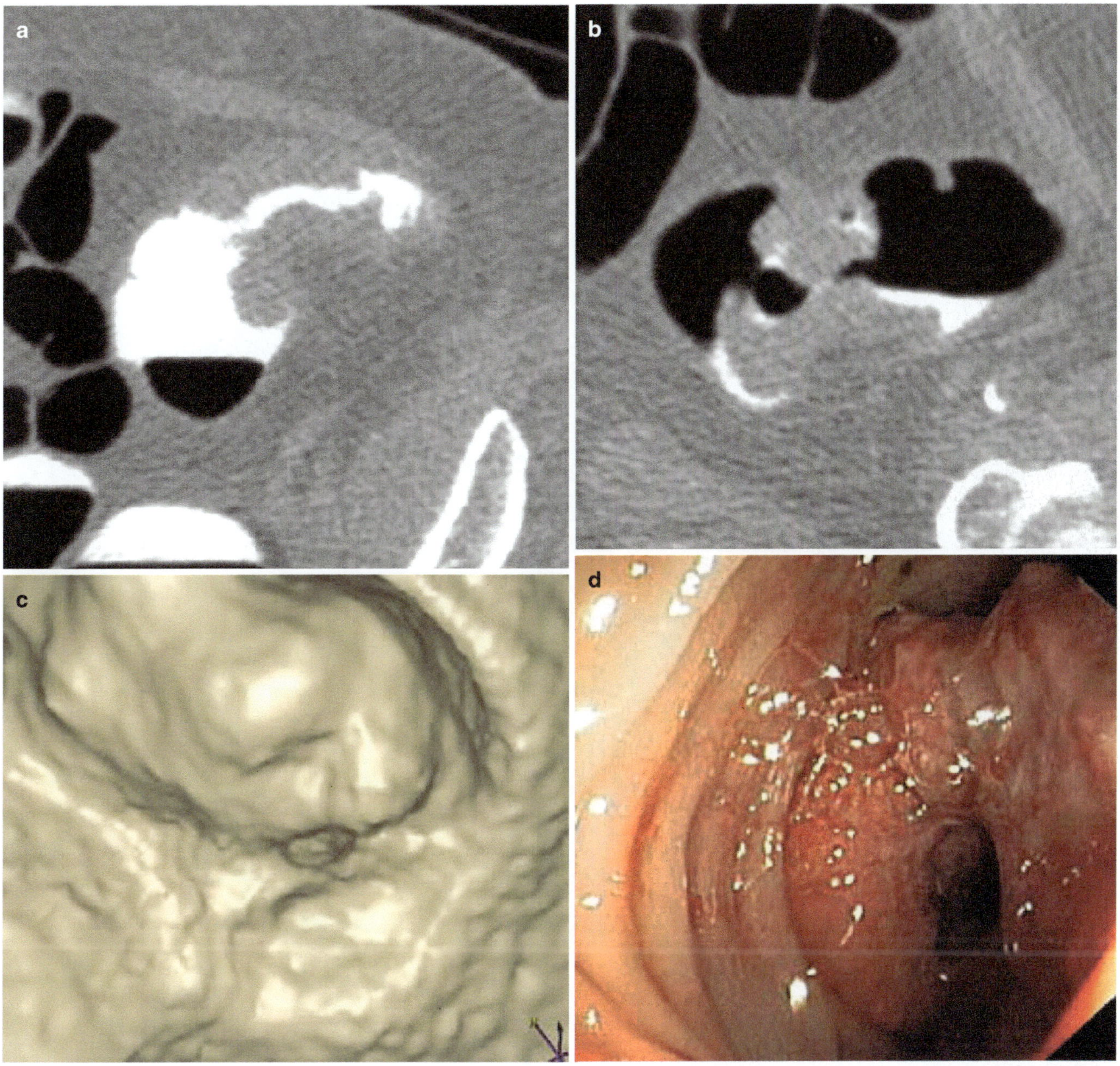

Fig. 5 A 74-year-old woman tested positive in FOBT screening. A vegetating mass in the sigmoid colon was found (adenocarcinoma). (**a**) Prone image, axial view. (**b**) Supine image, axial view. (**c**) Three-dimensional image. (**d**) Colonoscopy image

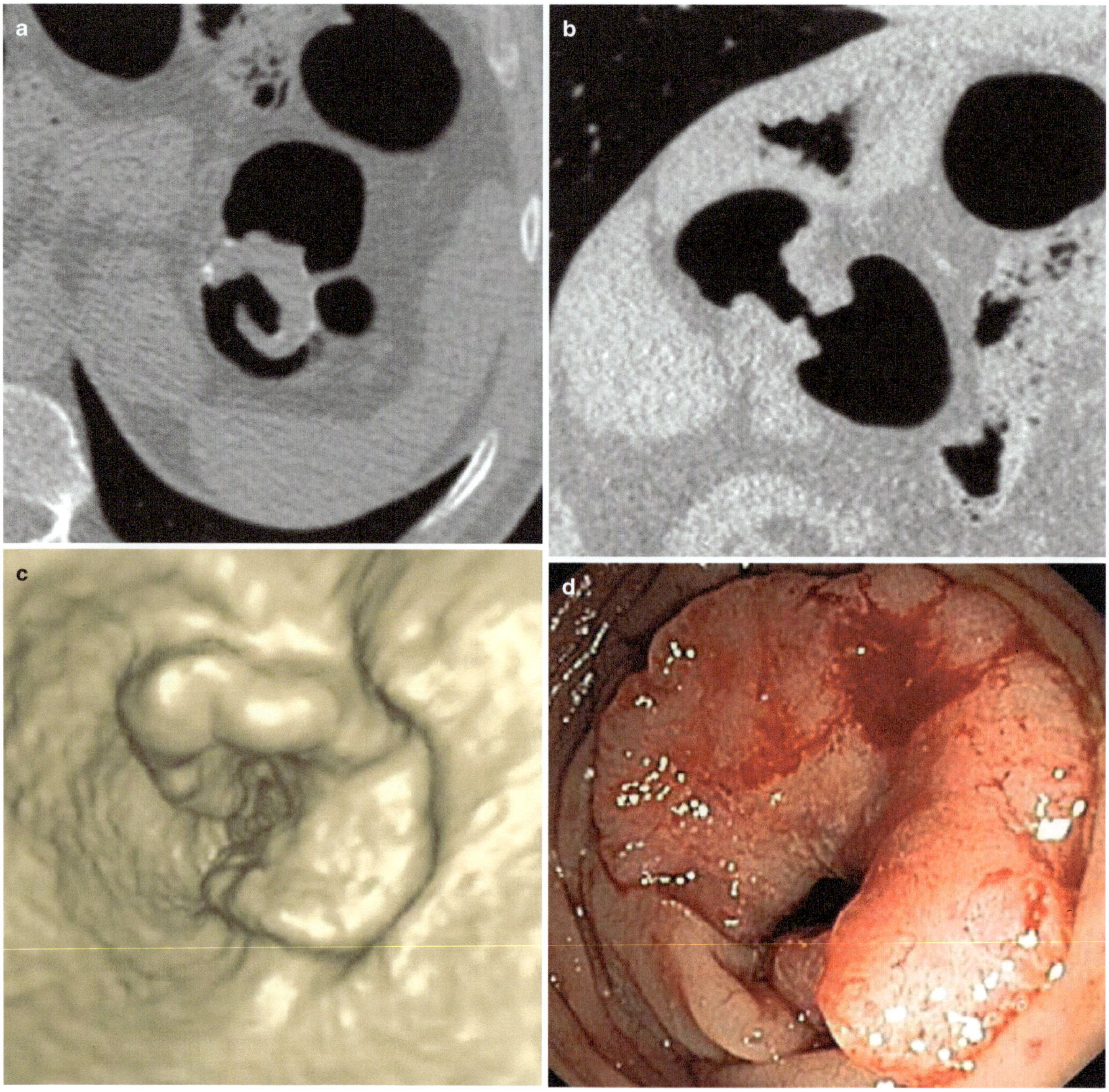

Fig. 6 A 66-year-old man tested positive in FOBT screening. Colorectal carcinoma in the descending colon. (**a**) Prone image, axial view. (**b**) Prone image, MPR sagittal view. (**c**) Three-dimensional image. (**d**) Colonoscopy image

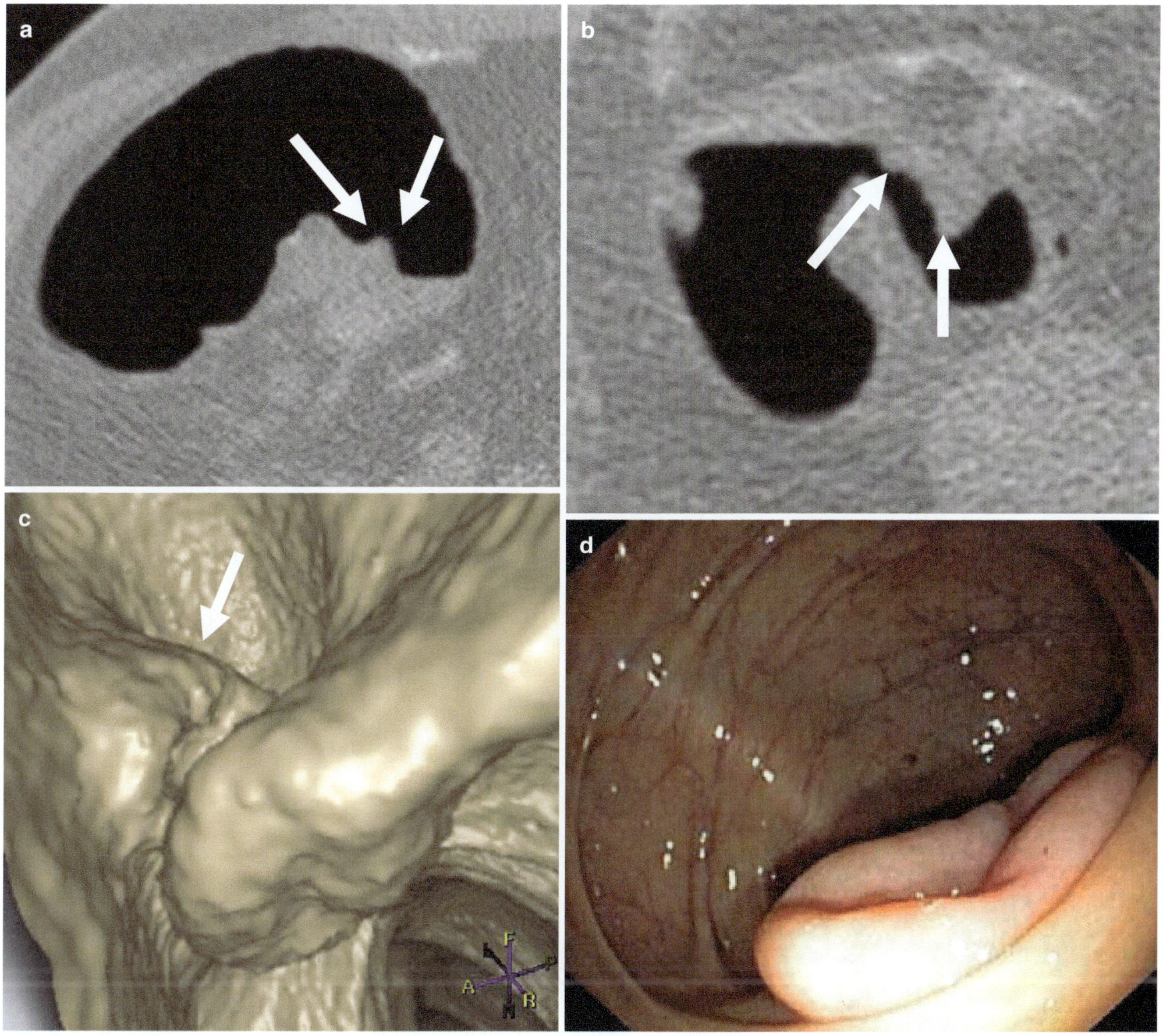

Fig. 7 A 64-year-old man tested positive in FOBT screening. Colorectal carcinoma in the cecum, just behind the ileocecal valve. The tumor was initially missed at CT colonography and colonoscopy, but 1 year later the patient became symptomatic for bowel cancer and a mass was found behind the ileocecal valve. (**a**) Supine image, axial view. Mass just behind the valve, *white arrows* indicate the tumor. Because of the poor tagging quality, the mass is hardly visible. (**b**) Prone image, axial view. (**c**) Three-dimensional image of the valve and the mass behind the valve. (**d**) Colonoscopy image of the valve, the mass behind it was missed

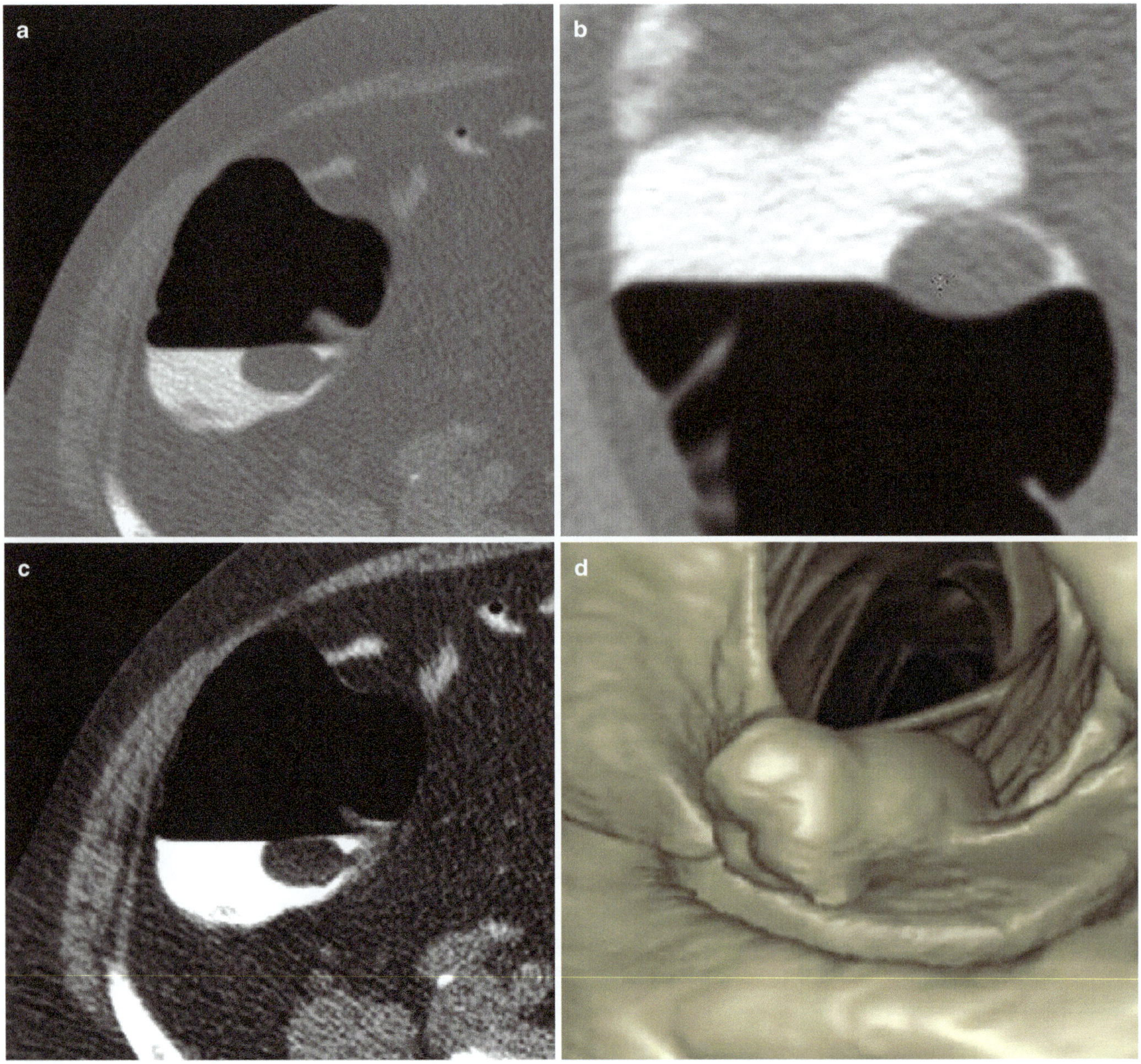

Fig. 8 A 69-year-old woman tested positive in FOBT screening. A lipoma in the cecum was found. (**a**) Supine image, axial view. (**b**) Prone image, axial view. (**c**) Supine axial image in soft-tissue window setting demonstrates that the mass has fat density. (**d**) Prone image, three-dimensional view after electronic cleansing. (**e**) Colonoscopy image

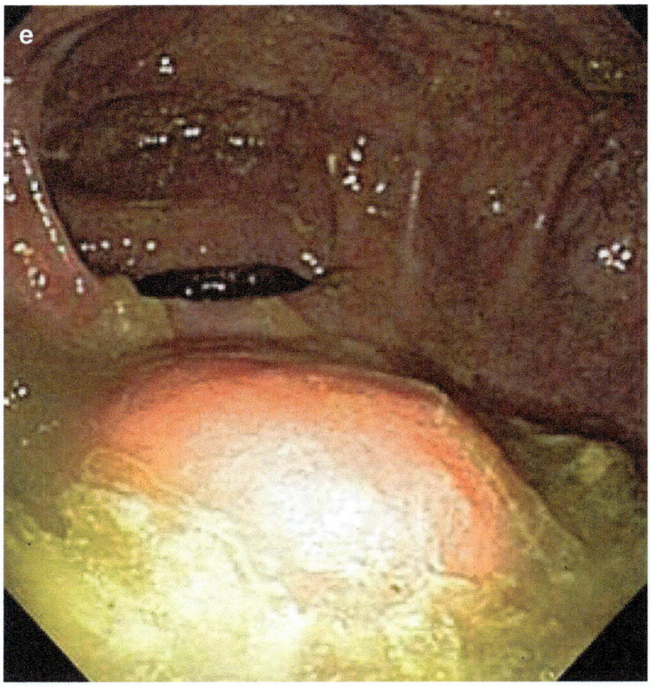

Fig. 8 (continued)

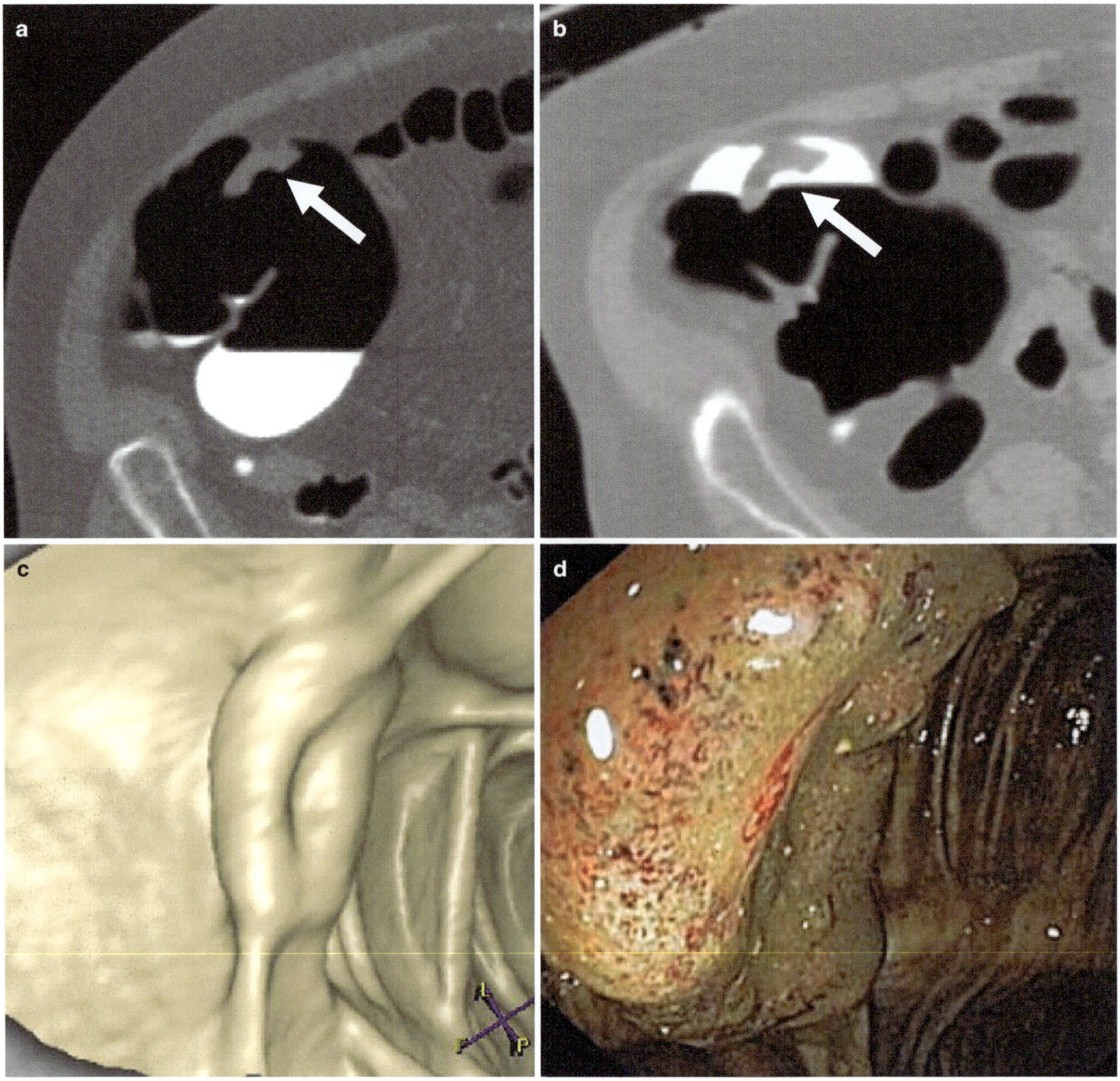

Fig. 9 A 92-year-old man with changed bowel habits. A vegetating mass in the cecum was found mimicking the ileocecal valve. (**a**) Supine image, axial view, *white arrow* indicates the tumor. (**b**) Prone image, axial view. (**c**) Three-dimensional image. (**d**) Colonoscopy image

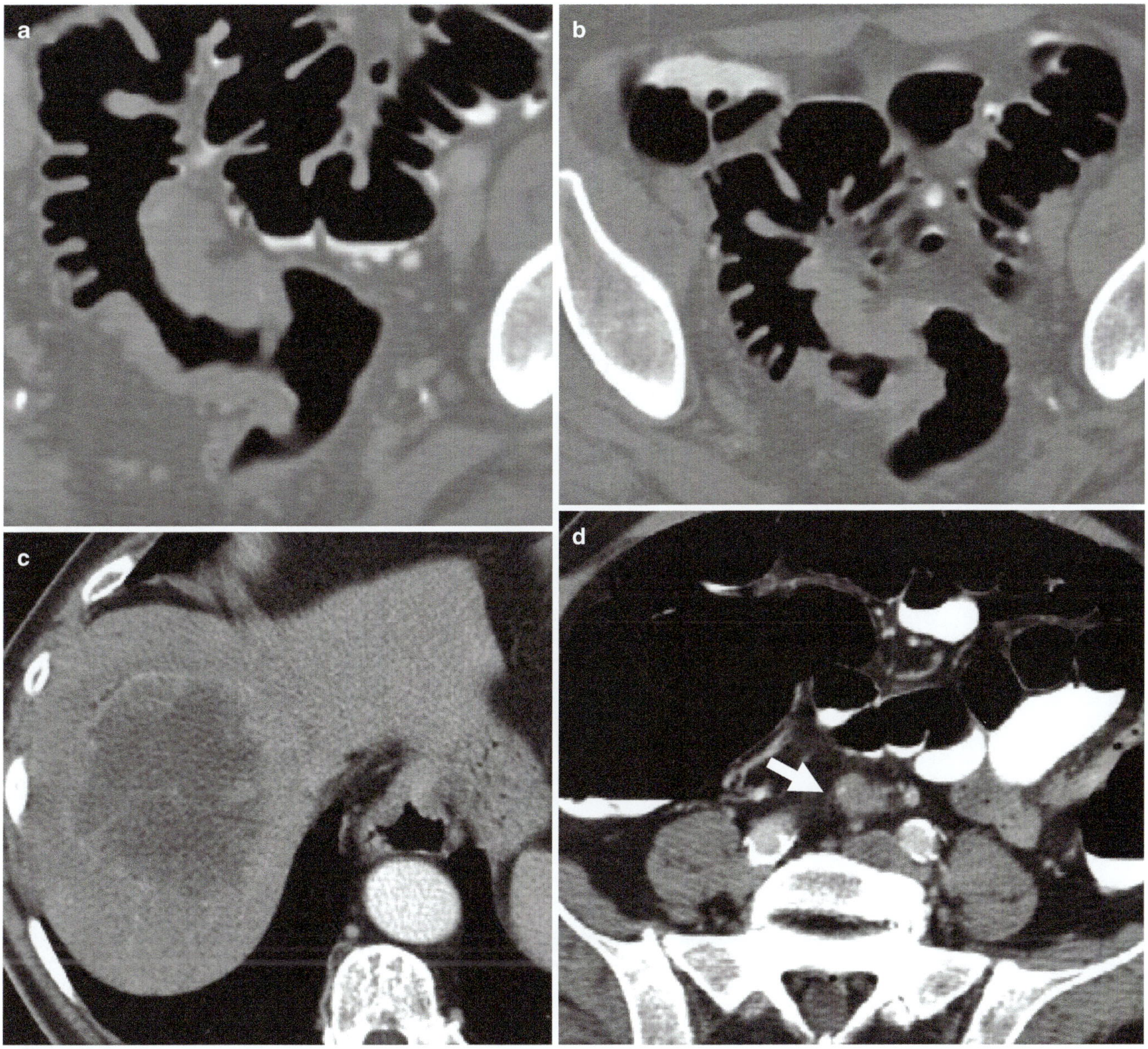

Fig. 10 A 75-year-old man with weight loss and changed bowel habits. A vegetating mass in the sigmoid was found. It could not be passed by the endoscope. (**a**) Supine image, axial view. (**b**) Prone image, axial view. (**c**) 9-cm liver metastasis in the right liver lobe. (**d**) Enlarged para-iliac lymph node is visible (see *white arrow*)

References

1. Bokemeyer B, Rambow A, Hüppe D et al (2009) Screening colonoscopy for colorectal cancer prevention – results from a German online registry on 269000 cases. Eur J Gastroenterol Hepatol 21(6):650–655
2. Bond JH (2000) Clinical evidence for the adenoma-carcinoma sequence, and the management of patients with colorectal adenomas. Semin Gastrointest Dis 11(4):176–184
3. Halligan S, Altman DG, Taylor SA et al (2005) CT colonography in the detection of colorectal polyps and cancer: systematic review, meta-analysis, and proposed minimum data set for study level reporting. Radiology 237(3):893–904
4. Jemal A, Siegel R, Ward E et al (2007) Cancer statistics, 2007. CA Cancer J Clin 57:43–66
5. Johnson CD, Chen MH, Toledano AY et al (2008) Accuracy of CT colonography for detection of large adenomas and cancers. N Engl J Med 359(12):1207–1217
6. Kim DH, Pickhardt PJ, Taylor AJ et al (2007) CT colonography versus colonoscopy for the detection of advanced neoplasia. N Engl J Med 357(14):1403–1412
7. Levin B, Lieberman DA, McFarland B et al (2008) Screening and surveillance for the early detection of colorectal cancer and adenomatous polyps, 2008: a joint guideline from the American Cancer Society, the US Multi-Society Task Force on Colorectal Cancer, and the American College of Radiology. Gastroenterology 134(5):1570–1595
8. Stewart SL, Wike JM, Kato I, Lewis DR, Michaud F (2006) A population-based study of colorectal cancer histology in the United States, 1998–2001. Cancer 107(5 Suppl):1128–1141
9. Vogelstein B, Fearon ER, Hamilton SR et al (1988) Genetic alterations during colorectal-tumor development. N Engl J Med 319(9):525–532
10. Zalis ME, Barish MA, Choi JR et al (2005) CT colonography reporting and data system: a consensus proposal. Radiology 236(1):3–9

Rectal Cancer

Darren Boone, Stuart A. Taylor, and Steve Halligan

Contents

Abstract
The rectum's anatomical location and proximity to pelvic structures demand that diagnosis and management of rectal cancer differ from that elsewhere in the colon. Surgery is technically challenging because the rectum is buried deep in the pelvis, and residual tumour can lead to local recurrence with devastating effects for the patient. The advent of total mesorectal excision (TME), which aims to remove the rectum and surrounding mesorectal tissues en-bloc, and adjuvant chemoradiotherapy therapy has led to dramatic reductions in local tumour recurrence and consequently improved survival. Fundamental to these advances is accurate radiologic staging. Given that approximately half of all colorectal cancers develop in the rectum and CT colonography will be the first investigation in many cases, knowledge of the strengths and weaknesses of CT are paramount. We discuss rectal tumours of varying stages, followed by examples of interpretative pitfalls and how best to avoid them. Finally, we provide recommendations based upon our personal experience.

Abbreviations

CRM	Circumferential resection margin
CTC	Computed tomographic colonography
FSE	Fast spin echo
MRI	Magnetic resonance imaging
TNM	Tumour, nodes, metastases

Introduction

Rectal cancer accounts for approximately half of all colorectal malignancy. Histologically, the vast majority of rectal tumours are carcinomas arising from adenomatous polyps, a situation paralleled throughout the colon [1]. However, the rectum's location and intimate relationship to surrounding structures complicate diagnosis and surgery.

D. Boone • S.A. Taylor • S. Halligan (✉)
Centre for Medical Imaging,
University College, London, UK
e-mail: s.halligan@ucl.ac.uk

E. Neri et al. (eds.), *CT Colonography Atlas*, Medical Radiology,
DOI 10.1007/978-3-642-11149-5_11,

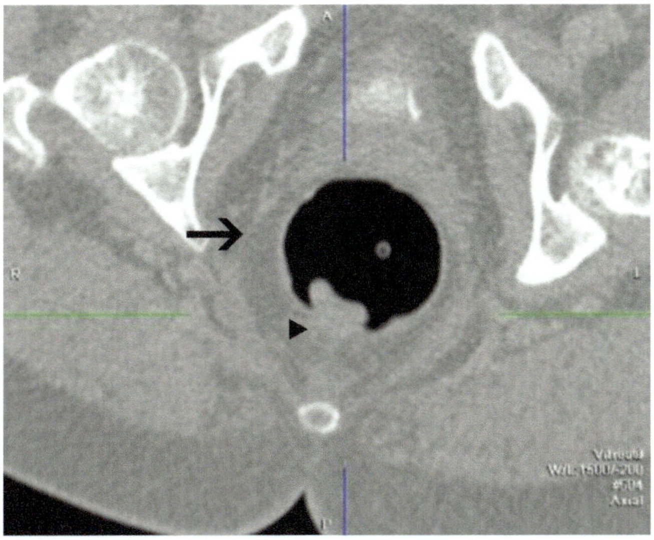

Fig. 1a Supine, axial colonography. The mesorectal fascia (*black arrow*) is seen as a circumferential, pencil-thin structure, iso-attenuating with skeletal muscle. Note the small, polypoid tumour at 6 o'clock and adjacent mesorectal fat stranding (*arrowhead*)

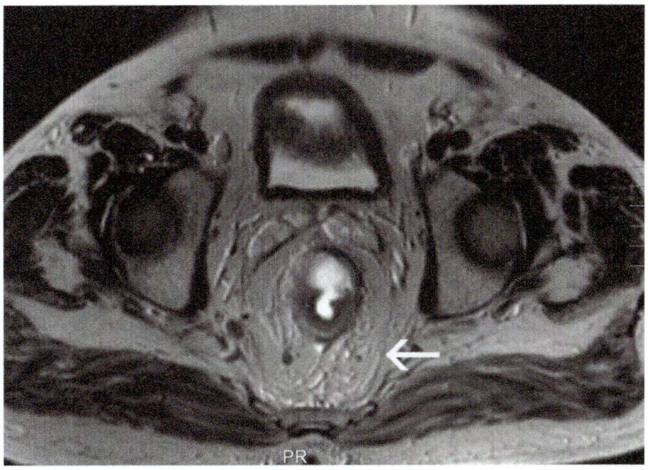

Fig. 1b Axial, T2-weighted, fast spin echo MRI. The mesorectal fascia (*white arrow*) is also well seen using MRI where it is iso-intense to skeletal muscle on this sequence

Consequently, there is a risk of incomplete tumour resection consequently resulting in local recurrence [2], which is often incurable and notoriously difficult to palliate. Thankfully, therapeutic and surgical advances over recent years have revolutionised rectal cancer treatment. Moreover, these improvements rely upon accurate radiologic staging of the primary tumour.

Rectal Anatomy

The rectum comprises the distal large intestine, constrained superiorly by the rectosigmoid junction, inferiorly by the sphincter complex and radially by the mesorectum. The mesorectal fascia envelops the mesorectal tissues (Fig. 1a, b) and so provides a natural boundary and surgical plane for en-bloc rectal resection. When performing total mesorectal excision (TME), the surgeon aims to dissect along the mesorectal fascia, which thus becomes the 'circumferential resection margin' (CRM) of the specimen. The distance between the tumour and the circumferential resection margin is crucial for planning potentially curative resection or guiding (neo)adjuvant therapy [3].

Anteriorly, the superior one-third of the rectum lies above the peritoneal reflection. Therefore, tumour invasion at this level may result in transcoelomic peritoneal metastasis.

Rectal Cancer: Pathological Staging

Consistent with all colonic tumours, rectal cancer can be staged in terms of local, nodal and metastatic extent, i.e. the TNM classification which is described in more detail in Table 1.

Local stage is determined by the tumour's relationship to the rectal wall; in particular, the inner circular and outer longitudinal muscles which together comprise the muscularis propria (Fig. 2a, b). T1 tumours are confined to the submucosa (i.e. they do not involve the muscularis propria at all), whereas T2 tumours invade the muscularis propria, but do not penetrate beyond it.

All T3 tumours breach the lateral aspect of the muscularis propria to reach the mesorectal tissues beyond the rectal wall. However, the degree to which they do this is highly variable, and so, these tumours constitute a very heterogeneous group which differ substantially in their prognosis and treatment despite sharing the same local 'T3' stage. For example, the management of tumours that penetrate just a few millimetres beyond the muscularis propria is very different to those that cross the mesorectal fascia – in the latter case, dissection along the CRM will leave residual tumour in the pelvis. Thus, local T-staging is limited for rectal cancer since it does not consider the relationship between the tumour and CRM despite its importance for patient management. Consequently, T3 tumours are often subclassified in terms of the presence/absence of 'poor prognostic features' such as a threatened CRM or vascular invasion.

Invasion of adjacent pelvic organs or musculature denotes T4 disease.

Surgical Approach

The decision whether or not to attempt potentially curative resection of the primary tumour is complex and depends upon the patient's fitness, the presence of distant metastases

Table 1 TNM rectal cancer staging

Primary tumour	
TX	Primary tumour cannot be assessed
T0	No evidence of primary tumour
Tis	Carcinoma in situ: intraepithelial or invasion of lamina propria
T1	Tumour invades submucosa
T2	Tumour invades muscularis propria
T3	Tumour invades through the muscularis propria into pericolorectal tissues
T4a	Tumour penetrates to the surface of the visceral peritoneum
T4b	Tumour directly invades or is adherent to other organs or structures
Regional lymph nodes (N)	
NX	Regional lymph nodes cannot be assessed
N0	No regional lymph node metastasis
N1	Metastases in 1–3 regional lymph nodes
N1a	Metastasis in 1 regional lymph node
N1b	Metastases in 2–3 regional lymph nodes
N1c	Tumour deposit(s) in the subserosa, mesentery, or nonperitonealized pericolic or perirectal tissues without regional nodal metastases
N2	Metastases in ≥4 regional lymph nodes
N2a	Metastases in 4–6 regional lymph nodes
N2b	Metastases in ≥7 regional lymph nodes
Distant metastasis (M)	
M0	No distant metastasis
M1	Distant metastasis
M1a	Metastasis confined to 1 organ or site (e.g. liver, lung, ovary, nonregional node)
M1b	Metastases in >1 organ/site or the peritoneum

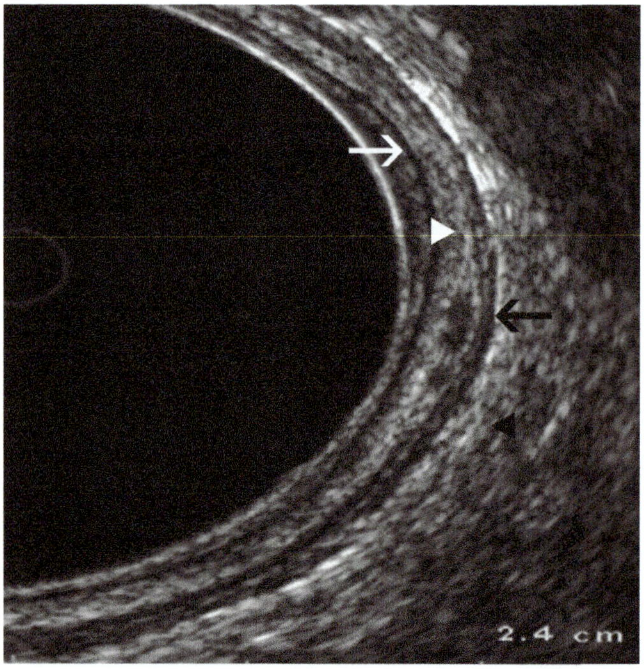

Fig. 2a Endoscopic ultrasound at mid-rectal level. The relationship between normal muscularis mucosae (*white arrow*), submucosa (*white arrowhead*), muscularis propria (*black arrow*) and mesorectal fat (*black arrowhead*) are illustrated

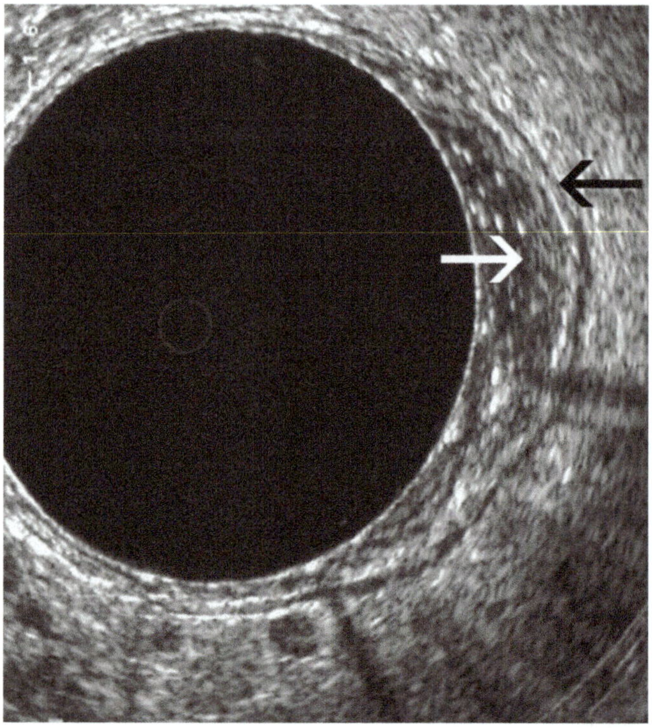

Fig. 2b The integrity of the muscularis propria is central to planning surgical and therapeutic management (see text). In this example, T1 tumour (*white arrow*) invades the submucosa and displaces, but does not invade the muscularis propria (*black arrow*)

and the local tumour stage. It is widely accepted therefore that management should involve multidisciplinary collaboration [4]. Total mesorectal excision (TME) is usually the procedure of choice for cure. During TME, the surgeon dissects around the CRM, removing the mesorectal tissues en-bloc, with the rectum, tumour and nodes 'buried' within the specimen. TME was made possible by the advent of stapling guns that permit a very low stapled anastamosis, almost to the level of the anus [5]. TME has been shown to substantially reduce local recurrence rates since en-bloc dissection aims to avoid leaving residual disease in the pelvis [6, 7]. For example, TME introduction in Stockholm reduced local recurrence from 15 to 6 % and cancer related death from 16 to 9 % [8].

However, not all patients will benefit from TME. For example, if the primary tumour or an involved node has already breached the mesorectal fascia, dissection along the CRM will inevitably dissect through tumour and so leave viable disease in the pelvis. Consequently, the resected specimen will have tumour at its surface, known as 'positive margins' pathologically. Supporting this, a study of 686 patients undergoing TME (without neoadjuvant therapy) found 22 % of patients whose specimens have positive margins developed local tumour recurrence compared to only 5 % of those who were negative [9].

Adjuvant and Neoadjuvant Therapy

If tumour is at or beyond the CRM, how can it be dealt with? Both radiotherapy and chemotherapy can reduce local recurrence, although their precise timing and delivery remain subjects of debate. Neoadjuvant therapy (administered preoperatively) aims to 'shrink' the primary tumour away from the mesorectal fascia, thus converting a potentially positive CRM into a negative one. On the other hand, adjuvant therapy (delivered postoperatively) aims to destroy residual tumour cells that may be left behind in the pelvis. Short-term neoadjuvant radiotherapy combined with TME has been shown to decrease the local recurrence rate in early T3 tumours [10], and longer-term preoperative radiotherapy has been shown to 'down-stage' more advanced T3 tumours, allowing potentially curative TME [11, 12]. Furthermore, long-term follow-up (median 13 years) of 1,168 patients with T3 disease, who were randomly assigned to preoperative radiotherapy or not showed the cancer-specific survival rate in the irradiated group, was 72 % compared to 62 % in the nonirradiated group [13].

Sauer et al. compared pre- and postoperative chemoradiotherapy for locally advanced rectal cancer. Preoperative chemoradiotherapy improved local control, but did not improve overall survival [14]. Furthermore, in a randomised trial of 1,011 patients with operable T3 or T4 rectal cancer, Bosset et al. demonstrated a significant reduction in local recurrence when preoperative radiotherapy was combined with chemotherapy, regardless of whether it was administered before or after surgery [15]. Therefore, adjuvant therapy is likely most beneficial in patients with locally advanced tumours that threaten the CRM, although there is an increasing tendency to employ it for T3 tumours of any stage.

Radiological Staging

From the discussion above, it is apparent that tumour stage is central to prognosis, operative approach and the decision whether to administer neoadjuvant therapy. Therefore, the aim of preoperative imaging is to stratify patients into two broad groups:

(a) Patients who are likely to be cured by surgery alone, which avoids unnecessary adjuvant treatment and so reduces morbidity, cost and inconvenience.
(b) Patients with more extensive tumours who are likely to have positive resection margins. These patients should benefit from down-staging with adjuvant therapy, possibly allowing TME to be carried out subsequently.

Therefore, radiological assessment of local tumour stage is now pivotal for patient management, both for anticipating the histological tumour extent and for identifying the relationship between mesorectal fascia and tumour.

Endosonography (EUS), magnetic resonance imaging (MRI) and multi-detector CT (MDCT) have varying merits in preoperative staging. An exhaustive review is outside the scope of this chapter but within-subject comparisons [16], the prospective MERCURY (Magnetic Resonance Imaging in Rectal Cancer European Equivalence) study [17], and a recent meta-analysis [18] all confirm preoperative MRI can predict the extent of the primary tumour and the involvement of the mesorectal fascia with very high accuracy.

However, not all patients are suitable for MRI because of claustrophobia or other contraindications. Moreover, internationally, access to MRI remains limited.

Given that CT is more readily available and well-established for staging distant metastases, there has been anticipation that technical advances could improve local staging to the point where CT can be used as the sole investigation. Although, currently, CT does not have sufficient contrast resolution to identify the muscularis propria, the mesorectal facia tends to be well visualised. The Dutch TME study [19] used conventional CT to assess preoperative CRM involvement, but even the most experienced observer achieved a sensitivity of only 47 %. Nevertheless, a more recent study using preoperative MDCT achieved a sensitivity of 74 % for predicting fascial involvement. However, sensitivity fell to 65.6 % for low rectal tumours [20]. Therefore, because MRI is superior for assessment of local disease extent, the role of CT colonography is largely restricted to diagnosis and distant staging.

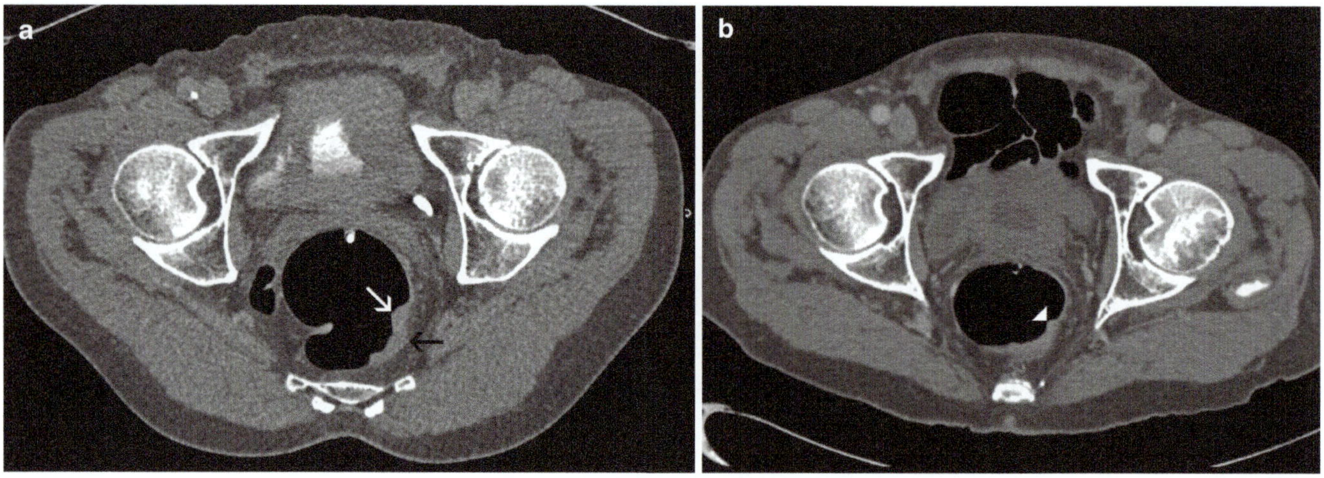

Fig. 3 (**a**, **b**) Contrast-enhanced, prone and supine axial colonography. This flat, ampullary tumour (*white arrow*) results in a luminal irregularity with little mural thickening. A trace of presacral fluid (*black arrow*) simulates tumour extension into mesorectal fat however T2 stage was confirmed at operation. Note the tumour's subtle luminal impression on the supine acquisition (*white arrowhead*)

Examples of Rectal Tumours

The examples listed below are grouped by local T-stage and ranged from small flat tumours to bulky, locally advanced disease. However, as described above, we consider CT colonography's role is not for accurate local staging but for sensitive tumour detection and simultaneous assessment of metastatic disease. Therefore, the aim of this section is to provide examples to improve diagnosis. Always bear in mind that nearly 50 % of all large bowel tumours are rectal.

T1 Rectal Tumours

It is predictable that T1 tumours are likely to pose the greatest diagnostic challenge. By definition, transmural extension is absent; therefore, detection relies purely upon an intraluminal mass. Poor distension or faecal residue can render a T1 lesion undetectable or indistinguishable from a bulky haustral fold. Therefore, detection of small tumours relies on meticulous technique, both in terms of performing and interpreting the CT colonography examination. Moreover, because there is, by definition, no substantial invasive component, the distinction between a T1 cancer and a large adenoma is not usually possible on imaging alone.

In general, the rectum is particularly well distended in the prone position, and this is a good place to start. Figure 3a, b shows a broad-based, flat neoplasm which is visible owing to optimal distension.

It is our routine practice to administer iodine-based faecal tagging (Fig. 4a). In addition to aiding diagnosis of submerged tumours, tagging solution has an affinity for some villous tumours. In an otherwise well-cleansed case, adherent tagging can draw attention to a subtle cancer. Small tumours around the rectal valves (of Houston) can be particularly difficult to detect, but routine review in the coronal plane (Fig. 4b, c) is often diagnostic.

Rectal Tumours: T2

T2 tumours involve the muscularis propria, but do not reach the mesorectal tissues. Consequently, mural thickening tends to be limited and there is no extramural component. Therefore, as for T1 tumours, a search for luminal irregularity is best able to detect these tumours, often achieved using wide 'colon' windows settings. Routine use of intravenous contrast during CT colonography is controversial, and a full discussion is outside the scope of this chapter; however, differential mural enhancement between prone and supine acquisitions can sometimes aid small tumour detection.

As with T1 tumours, the absence of frank extramural disease makes adequate rectal insufflation mandatory. Figure 5a, b shows subtle thickening between 9 and 11 o'clock on the prone acquisition with rectal collapse on the supine scan. The absence of extramural disease makes detection very challenging. Closer inspection of the tumour using narrow 'abdominal' window settings reveals subtle enhancement allowing a confident diagnosis to be made.

Figure 6a shows a larger polypoid rectal tumour which is conspicuous on the 2D images, and its intraluminal extension renders it easily visualised on the endoluminal flythrough (Fig. 6b).

Cancer arising on a haustral fold poses a particular problem as bulky folds around the rectosigmoid junction are common, particularly in the setting of diverticulosis. Figure 7a–c shows one such tumour with MRI correlation.

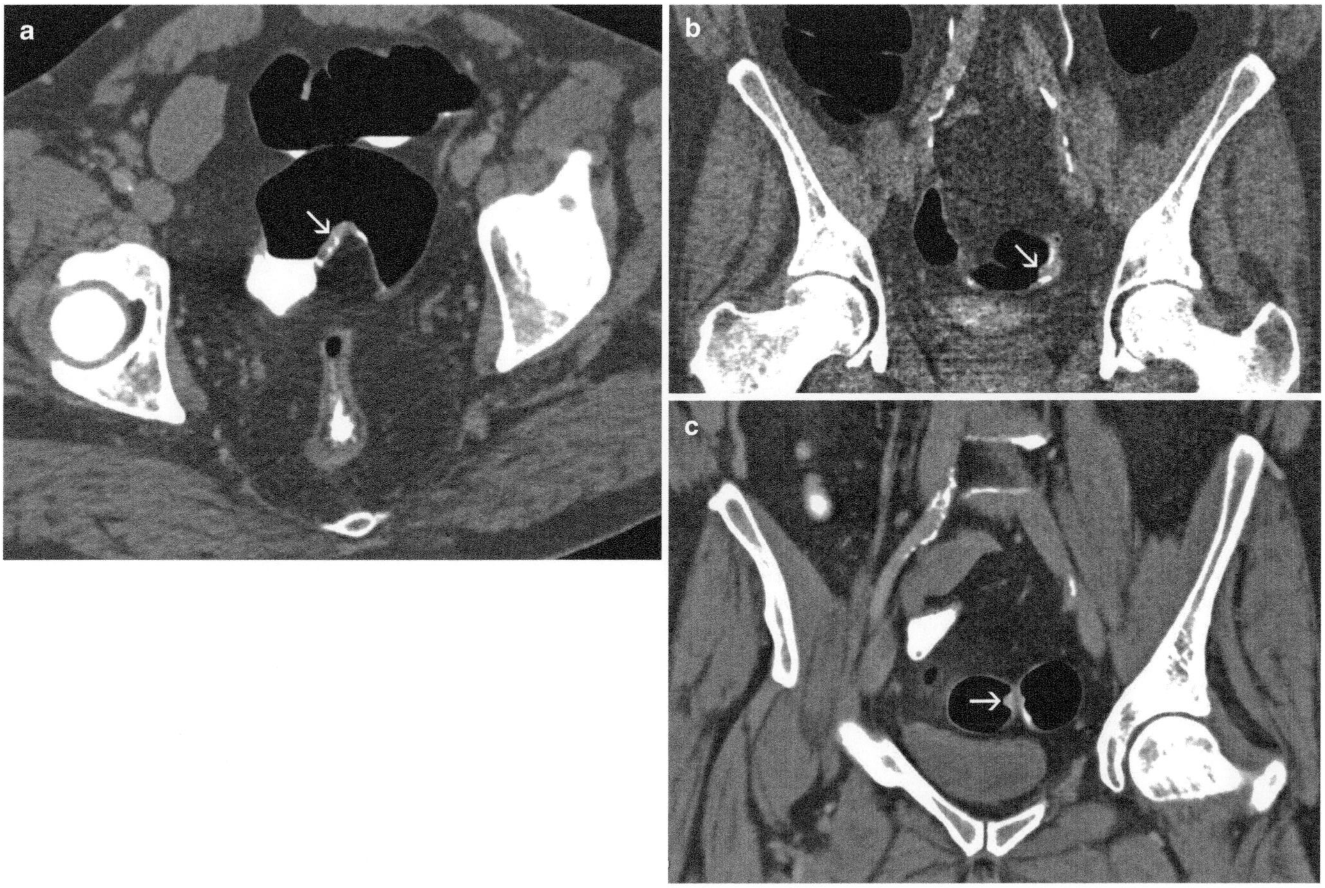

Fig. 4 (**a**–**c**) Supine axial, prone coronal and supine coronal reconstructions. A subtle tumour is present at the base of the third rectal valve (*white arrows*). Note the residual tagged fluid; in a well-cleansed case, adherent iodine solution can and draw attention to a subtle villous tumour

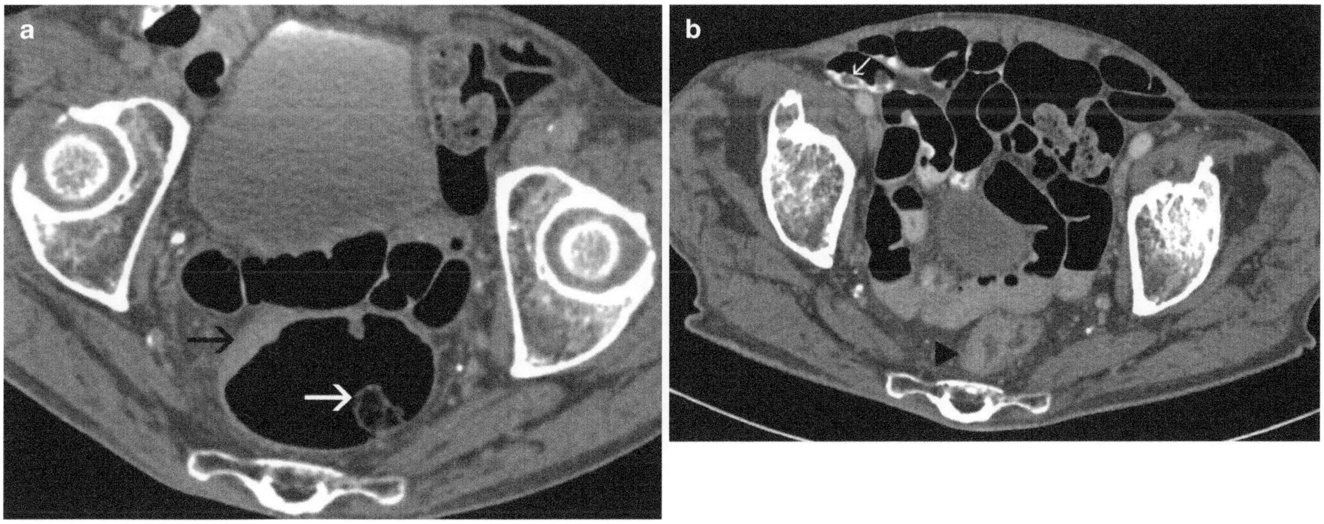

Fig. 5 (**a**, **b**) Enhanced supine axial colonography. Bowel preparation has been suboptimal in this cachectic elderly patient, and although oral iodine solution has been taken, there remains considerable untagged residue (*white arrows*). The supine acquisition shows a collapsed, fluid-filled rectum (*black arrowhead*). Prone repositioning allows further rectal insufflation and demonstrates a shallow tumour between 9 and 11o'clock (*black arrow*)

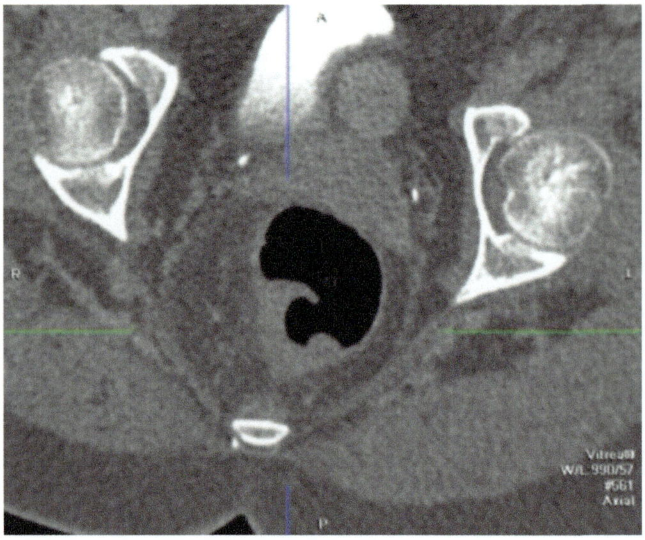

Fig. 6a Axial enhanced prone colonography. There is a relatively large intraluminal component to this early T3 tumour. The polypoid 'tongue' of tissue is characteristic and aids detection

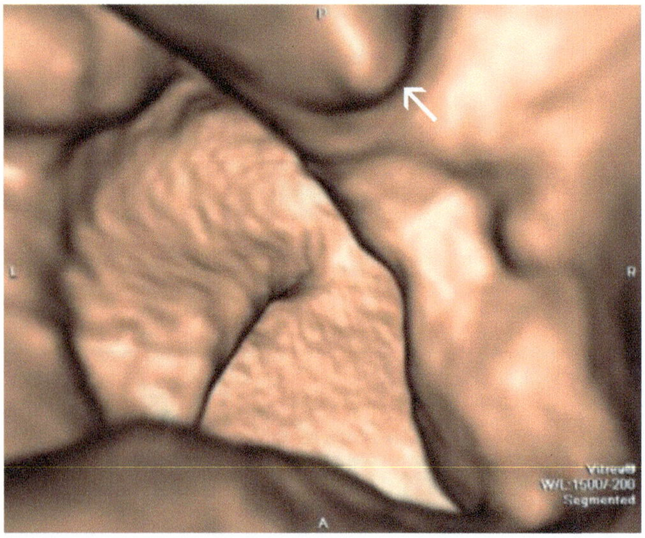

Fig. 6b Endoluminal reconstruction, prone colonography. The polypoid nodule (*white arrow*) draws attention to this tumour but its full extent is underestimated

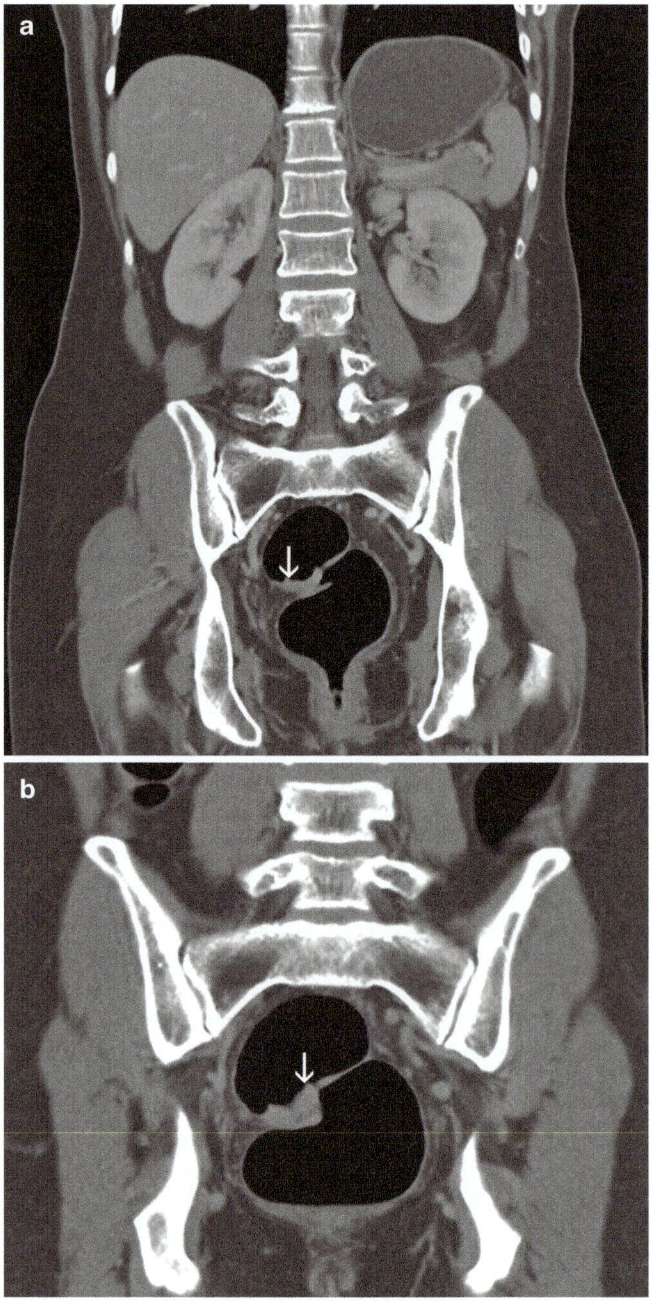

Fig. 7a and b Coronal, enhanced, supine and prone CT colonography. There is relatively subtle thickening of the inferior valve of Houston (*white arrows*), seen best on these coronal reconstructions. There is no CT evidence of transmural involvement

CT is relatively insensitive and non-specific for nodal involvement but generally, mesorectal nodes are considered likely involved when their short axis diameter exceeds 10 mm [21]. There are additional morphological features on MR that may allow smaller involved nodes to be diagnosed with reasonable certainty [22, 23]. Nodal involvement, particularly when close to the mesorectal facia, is an independent poor prognostic indicator. Therefore, mesorectal nodes should still be viewed with suspicion even when not significantly enlarged by 'standard' CT criteria. Although only 6 mm, the nodes in Fig. 8 do not show chemical shift artefact on MRI and, indeed, were involved at operation.

Rectal Tumours: T3

T3 tumours comprise a very heterogeneous group for the reasons explained in the sections above.

Also as noted above, the sensitivity of CT for mesorectal invasion is poor [16], and meta-analysis confirms MRI to be the preferred investigation [18].

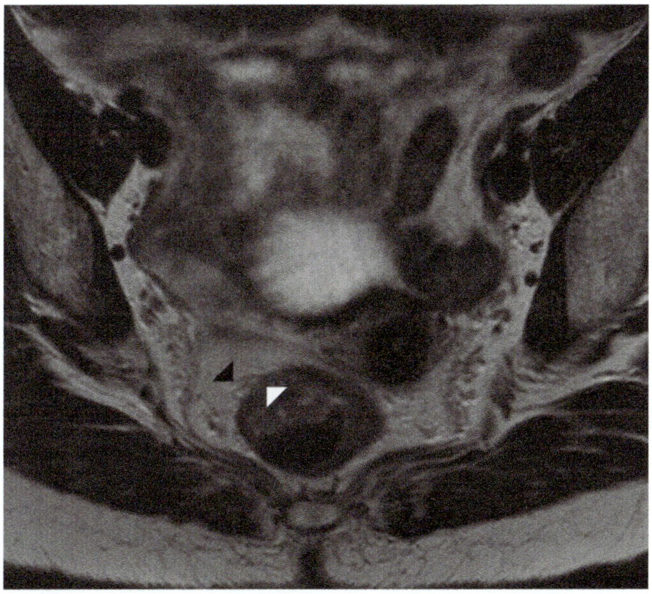

Fig. 7c Angled axial, high resolution, T2-weighted and fast spin echo MRI shows the tumour epicentre at 10 o'clock just breaching the muscularis propria (*white arrowhead*). There is adjacent desmoplastic reaction (*black arrowhead*) and no discrete extraluminal tumour nodule suggesting T2 disease. An early T3 tumour was confirmed at operation

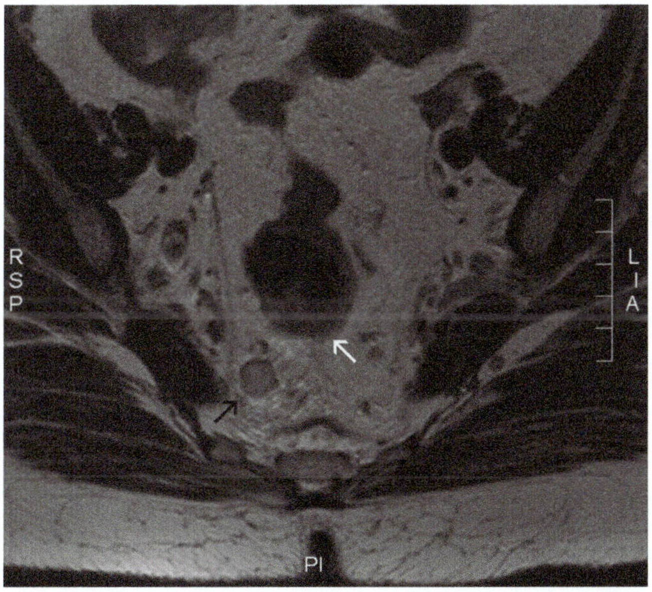

Fig. 8 High resolution, angled axial, T2-weighted fast spin echo MRI. Circumferential tumour is present with an epicentre at 5 o'clock (*white arrow*). Careful examination of the adjacent mesorectum confirms early T3 extension. However, note the large irregular right posterior mesorectal node which abuts the circumferential excision margin (*black arrow*)

However, once tumours have obvious extramural extension, their imaging characteristics lend themselves to detection with CT; in addition to luminal filling defects,

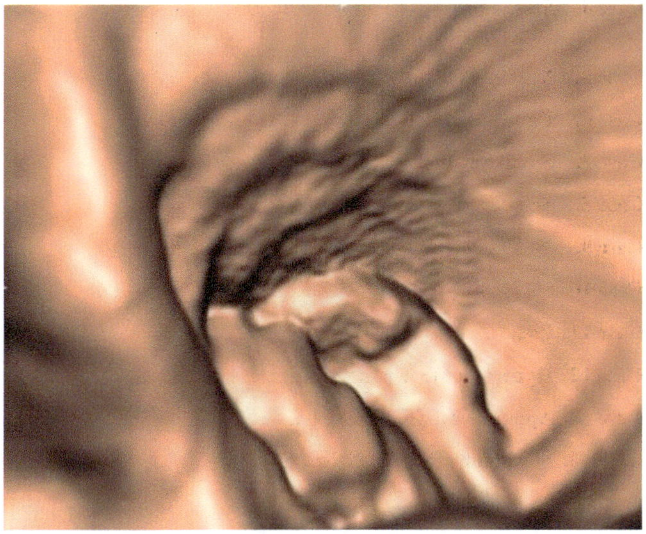

Fig. 9a *Endoluminal* reconstruction facing the rectum. Note the thickened, irregular and circumferential tumour causing malignant stricture. The 'rolled edge' and irregular appearance helps differentiate this from annular spasm

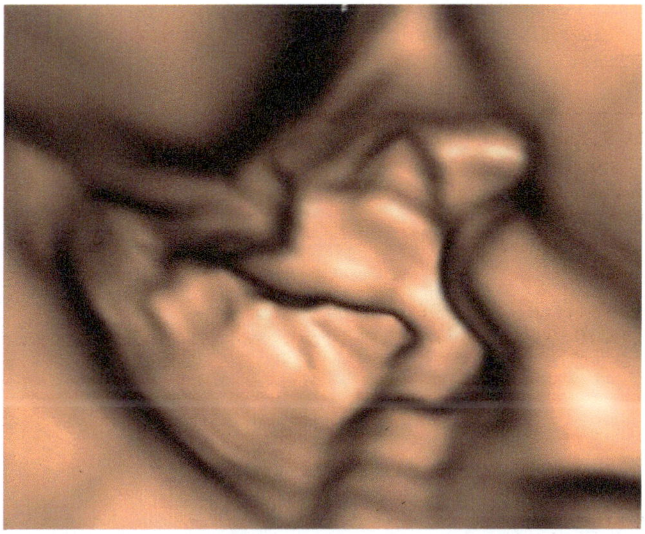

Fig. 9b Endoluminal view from within the tumour stricture facing the rectum. Most strictures are too narrow for endoluminal navigation, but when possible, the appearance from within the tumour is characteristic

there is conspicuous mural thickening and often soft tissue stranding of the adjacent mesorectal fat. For example, Fig. 9a illustrates an unmistakeable stenosing 'apple-core' cancer. The endoluminal appearances (Fig. 9b, c) confirm the characteristic, shouldered stricture. However, the relative insensitivity of endoluminal reconstruction (Fig. 10a, b) is worth noting even for large polypoid tumours. Furthermore, although a unidirectional 3D flythrough has been shown to provide equivalent mucosal

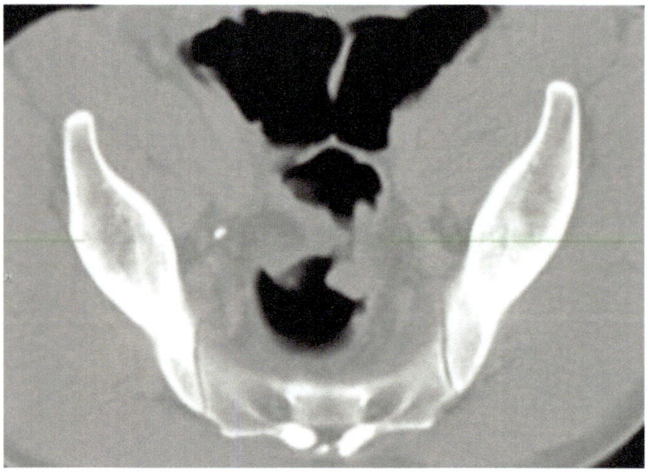

Fig. 9c *Supine* axial and unenhanced CT colonography. A familiar 'apple-core' stricture is well demonstrated using 2D images

visualisation as bidirectional fly-throughs, there are occasions when rectal tumours are only visible when approached from the sigmoid (Fig. 10c–e).

Also of considerable importance for surgical planning is the tumour's distal relationship to the sphincter complex since this will decide whether an anterior-posterior resection (i.e. anal excision) is needed.

In Fig. 11a–c, the coronal reformat demonstrates the tumour's distal margin relative to the sphincter complex while the sagittal reformat illustrates the proximal margin's position above the peritoneal reflection.

T3 Tumours with Poor Prognostic Features

In addition to the local T-stage, nodal status, integrity of the mesorectal facia, vascular invasion and peritoneal involvement are also important independent prognostic indicators which may be demonstrated using CT. For example, the annular tumour in Fig. 12a, b clearly threatens the CRM, and a large extramural tumour nodule was confirmed on MRI.

Furthermore, although nodal status is underestimated with CT, particularly when using a 10-mm threshold [21], mesorectal lymphadenopathy and its proximity to the CRM is often adequately demonstrated (Fig. 13a, b).

Rectal Tumours: T4

Direct tumour invasion into local structures such as the seminal vesicles, bladder, vagina, ovary and bladder (all of which convey a T4 stage) are usually well delineated with CT colonography. Figure 14a, b shows a bulky T4 tumour invading the CRM and extending cranially into the presacral space, left pelvic sidewall and sacrum.

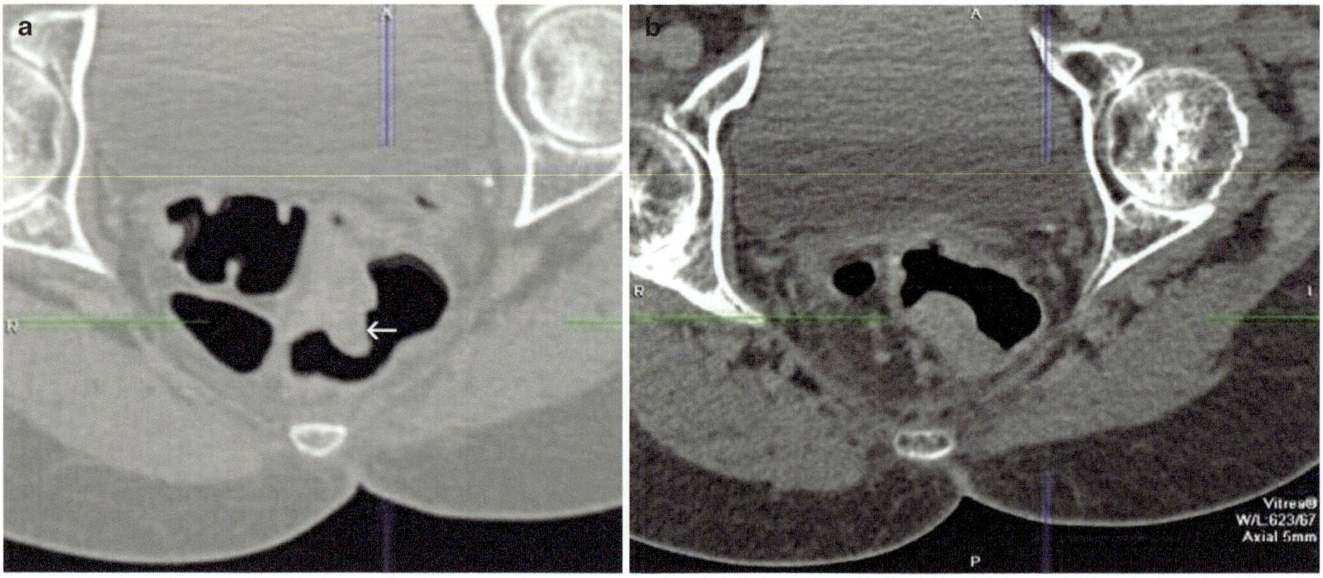

Fig. 10a and b Axial, supine and enhanced CT colonography. A large intraluminal filling defect in the superior rectum is well visualised on standard colonography window settings (*white arrow*), and its enhancing homogenous attenuation pattern is diagnostic on soft tissue windows

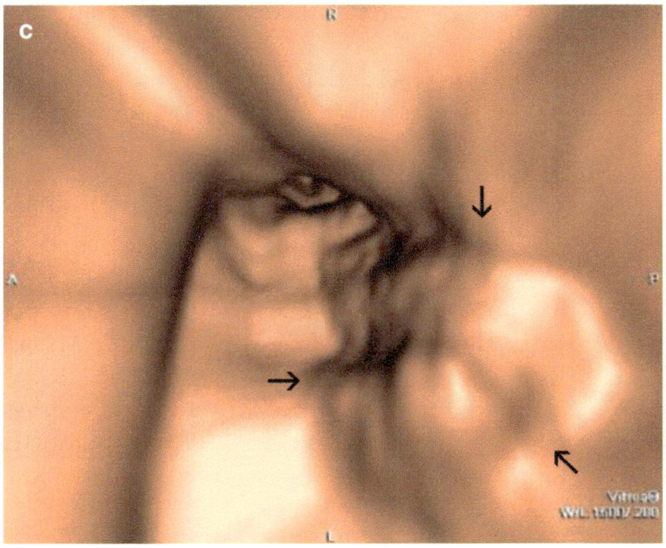

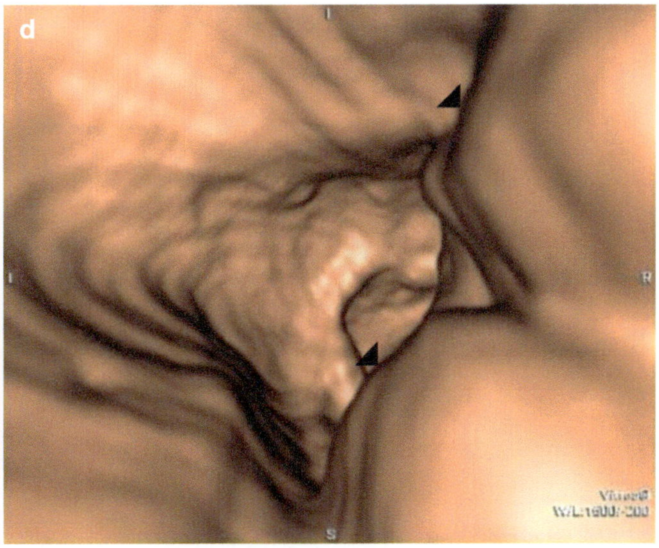

Fig. 10c and d *Endoluminal* CT colonography facing the cecum from the rectal ampulla. There is ill-defined, lobulated mural indentation between 3 to 6 o'clock (*black arrows*). This appearance is characteristic. The smooth, lobulated mural impression indicates the large underlying polypoid tumour (*black arrowheads*)

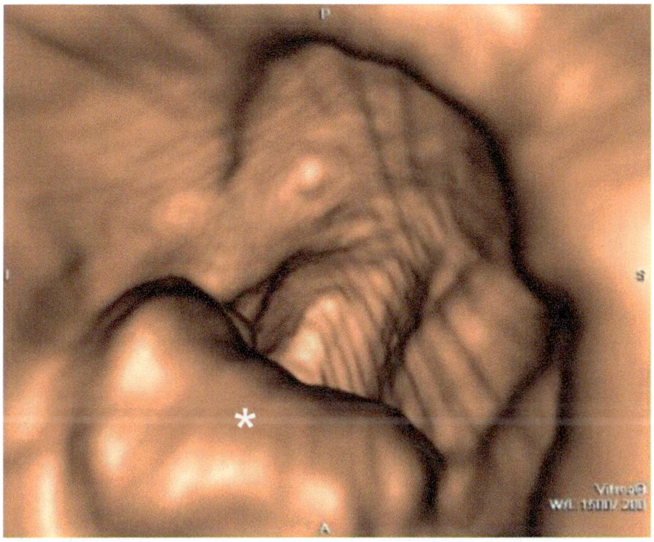

Fig. 10e Endoluminal CT colonography facing the rectum. The large polyp partially occludes the lumen. The 3D reconstruction is very clearly seen and reflects the 2D findings (*asterisk*)

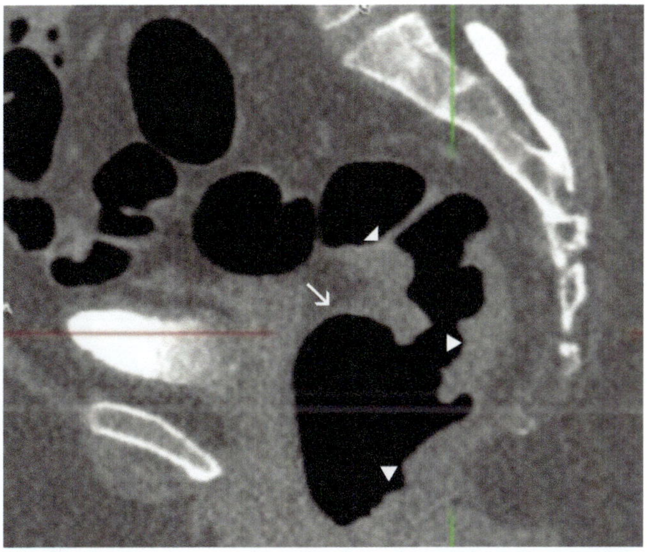

Fig. 11a Enhanced, prone mid-sagittal colonography. There is a 5-cm stricture extending from mid-rectum to the rectosigmoid junction (*white arrowheads.*) The sagittal reconstruction demonstrates the tumour's extension above the peritoneal reflection (*white arrow*)

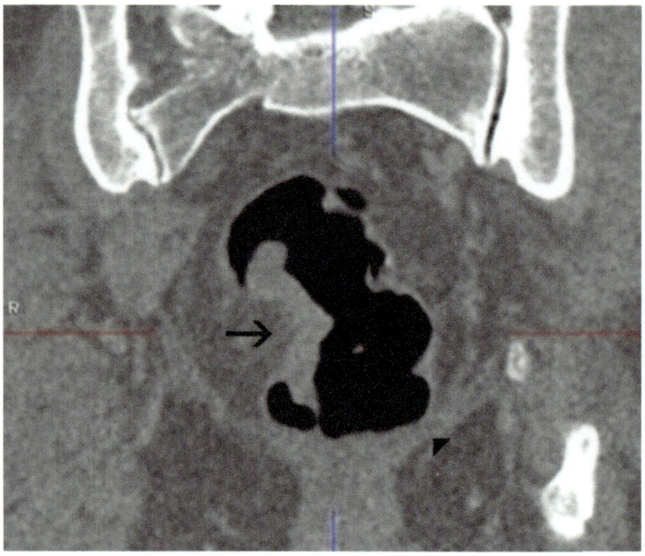

Fig. 11b *Coronal* and prone CT colonography. The relationship to the levator (*black arrowhead*) is best demonstrated in the coronal plane. Note the desmoplastic reaction within mesorectal fat (*black arrow*)

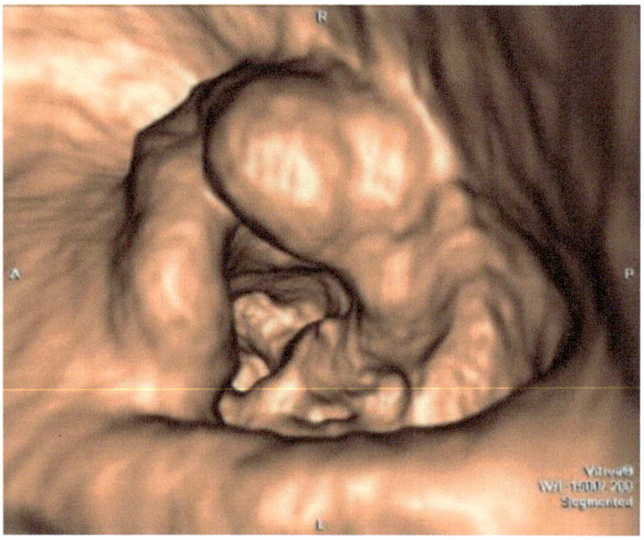

Fig. 11c Endoluminal reconstruction of prone colonography from the distal rectum, facing the sigmoid. Note the relative lack of stenosis for a tumour of this size and the shouldered leading edge

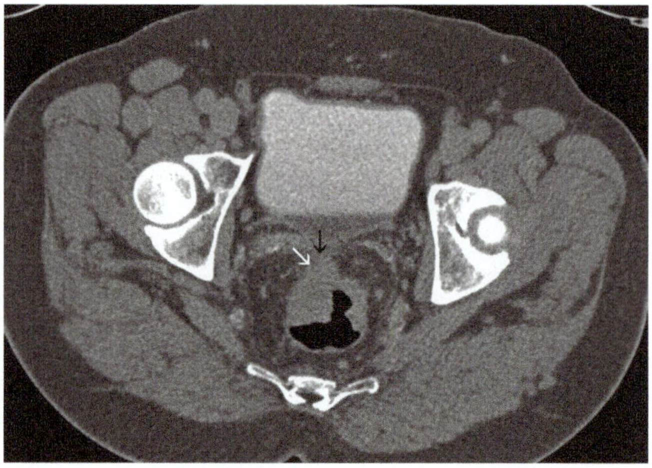

Fig. 12a Prone, axial and enhanced colonography. The endoluminal mass and stenotic effect of a large tumour such as this requires good insufflation to avoid luminal collapse. The tumour's epicentre is at 12 o'clock, and careful examination of the adjacent mesorectum suggests extraluminal extension (*white arrow*) in close proximity to the circumferential excision margin (*black arrow*)

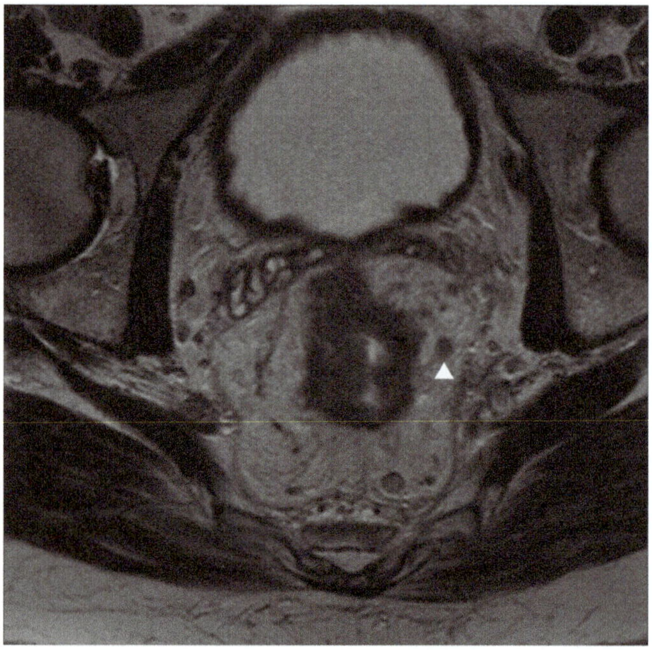

Fig. 12b Angled axial, T2 weighted fast spin echo MRI. The muscularis propria is breached anteriorly with a large tumour nodule within 1 mm of the anterior CRM. Note also multiple nodes seen on both CT and MRI. Although the largest (*white arrowhead*) measures only 6 mm and therefore is not considered significant by CT size criteria, MRI shows the nodal signal intensity matches that of the primary tumour

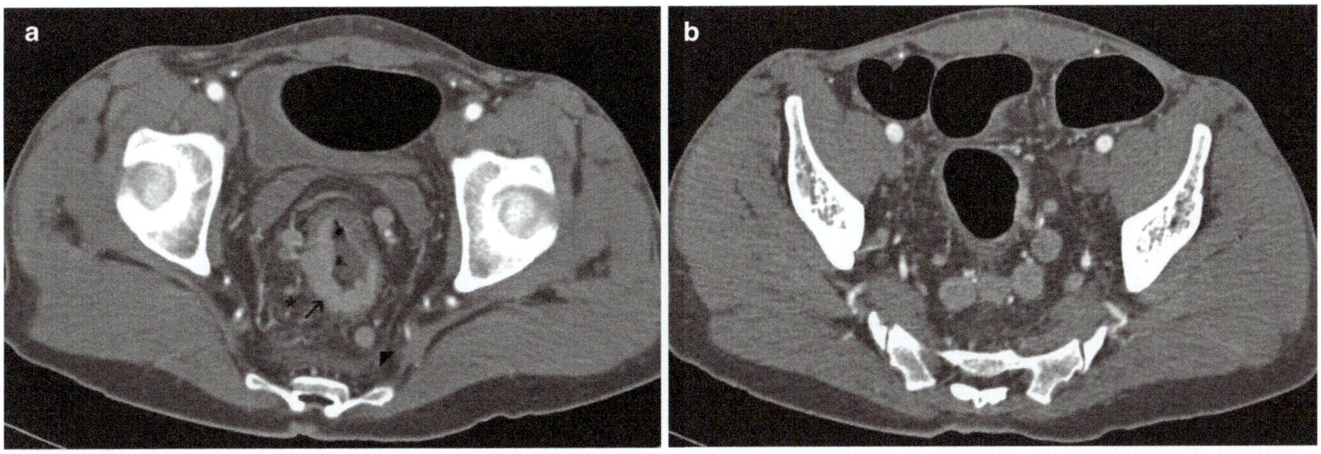

Fig. 13 (**a**, **b**) Axial, enhanced supine colonography at mid-rectal and superior rectal levels. Avidly enhancing circumferential tumour is present with convincing extramural tumour extension in the right posterior quadrant (*black arrow*) and considerable soft tissue changes in the adjacent mesorectum (*asterisk*). Several rounded, mesorectal lymph nodes are present, at least one of which threatens the CRM (*black arrowhead*)

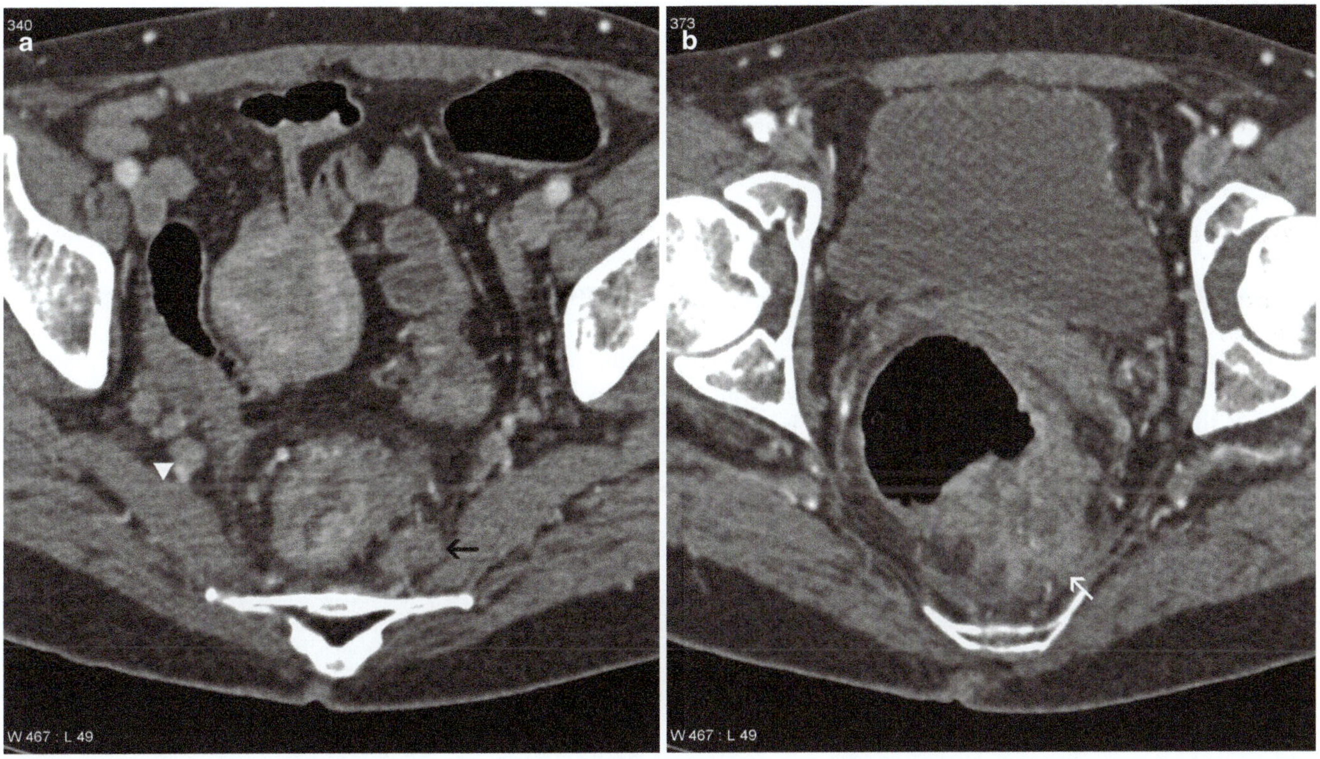

Fig. 14 (**a**, **b**) Axial, enhanced supine colonography at superior and mid-rectal levels. The CRM is clearly breached by a large tumour nodule (*black arrow*) while more superiorly, tumour invades the presacral space and left hemi-sacrum (*white arrow*). Also note right pelvic sidewall nodal enlargement (*arrowhead*)

Interpretative Pitfalls

Incorrect diagnoses are often due to poor technical implementation. Poor insufflation, inadequate faecal tagging and poor bowel preparation will reduce diagnostic accuracy. However, even in well-distended cases, there are several interpretative pitfalls which should be recognised and avoided.

Heterogeneous Tumour Enhancement

Routine intravenous contrast enhancement during CT colonography is controversial, and opinions vary in both screening and symptomatic settings. Nevertheless, enhancement is often useful when differentiating tumour from faecal residue. However, when enhancement is heterogeneous, it can have the opposite effect and cause large tumours to resemble stool. Figure 15a illustrates a 4-cm rectal ampullary mass which forms an acute angle with the rectal wall and has a heterogeneous attenuation pattern. This case is poorly cleansed and the mass could be mistaken for a large faecal ball. Closer inspection of perirectal soft tissue shows the mass is mural in origin with mesorectal invasion. Moreover, Fig. 15b confirms that it does not move during prone positioning.

Suboptimal Residual Fluid Tagging

Residual faecal fluid and incomplete tagging are troublesome wherever they occur. Submerged tumours can be difficult to see, particularly when distension is suboptimal. The problem is accentuated by routine use of wide 'colonic' window settings (Fig. 16a) which are particularly helpful when looking for small polyps, but minimise the contrast resolution between untagged stool and abnormal mural thickening. We advise reviewing the rectum using routine 'soft tissue' window settings, preferably in the coronal plane (Fig. 16b), when fluid tagging is incomplete.

Sigmoid Diverticulosis

Sigmoid diverticulosis is present in up to 50 % of American and European patients. Muscular hypertrophy leads to reduced luminal distension, which in turn complicates interpretation [24]. Research suggests primary 3D endoluminal navigation can alleviate the difficulties inherent in examining a diverticular segment [25]. However, the abrupt transition between normal rectum and narrowed sigmoid colon can pose a unique problem for diagnosis of rectal tumours in the proximal third. For example, Fig. 17a shows extensive sigmoid hypertrophy obscuring a stenosing, annular carcinoma at the rectosigmoid junction. Figure 17b, c illustrates mural enhancement in a thickened segment which further reduces the contrast between tumour and diverticulosis. In Fig. 17d, review of the 2D data in an alternative plane clearly shows the tumour, and we suggest this approach is particularly useful in this setting.

Sigmoid Diverticulitis

Although it is not our usual practice to perform CT colonography in the presence of active diverticulitis, it is not unusual to find incidental colonic inflammation during an apparently routine examination. The presence of enhancing mural thickening with pericolonic inflammatory change can impair

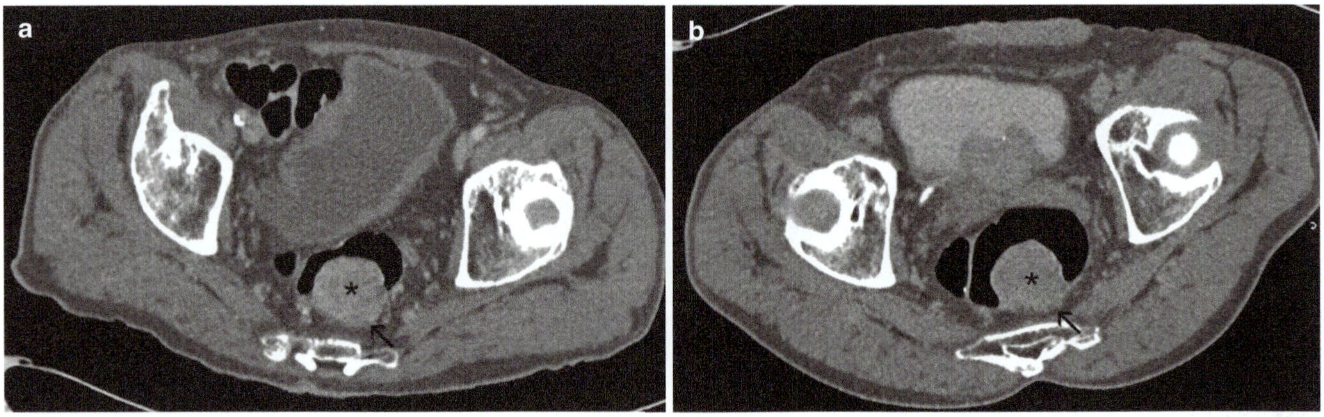

Fig. 15 (**a**, **b**) Supine and prone, axial, enhanced colonography. There is a 4-cm diameter superior rectal mass (*asterisks*) which has a heterogeneous attenuation pattern and forms an acute angle with the bowel wall. In the context of incomplete bowel preparation this could be misinterpreted as a large faecal ball. However the mass remains suspended during prone positioning, has differential enhancement between scans and lacks gas within. Furthermore, careful examination confirms transmural extension (*black arrows*)

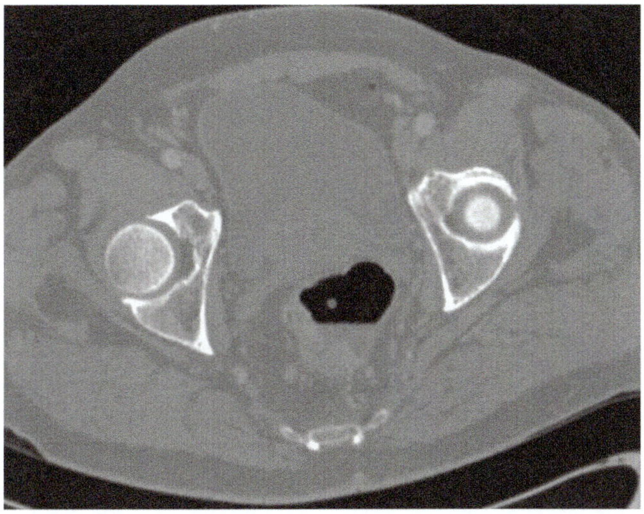

Fig. 16a Axial colonography using standard window settings. Untagged residue forms a fluid level in the rectal ampulla

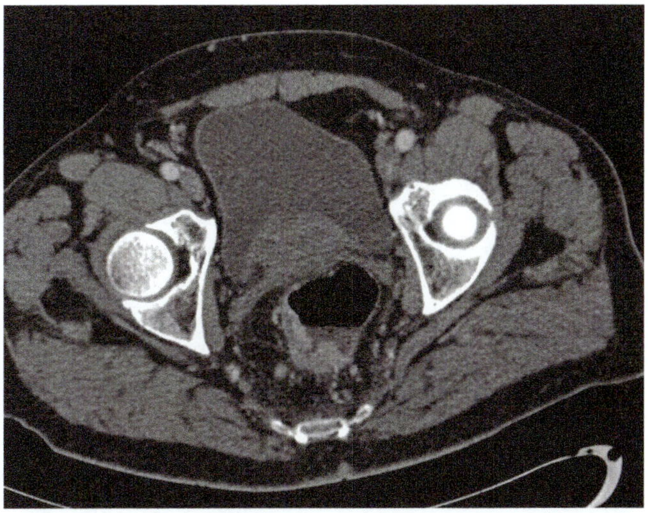

Fig. 16b Narrow 'soft tissue' window settings increase the contrast between residual fluid and enhancing tissue, allowing a large, T3 tumour to be clearly seen. Also note the rounded mesorectal nodes which, although small, are infiltrated

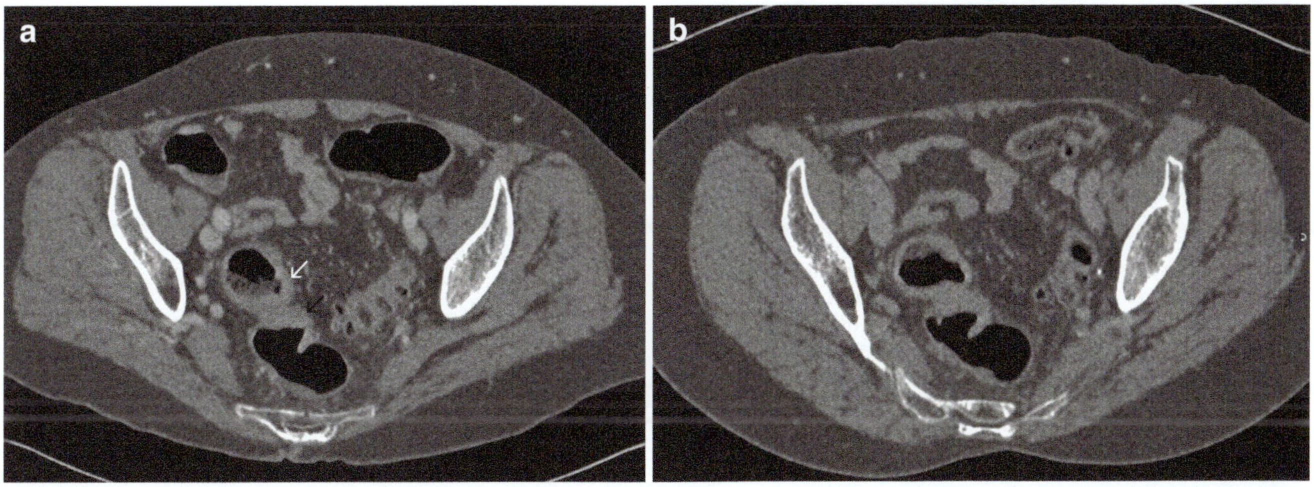

Fig. 17a and b Enhanced supine and prone axial colonography. There is mild circumferential sigmoid thickening (*white arrow*) which extends to the rectosigmoid junction associated with numerous diverticula. There is relative narrowing at the rectosigmoid junction and thickening of the adjacent haustral fold (*black arrow*). The bowel is poorly prepared. Endoluminal reconstruction is hampered by collapse and faecal residue

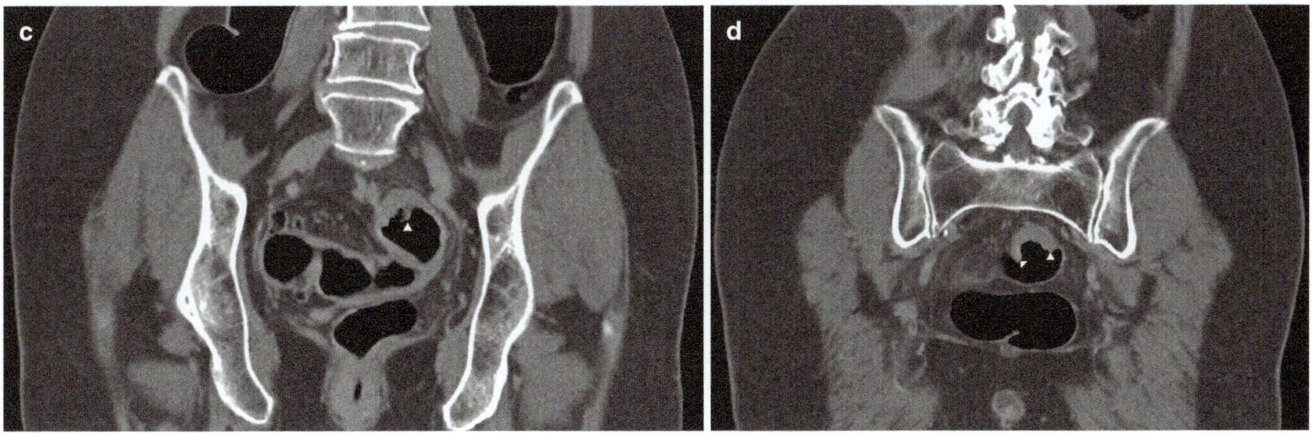

Fig. 17c and d Coronal reconstruction. There is circumferential sigmoid thickening. Only the supine coronal reconstruction adequately demonstrates the asymmetrical, crescenteric tumour at the rectosigmoid junction (*white arrowheads*)

the visibility of a synchronous cancer, and the distinction between diverticulitis and a perforated cancer can be extremely challenging. Although various attempts have been made to differentiate tumour from diverticulitis by assessing the degree of mesenteric stranding and lymphadenopathy on CT, it is our contention that these patients must have direct visualisation by endoscopy if at all possible (and even then differentiation between the two diagnoses may be impossible). Indeed, even at open operation, it can be difficult to exclude tumour in a diverticular segment. Figure 18 illustrates this challenge. A combination of circumferential mural thickening, inflammatory change and luminal collapse obscure the 5-cm annular tumour. Scrutiny of the rectosigmoid junction shows an asymmetric shouldered mass.

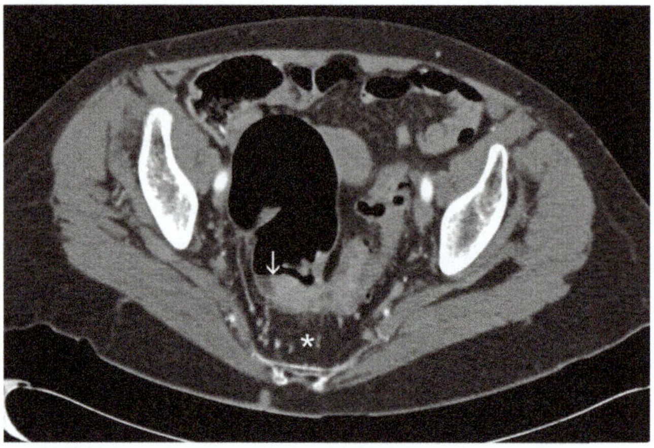

Fig. 18 Enhanced supine colonography performed for altered bowel habit and a left iliac fossa mass. There is a long segment of collapsed, thickened sigmoid with diverticula and surrounding inflammatory change (*asterisk*). However, careful inspection of the posterior rectosigmoid junction reveals an enhancing 'rolled edge' at the distal extent of the rectosigmoid tumour (*white arrow*). Extreme caution must be exercised when attempting to exclude cancer in the presence of diverticulosis or diverticulitis

Insufflation Tube Artefacts

Although it is considered good practice to remove the insufflation tube before acquiring rectal radiographs during barium enema, this practice is not specifically recommended for CT colonography [26]. The requirement to introduce more gas following repositioning and the use of automated insufflators encourages the rectal tube to be left in situ. Nevertheless, Fig. 19a, b illustrates a case where a small, flat cancer was obscured until removal of the tube prior to the prone acquisition. When a rectal balloon catheter is inflated, this too may efface a small rectal tumour (Fig. 20a, b), particularly when there is poor rectal distension or residue. Again, meticulous technique in terms of both carrying out and reporting the examination is recommended.

Limitations of Endoluminal Reconstruction

Virtual endoscopic reconstruction is now almost universally adopted by those reading CT colonography, either for the primary interpretation or for 'problem solving' following initial 2D review.

Much research has compared 3D and 2D interpretation, but suffice it to say that the vast majority of studies concentrate on sensitivity for polyps rather than cancer. Furthermore, the emphasis of training tends to focus on polyp detection and cancer detection may even be considered 'trivial' by some readers who believe that cancers are obvious by dint of their size. However, the 3D endoluminal appearances of

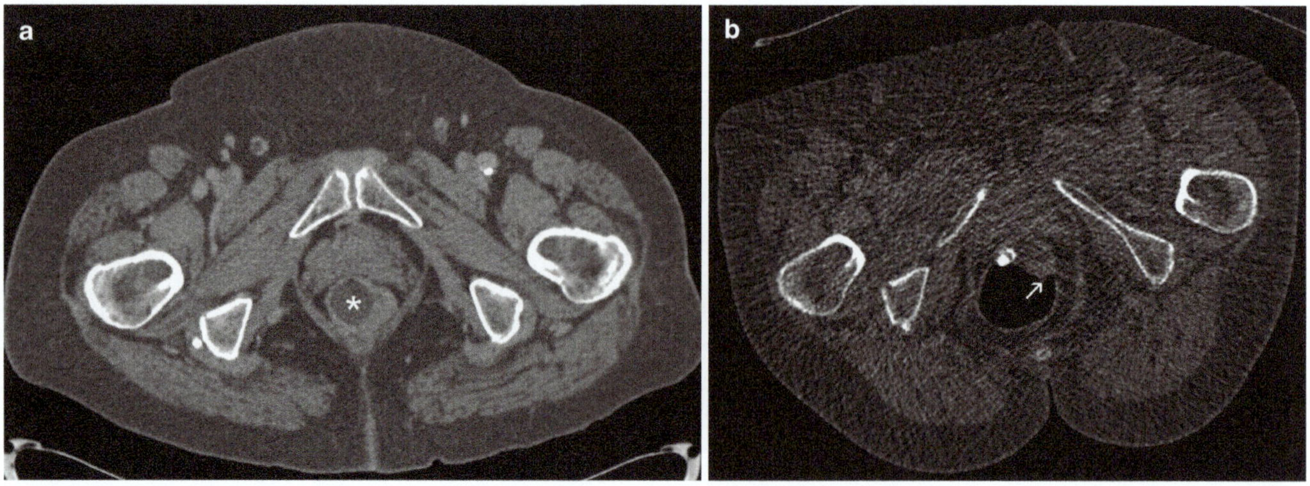

Fig. 19a and b Enhanced supine and prone axial colonography with a water-filled balloon catheter in situ (*asterisk*). The rectum is collapsed on the supine projection impairing detection of the small, rounded anterior ampullary tumour. Furthermore, the luminal filling defect on the well-distended prone scan is not typical of tumour (*white arrow*)

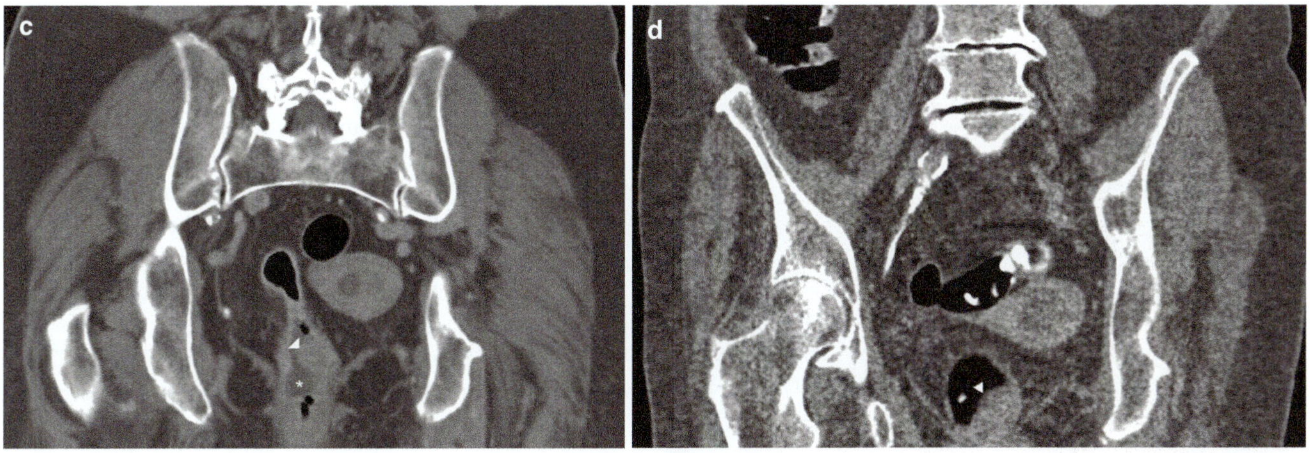

Fig. 19c and d Prone and supine coronal reconstructions illustrate the water-filled rectal balloon (*asterisk*) effacing the left lateral rectal tumour (*white arrowhead*)

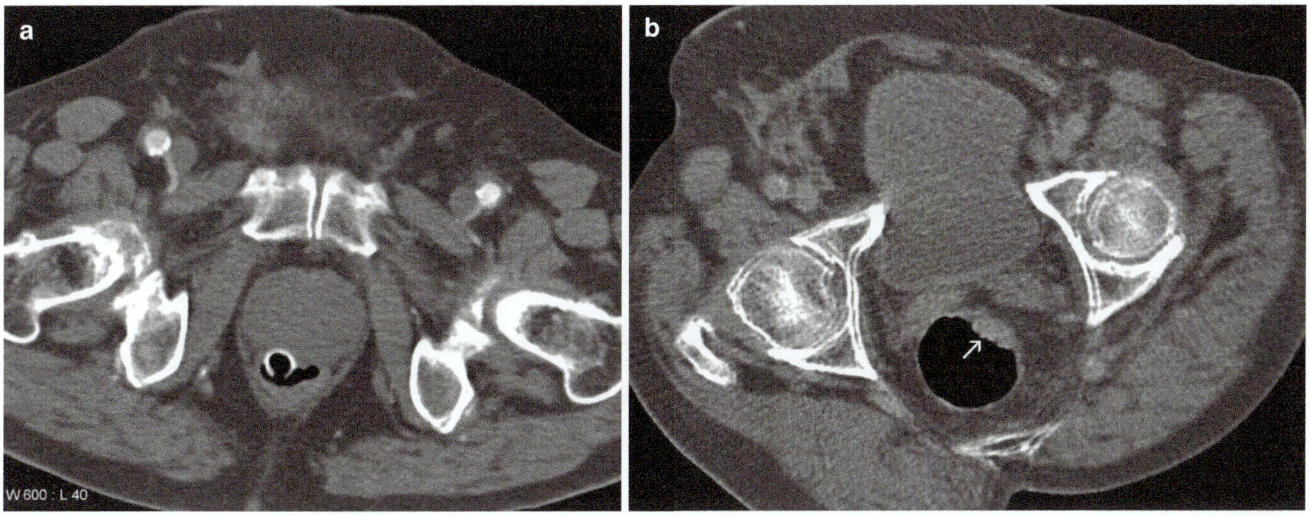

Fig. 20 (**a**, **b**) Supine and prone axial colonography with a rectal insufflation tube in situ. The rectum is collapsed in the supine position, allowing the rectal tube to efface the small tumour. Prone repositioning reveals the small, crenulated T1 cancer (*white arrow*)

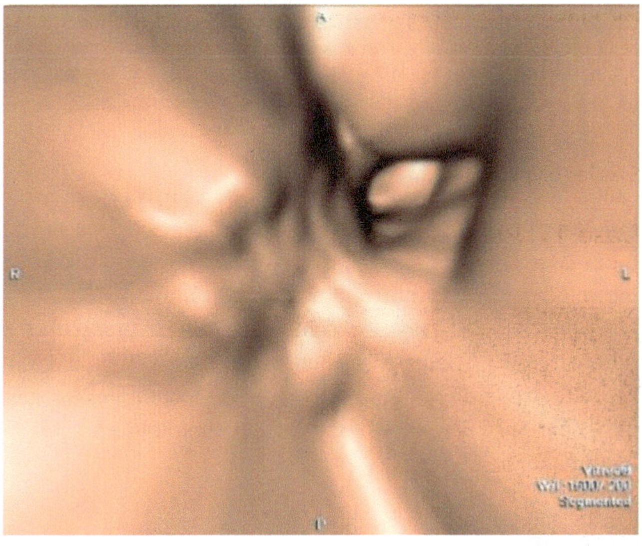

Fig. 21a This endoluminal reconstruction demonstrates the potential difficulty in diagnosing large circumferential tumours using a primary 3D technique. The lumen is circumferentially narrowed as one would expect with spasm. Only the surface irregularity between 6 and 9 o'clock suggests the presence of underlying malignancy

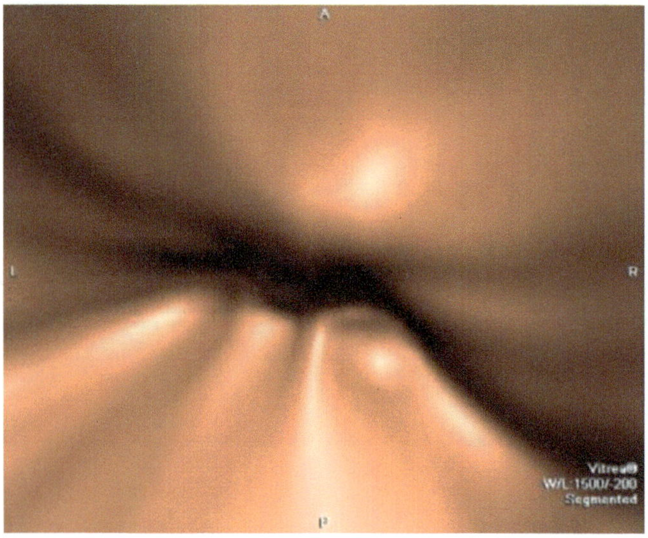

Fig. 21b Endoluminal reconstruction facing from the sigmoid into the stenosed rectal ampulla. Note the smooth, circumferential narrowing which could be misinterpreted as sigmoid muscular thickening and spasm

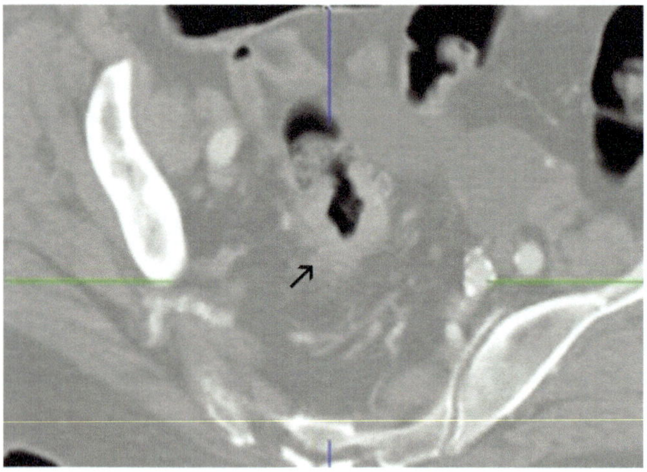

Fig. 21c Enhanced, supine, axial reconstruction through the cranial extent of the large partially obstructing tumour. Bowel preparation has been incomplete and a fluid level is present within the stenosed lumen. A large polypoid luminal filling defect is present. There is peritumoural fat stranding and likely extramural extension (*black arrow*)

cancer can be surprisingly subtle, even with very extensive tumours. Figure 21a, b shows one example where a bulky, 6-cm stenosing tumour could be mistaken for spasm when viewed from the rectum, and neither is it immediately obvious when viewed from the sigmoid. Contrast this with the relative ease of diagnosis when using the 2D sequence in Fig. 21c. Regardless of preferred reading technique, we suggest a careful 2D review of the rectum should be carried out in all patients.

Conclusion

Approximately 50 % of all colorectal cancers will be present in the rectum, and management of rectal cancer differs markedly to colonic tumours elsewhere. Meticulous radiological assessment is required to determine the local tumour extent, in particular its relationship to the CRM, and current evidence suggests this is best performed with MRI. Nevertheless, CT colonography has the advantage of detecting rectal tumours and simultaneously assessing distant metastases.

Rectal tumours are usually well visualised using a combination of 2D multiplanar reformats, providing there is good bowel preparation and distension in accordance with European consensus guidelines [26]. Endoluminal reconstructions are invaluable for problem solving, especially around the valves of Houston, but it must be remembered that collapsed segments or those containing residual fluid will obscure tumours when using a primary 3D approach. Particular care must be exercised in the presence of sigmoid diverticulosis, particularly at the rectosigmoid junction.

Regardless of preferred reading paradigm, we recommend a thorough review of the rectum using a combination of multiplanar reformats, preferably using narrow 'abdominal' window settings.

References

1. Atkin WS et al (2010) Once-only flexible sigmoidoscopy screening in prevention of colorectal cancer: a multicentre randomised controlled trial. Lancet 375(9726):1624–1633
2. Quirke P et al (1986) Local recurrence of rectal adenocarcinoma due to inadequate surgical resection. Histopathological study of lateral tumour spread and surgical excision. Lancet 2(2430152): 996–999
3. Adam IJ et al (1994) Role of circumferential margin involvement in the local recurrence of rectal cancer. Lancet 344(7915774):707–711
4. Palmer G et al (2010) Preoperative tumour staging with multidisciplinary team assessment improves the outcome in locally advanced primary rectal cancer. Colorectal Dis (20958913)
5. Heald RJ, Husband EM, Ryall RD (1982) The mesorectum in rectal cancer surgery–the clue to pelvic recurrence? Br J Surg 69(6751457):613–616
6. Havenga K et al (1999) Improved survival and local control after total mesorectal excision or D3 lymphadenectomy in the treatment of primary rectal cancer: an international analysis of 1411 patients. Eur J Surg Oncol 25(10419706):368–374
7. MacFarlane JK, Ryall RD, Heald RJ (1993) Mesorectal excision for rectal cancer. Lancet 341(8094488):457–460
8. Martling AL et al (2000) Effect of a surgical training programme on outcome of rectal cancer in the County of Stockholm. Stockholm Colorectal Cancer Study Group, Basingstoke Bowel Cancer Research Project. Lancet 356(10963244):93–96

9. Wibe A et al (2002) Prognostic significance of the circumferential resection margin following total mesorectal excision for rectal cancer. Br J Surg 89(11872058):327–334
10. Kapiteijn E et al (2001) Preoperative radiotherapy combined with total mesorectal excision for resectable rectal cancer. N Engl J Med 345(11547717):638–646
11. Steele RJ, Sebag-Montefiore D (1999) Adjuvant radiotherapy for rectal cancer. Br J Surg 86(10540121):1233–1234
12. Gray R et al (2001) Adjuvant radiotherapy for rectal cancer: a systematic overview of 8507 patients from 22 randomised trials. Lancet 358(9290):1291–1304
13. Folkesson J et al (2005) Swedish Rectal Cancer Trial: long lasting benefits from radiotherapy on survival and local recurrence rate. J Clin Oncol 23(16110023):5644–5650
14. Sauer R et al (2004) Preoperative versus postoperative chemoradiotherapy for rectal cancer. N Engl J Med 351(15496622):1731–1740
15. Bosset J-F et al (2006) Chemotherapy with preoperative radiotherapy in rectal cancer. N Engl J Med 355(16971718):1114–1123
16. Beets-Tan RGH et al (2001) Accuracy of magnetic resonance imaging in prediction of tumour-free resection margin in rectal cancer surgery. Lancet 357(9255):497–504
17. Fowler JM et al (2007) Extramural depth of tumor invasion at thin-section MR in patients with rectal cancer: Results of the MERCURY Study. Radiology 243(1):132–139
18. Bipat S et al (2004) Rectal cancer: local staging and assessment of lymph node involvement with endoluminal US, CT, and MR imaging – a meta-analysis. Radiology 232(3):773–783
19. Wolberink S et al (2007) Conventional CT for the prediction of an involved circumferential resection margin in primary rectal cancer. Dig Dis 25(1):80–85
20. Wolberink SVRC et al (2009) Multislice CT as a primary screening tool for the prediction of an involved mesorectal fascia and distant metastases in primary rectal cancer: a multicenter study. Dis Colon Rectum 52(19502858):928–934
21. Pomerri F et al (2009) Prediction of rectal lymph node metastasis by pelvic computed tomography measurement. Eur J Surg Oncol 35(18359603):168–173
22. Brown G et al (2003) Preoperative assessment of prognostic factors in rectal cancer using high-resolution magnetic resonance imaging. Br J Surg 90(3):355–364
23. Brown G et al (2003) Morphologic predictors of lymph node status in rectal cancer with use of high-spatial-resolution MR imaging with histopathologic comparison. Radiology 227(2): 371–377
24. Gollub MJ et al (2005) CT colonography features of sigmoid diverticular disease. Clin Imaging 29(3):200–206
25. Sanford M, Pickhardt P (2006) Diagnostic performance of primary 3-dimensional computed tomography colonography in the setting of colonic diverticular disease. Clin Gastroenterol Hepatol 4(8):1039–1047
26. Taylor S et al (2007) European society of gastrointestinal and abdominal radiology (ESGAR): consensus statement on CT colonography. Eur Radiol 17(2):575–579

The Ileocecal Valve

Danielle Hock, Roxanne Ouhadi, Roland Materne, Isabelle Mancini, and Alain Nchimi

Contents

D. Hock, M.D. (✉) • R. Ouhadi, M.D.
R. Materne, M.D. • I. Mancini, M.Sc.
Department of Medical Imaging,
Centre Hospitalier Chrétien (CHC),
Rue de Hesbaye, 75, B-4000 Liège, Belgium
e-mail: danielle.hock@chc.be

A. Nchimi, M.D.
Department of Thoracic and Cardiovascular Imaging,
Centre Hospitalier Universitaire de Liège,
Domaine Universitaire du Sart-Tilman, Bâtiment B35,
B 4000 Liège, Belgium

Abstract

The ileocecal valve sits at the confluence between the terminal ileum and the colon and may thus be involved by number of pathologies linked to these two entities.

The normal ileocecal valve presents with two lips that may be open or closed, thin or large in accordance with their submucosal fatty content and with a smooth or slightly nodular surface, but they are always harmonious and symmetrical.

Its recognition is important not only to assess colonic distension and prove a complete study but also to avoid the misdiagnosis of a possible cecal or ascending colon tumor for the ileocecal valve.

Its two-dimensional thorough analysis is mandatory as the ileocecal valve may present with a normal external aspect but be nevertheless infiltrated by a submucosal process.

The ileocecal valve (ICV), also known as colic valve or valvula coli, constitutes a special entity because of its situation at the confluence between the terminal ileum and the colon: it may thus be involved in a variety of pathologies linked to the colon, the terminal ileum and even the appendix.

The Normal Ileocecal Valve

Situation

The ileocecal valve is situated in the colon at the level of the first complete haustral fold, usually on the medial or posterior colonic wall at the junction between the cecum and ascending colon. As the cecum is a very mobile structure (indeed subject to volvulus), the ICV may thus move with the patient's position and, for instance, shift from the medial aspect of the colon in supine position to its external aspect when the patient is set in prone position [1].

E. Neri et al. (eds.), *CT Colonography Atlas*, Medical Radiology,
DOI 10.1007/978-3-642-11149-5_12, © Springer-Verlag Berlin Heidelberg 2013

Anatomy

From an anatomical point of view, the ileocecal valve results from a kind of short intussusception of the small bowel into the cecum. Each lip is indeed composed by an internal layer born of the ileum and an external layer born of the large bowel. These layers are not complete as they only comprise the mucosa, the submucosa with a variable content of fat, and the internal circular muscle, but not the ileal external longitudinal muscle layer, serosa, and peritoneum that turn back and mix with those pertaining to the large bowel [2].

External Aspect

The ileocecal valve is an oblong protrusion within the colon representing the termination of the ileum. Its 10-mm long slit-like aperture is surrounded by two lips: the superior lip, also known as the superior valve or ileocolic lip, that is salient with a downward direction and the inferior lip, also known as the inferior valve or ileocecal lip, that is shorter and vertical. The superior lip thus covers the inferior, and the aperture of the valve faces downward in the direction of the cecum. The two lips join laterally and end on both sides in two narrow membranous ridges constituting the frenula of the valve.

Normal lips may be thin or thick, resulting from localized and sometimes massive accumulation of submucosal fat: this is known as fatty infiltration, lipohyperplasia or lipomatous infiltration. The lack of capsule differentiates this fatty proliferation from true lipoma [3]. Usually, lips have a smooth appearance but may occasionally present with stellate folds radiating toward their aperture [4]. A valve may be open in one acquisition and closed in the other (Fig. 1).

Function

The ileocecal valve function is double: to allow the thorough flow of the small bowel content into the cecum and to prevent the reflux from the large bowel into the ileum [5].

Thorough Flow from the Small Bowel

As the superior lip overlaps the inferior and the valve prolongs sideway with the frenula, it results in an incomplete and semilunar wall between the cecum and the right colon. In consequence, the ileal content has to flow into the cecum, filling first its internal side, and then moving to its external portion. The inward curvature of the cecum, increasing the internal depression of this organ, still emphasizes this motion. The action of the ileocecal valve is nevertheless not only passive. The circular muscle layer acts as a sphincter, as the flow of the ileal content is not continuous but split up.

Opposition to the Reflux

The ileocecal valve was long thought to be impassable: if this is not true in corpses, this is almost always the case in the living. The anatomy gives a partial explanation: feces are mashed in the right colon by numerous peristaltic and antiperistaltic contractions, squeezing thus the two ileocecal lips shut. As this closing apparatus reveals insufficient in some experiences performed on corpses, there is an additional effect linked to the ileocolic sphincter that is probably maneuvered by the autonomous nervous system, acting as in the opening and closing of the pylorus.

Competency of the valve may be of importance in case of colonic obstruction: an incompetent valve allows retrograde decompression into the small bowel without the risk of a closed loop.

1 mg of glucagon, which is a relatively potent spasmolytic agent in smooth muscle, has a relaxant effect on the ileocecal valve, while anticholinergics such as scopolamine butylbromide (Buscopan®) have little effect [6].

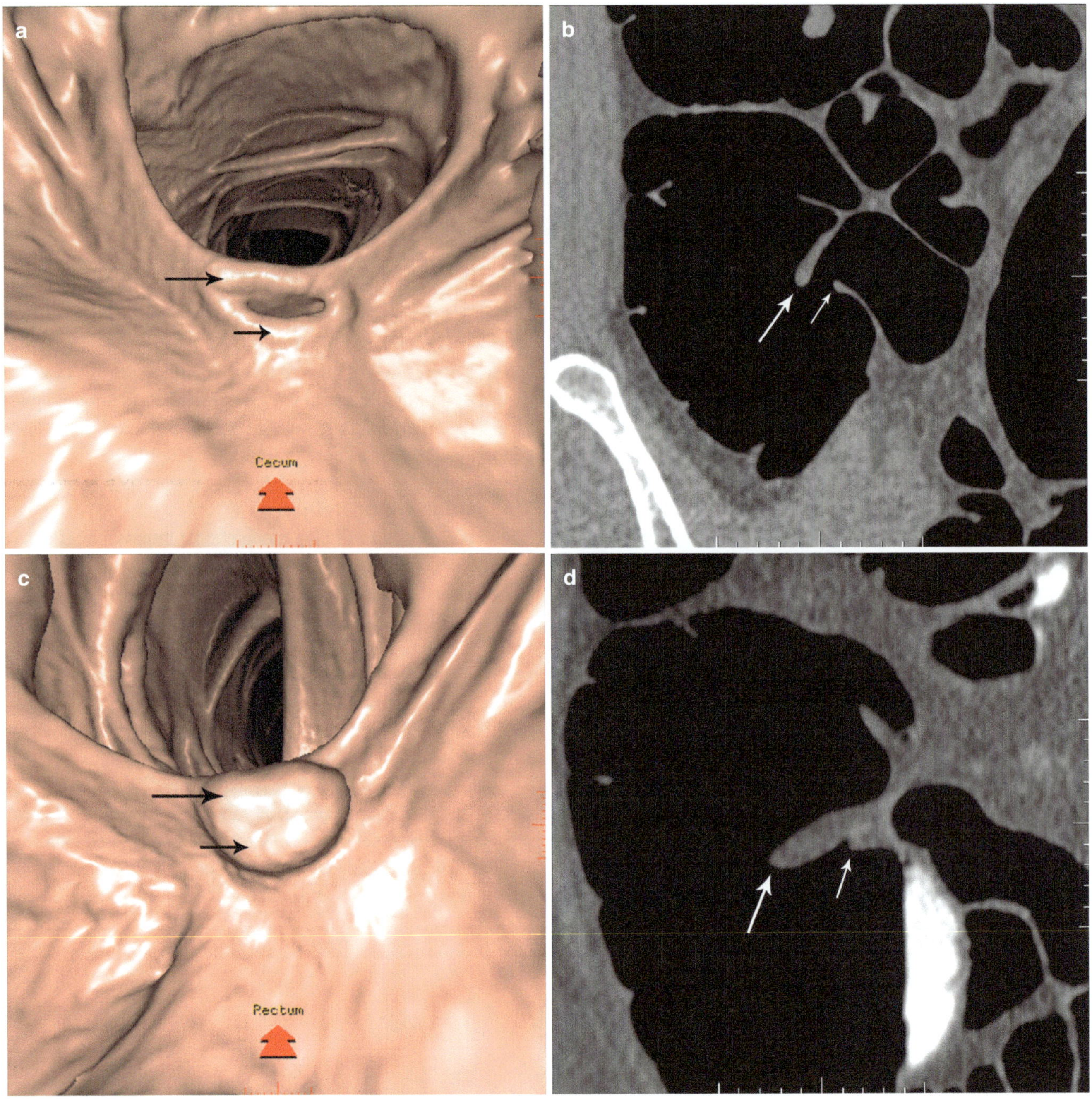

Fig. 1 Variety of normal ileocecal valves: the superior lip (*long arrow*) covers slightly the inferior lip (*short arrow*). (**a**, **b**) Endoluminal (**a**) and coronal view (**b**) of a thin-lipped open ileocecal valve: the lips present with soft tissue densities. (**c**, **d**) Endoluminal (**c**) and coronal (**d**) view of a closed lipomatous ileocecal valve: both lips present with a fatty content. (**e–g**) Endoluminal (**e**) and coronal (**f**, **g**) views of an ileocecal valve with stellate folds radiating toward its aperture; the valve is closed in supine acquisition (**f**) and open in prone acquisition (**g**)

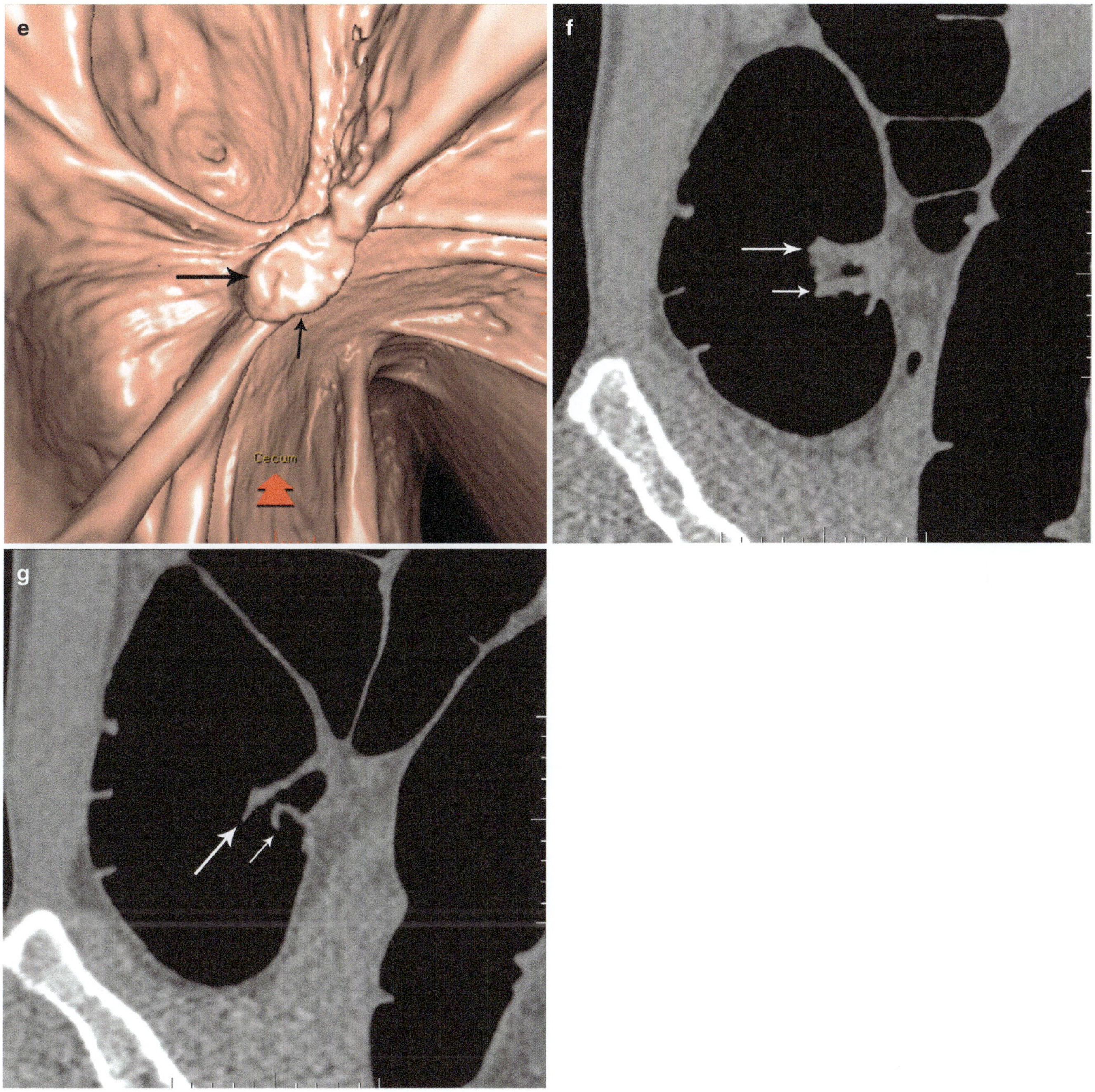

Fig. 1 (continued)

Pathology of the Ileocecal Valve

Even when the ileocecal valve is normal, it may not always be easy to recognize either in the fly-through mode or in axial sections. In those cases, the junction between small and large bowel is more obvious using the coronal views. Proceeding likewise allows avoiding common pitfalls for beginners. The first one is to misdiagnose a cecal tumor for the ileocecal valve (Fig. 2). The second one is to fail to recognize incomplete colonic insufflations with total or partial collapse of the right colon: as a matter of fact, the colon being a tortuous organ of variable length, the dead cert of a complete study by optical or virtual colonoscopy is only possible if the ileocecal valve (ICV) is clearly identified (Fig. 3).

Once the ileocecal valve has been localized, it deserves a close three-dimensional inspection as well as a dedicated two-dimensional analysis.

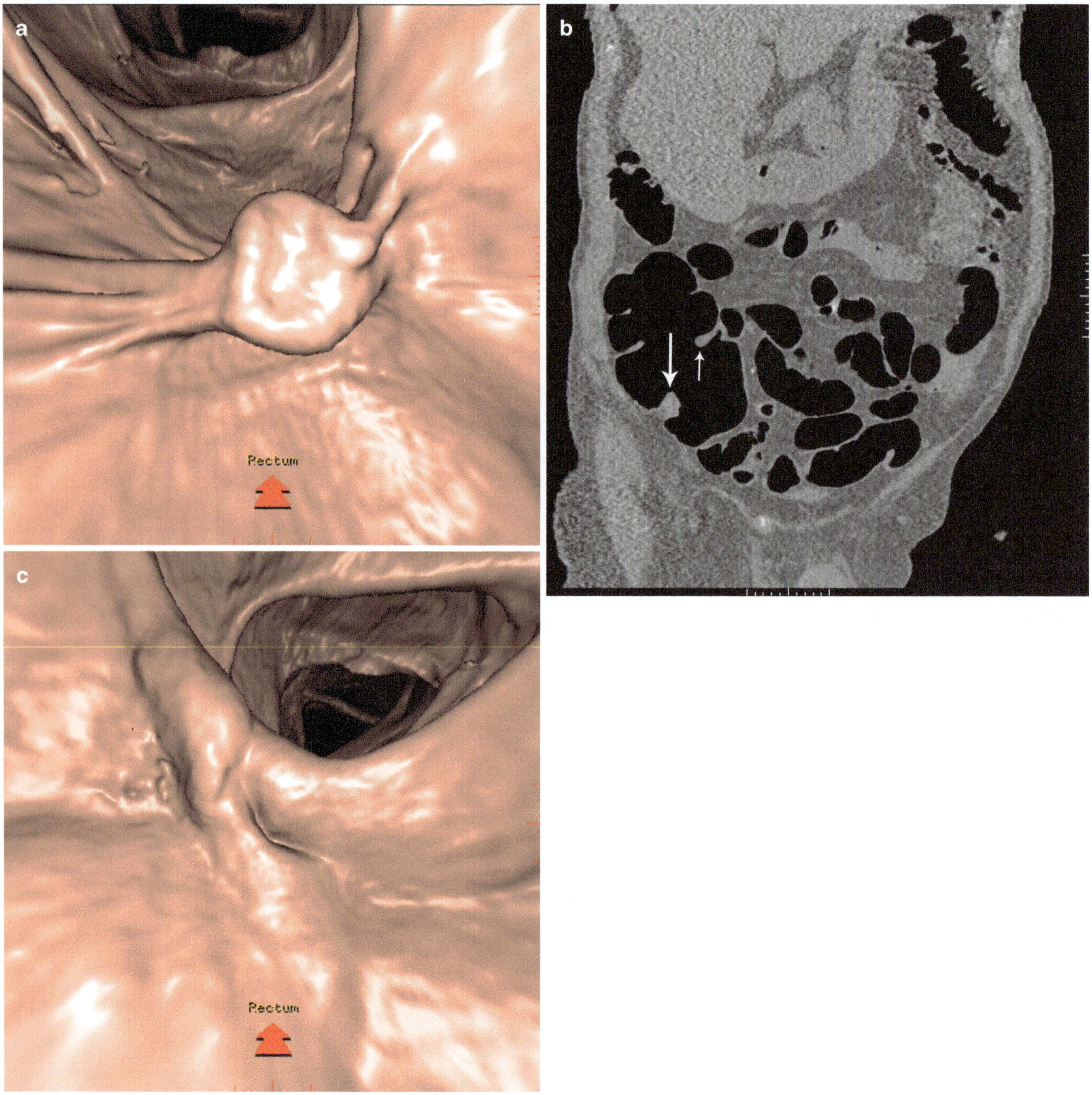

Fig. 2 Common pitfall for beginners: to misdiagnose a cecal tumor for the ileocecal valve. (**a**) Endoluminal view of a flat tumor resembling to an ileocecal valve. (**b**) Coronal view demonstrating the tumor (*long arrow*) and the ileocecal valve (*short arrow*). (**c**) Endoluminal view of the ileocecal valve

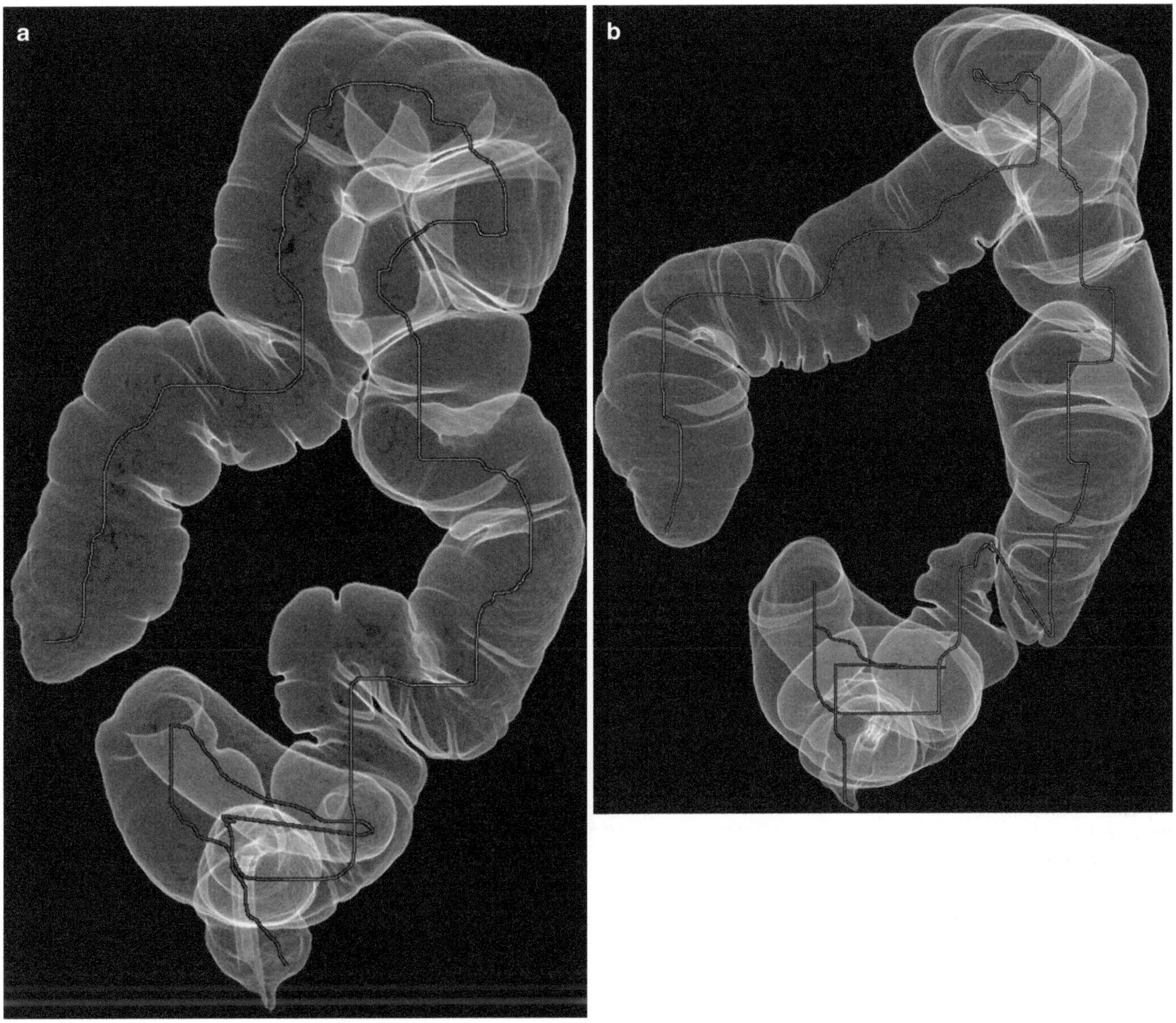

Fig. 3 Common pitfall: incomplete insufflations. (**a**, **b**) Supine (**a**) and prone (**b**) acquisitions showing seemingly complete insufflations with a short right colon. (**c**) Left lateral decubitus with complete insufflations. The ileocecal valve is recognized with a discrete reflux into the terminal ileum (*arrow*)

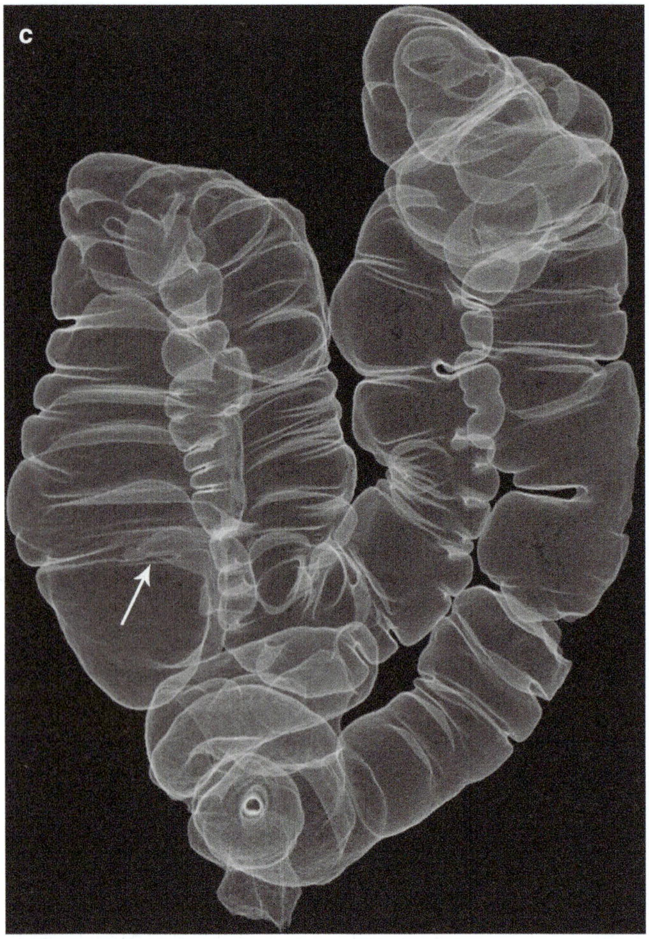

Fig. 3 (continued)

Tumors

Protruding Lesions

Lipoma

The colon is the most frequent site of gastrointestinal involvement by lipoma although colonic lipomas are uncommon lesions occurring at autopsy in less than 1 % of patients [7]. Most of these lipomas occur in the right colon and originate from the submucosa. Multiple tumors are found in 25 % of patients: these tumors are usually less than 3 cm in diameter, but those that cause symptoms such as abdominal pain and discomfort or bleeding and pain related to intussusception tend to be either larger lesions or lesion situated near or on the ileocecal valve, thus subject to prolapse into the terminal ileum [8] (Fig. 4). Colonic lipomas are encapsulated masses of mature adipose tissue usually confined to the submucosa and covered by normal colonic mucosa: they form obtuse angles with the adjacent colonic wall and their surface is smooth. Approximately two-thirds of them are pedunculated, with a broad-based pedicle. Because of the pliable nature of fat, lipomas change their shape according to the position of the patient or the degree of colonic distension [9]. Their CT diagnosis is definitive and simple: the mass is of uniform fatty density (−60 to −120 HU) without septa or other large areas of nonfatty tissue [10].

Polyps and Adenocarcinoma

The ileocecal valve is covered on its external surface by colonic mucosa and may thus harbor polyps or adenocarcinomas as any other area of the colon. Small lesions are recognized on 3-D endoluminal views when the ileocecal valve shows asymmetry in the shape of its lips (Fig. 5) or a mass in case of a large lesion. The 2D analysis demonstrates a soft tissue density protrusion arising from a valve. Malignant transformation is suspected when there is a soft tissue density infiltration with thickening of a valve (especially recognizable in case of fatty infiltration) as well as abnormal sharp or straight contours of the lips, eventually reaching the adjacent colonic wall that is thickened.

As for any malignant process, an advanced stage may be suspected by strands of soft tissue extending from the serosal surface into the pericolonic fat as well as by the presence of local lymph nodes.

Infiltrating Tumors

Neuroendocrine (Carcinoid) Tumor

Infiltration of the ileocecal valve by a carcinoid tumor may be either primary or secondary to a colonic or terminal ileum location as endocrine cells are scattered throughout the gastrointestinal tract: the most common sites of involvement include the appendix (35 %), ileum (16 %), lung (14 %), and rectum (13 %) [11]. Neuroendocrine tumors arising in the remainder of the colon constitute only 2–3 % of all the carcinoid tumors, and the most common colonic sites are the rectum and the cecum. Neuroendocrine tumors arising from right and transverse colon are of midgut origin and may synthetize serotonin (with thus possible but rare subsequent carcinoid syndrome) [12], while those arising from the left colon to the rectum are from hindgut origin, do not produce serotonin or cause carcinoid syndrome, and have a better prognosis [13]. Cecal or right colon neuroendocrine tumors are usually large and aggressive lesions associated with a poor prognosis (approximately 50 % of 5-year survival rate). They occur usually in the sixth decade of life with symptoms similar to those of colonic carcinoma, including abdominal pain, distension, and palpable abdominal mass [14]. These tumors originate in the submucosa: there is at first a wall thickening with desmoplastic retraction,

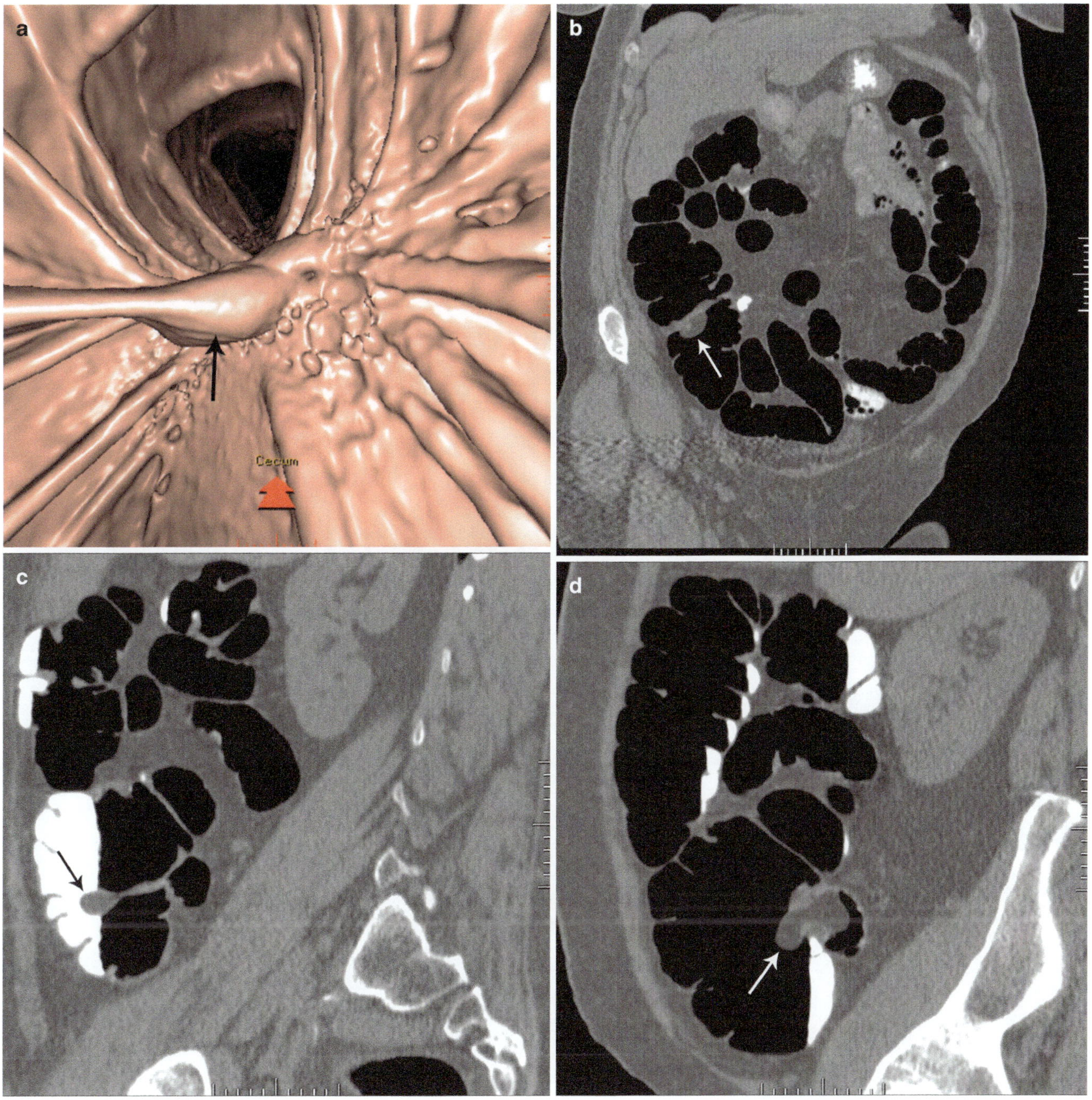

Fig. 4 Lipomas. (**a**, **b**) Endoluminal (**a**) and coronal (**b**) views of a centimetric sessile lipoma (*arrow*) located on the side of the ileocecal valve. (**c**, **d**) Oblique views of a pedunculated lipoma (*arrow*) of the ileocecal valve, floating freely in prone position (**c**) and prolapsing through the ileocecal valve in supine position (**d**)

stranding of the adjacent peritoneal fat and lymph nodes. Then they may evolve into a large submucosal polypoid mass and even an irregular annular lesion that may be indistinguishable from colonic adenocarcinoma [15].

At an early stage, this infiltration gives the ileocecal valve a bulging 3-D endoluminal aspect resembling a lipohyperplasia but with soft tissue density on cross-sectional study (Fig. 6).

Lymphoma

Malignant lymphoma involves the gastrointestinal tract either as primary neoplasm or as part of a disseminated disease. Disseminated systemic lymphoma, involving the entire colon or long segments, is relatively common and asymptomatic [16]. Non-Hodgkin's lymphoma, principally large cell lymphoma, accounts for almost all

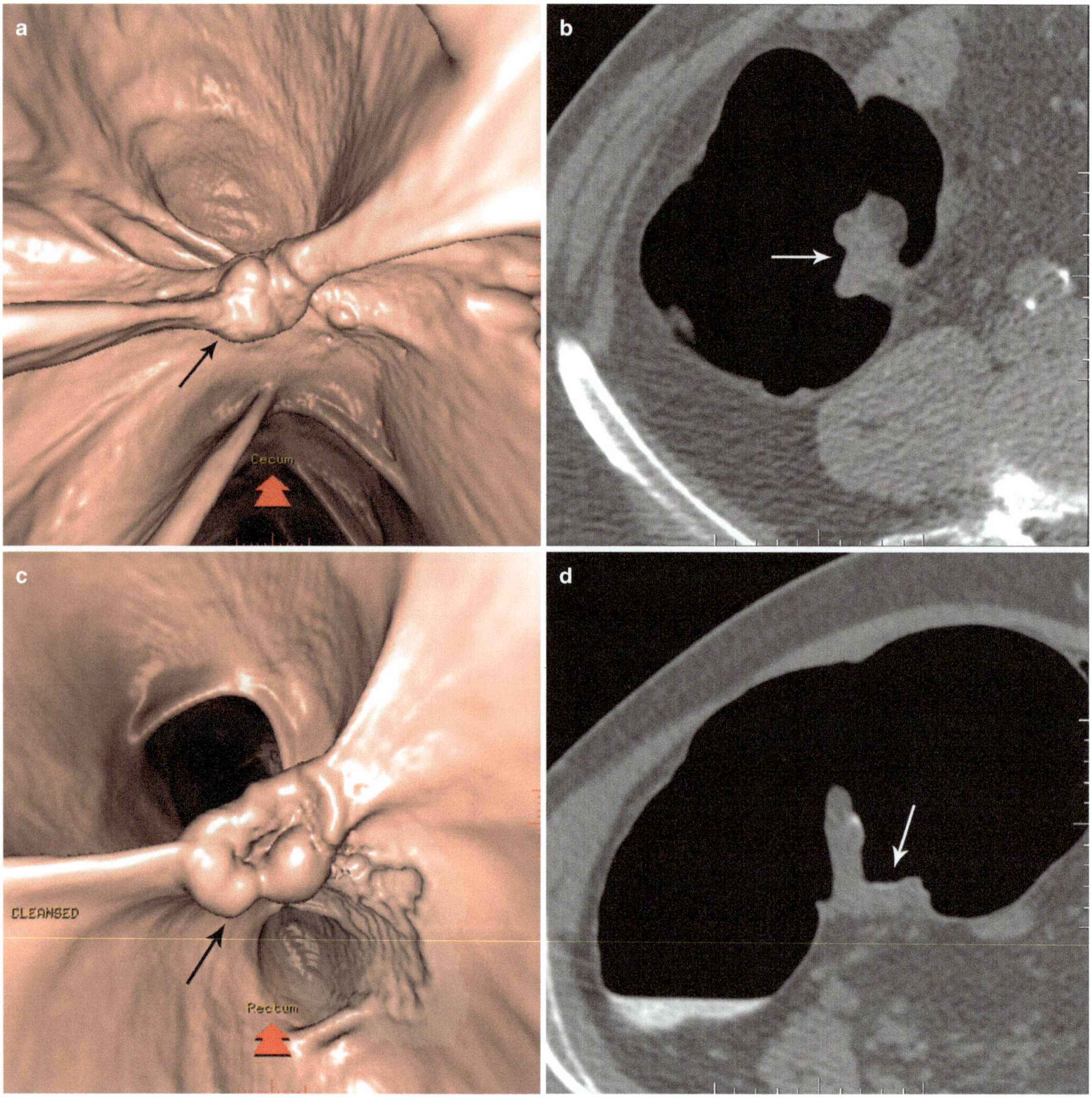

Fig. 5 Adenocarcinoma of the ileocecal valve (*arrow*). (**a**, **b**) Endoluminal view (**a**) of a distorted ileocecal valve where the two lips are not recognizable; axial view (**b**) demonstrating a soft tissue infiltration (tumor) of a lipomatous ileocecal valve with an abnormal flat, straight contour. (**c**, **d**) Endoluminal view (**c**) of an irregular and asymmetrical ileocecal valve; axial view (**d**) demonstrating a soft tissue infiltration (tumor) of the ileocecal valve with thickening and straightening of the adjacent colonic wall (Courtesy of Dr. Petrover)

colonic lymphomas [17] (representing less than 1 % of all primary tumors of the colon [4, 18]) and involves usually the ileocecal valve, cecum, and rectum [19]. Lymphoma has a submucosal origin and may present with a variety of forms. Commonly, it appears as bulky polypoid masses that are smooth-surfaced, broad-based, sessile lesions with or without central ulcerations or depressions [20]. These lesions vary from 4 to 20 cm and are most frequently located near the ileocecal valve [19]: extension into the terminal ileum is not uncommon. Other presentations include an annular infiltrating form, a large infiltrating mass that may extend into the

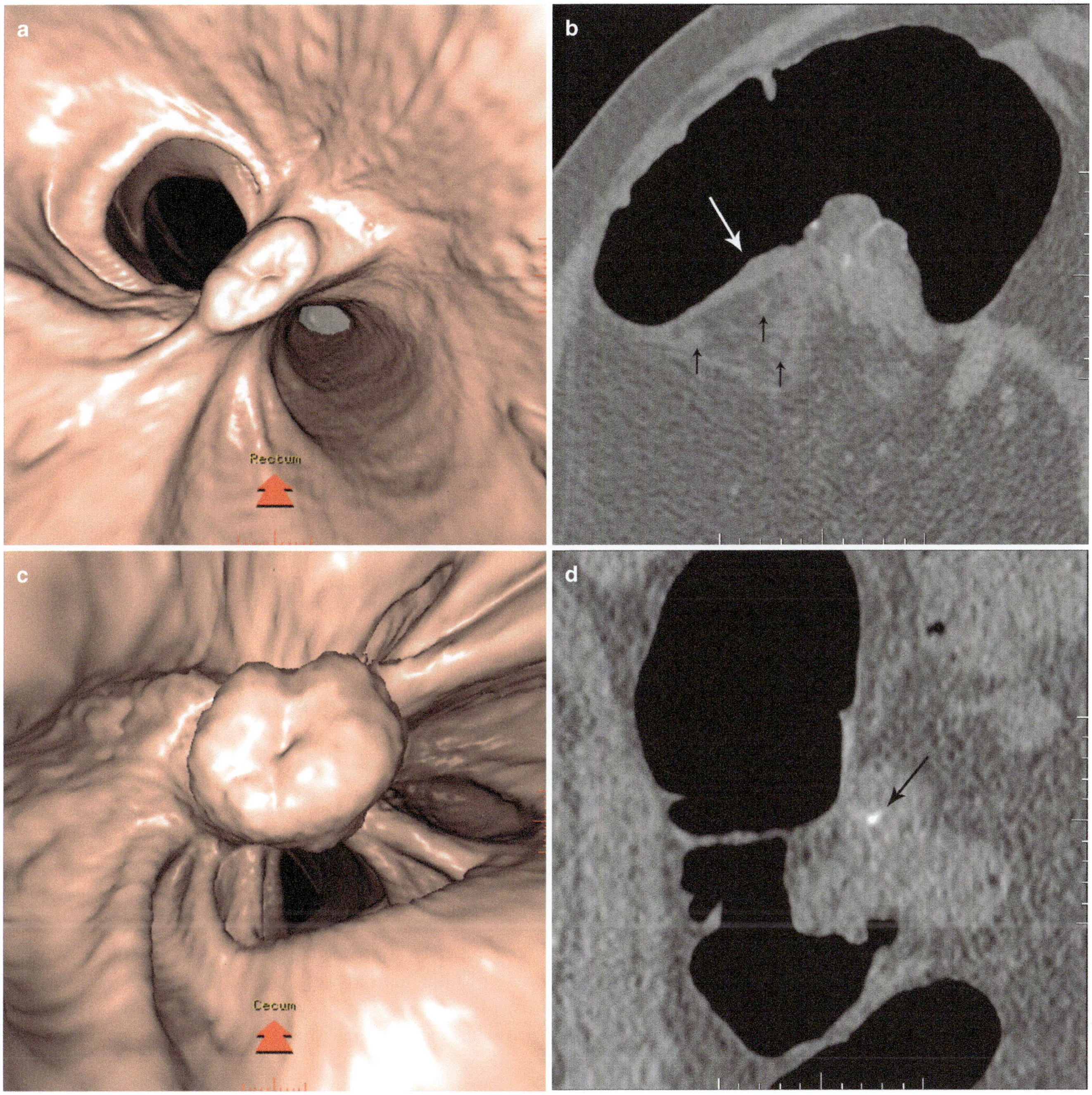

Fig. 6 Carcinoid tumor. (**a**, **b**) Endoluminal view (**a**) of a seemingly normal and symmetrical ileocecal valve; axial view (**b**) demonstrating a soft tissue infiltration of a lipomatous ileocecal valve and the adjacent colonic wall that is thickened (*long arrow*) with stranding of the neighboring peritoneal fat and small lymph nodes (*small arrows*). (**c**, **d**) Endoluminal view (**c**) of a bulging but symmetrical and seemingly normal ileocecal valve; coronal view (**d**) demonstrating a soft tissue infiltration with tiny calcification (*arrow*) of the terminal ileum reaching the ileocecal valve

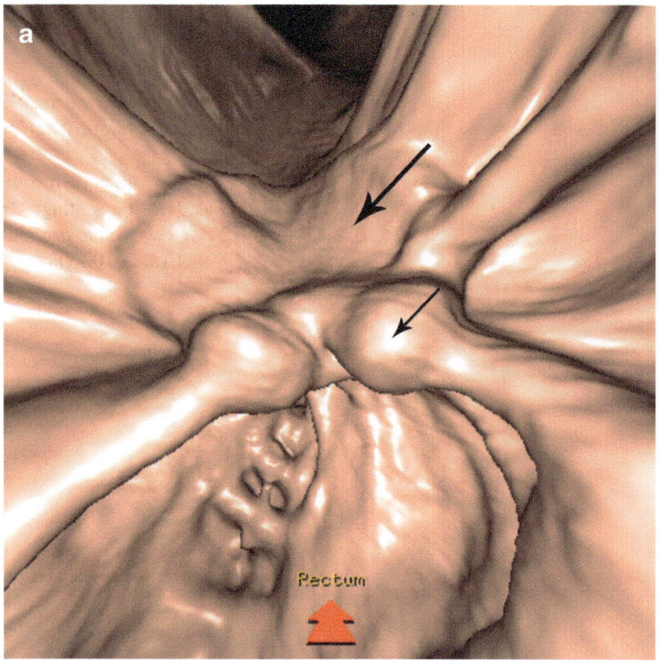

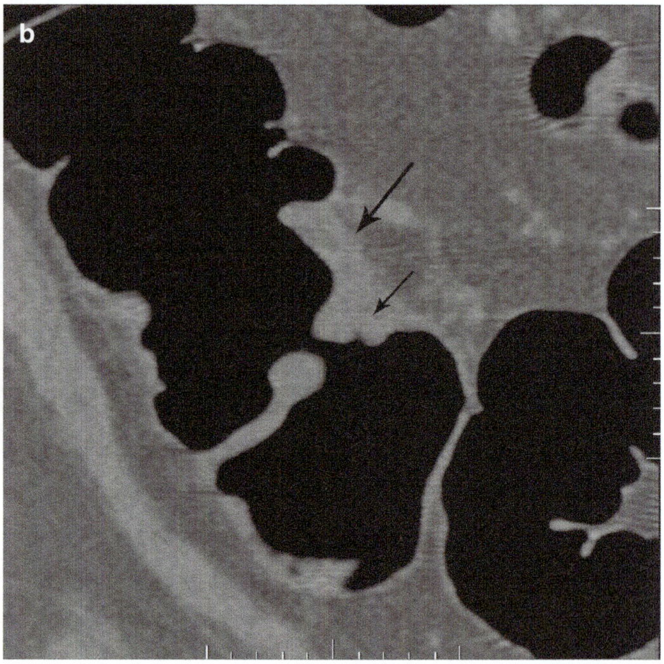

Fig. 7 Infiltration of the ileocecal valve by an adjacent tumor. (**a**) Endoluminal view of an asymmetrical ileocecal valve, with not recognizable lips (*short arrow*), and of a flat lesion (*long arrow*) of the adjacent colonic wall. (**b**) Axial view showing a thickening of the colonic wall (*long arrow*) with small lymph nodes in the adjacent fat and soft tissue infiltration of the ileocecal valve (*short arrow*)

mesentery or exhibit central cavitation [20] or a diffuse multinodular form (lymphomatous polyposis) usually associated with disseminated disease from a nodal primary lymphoma where a conglomerate cecal mass is seen in almost 50 % of cases [21].

Adjacent Adenocarcinoma

The ileocecal valve may be infiltrated by an adjacent tumor, resulting in an asymmetry and thickening of the involved lip (Fig. 7) which then presents with soft tissue densities.

Metastasis

Peritoneal metastatic dissemination may exceptionally involve the ileocecal valve by serosal seeding.

Inflammatory Diseases

Crohn's Disease

In case of Crohn's disease involvement of the terminal ileum, the ileocecal valve may appear enlarged, either by submucosal edema in acute disease or by fibrofatty proliferation in case of chronic disease [22]. The adjacent mesenteric fat may show "smudgy" or "streaky" appearance in case of phlegmon as well as small lymph nodes (these are usually larger in case of lymphoma or carcinoma). The ICV valve may also be narrowed by fibrosis at the scared over stage of the disease.

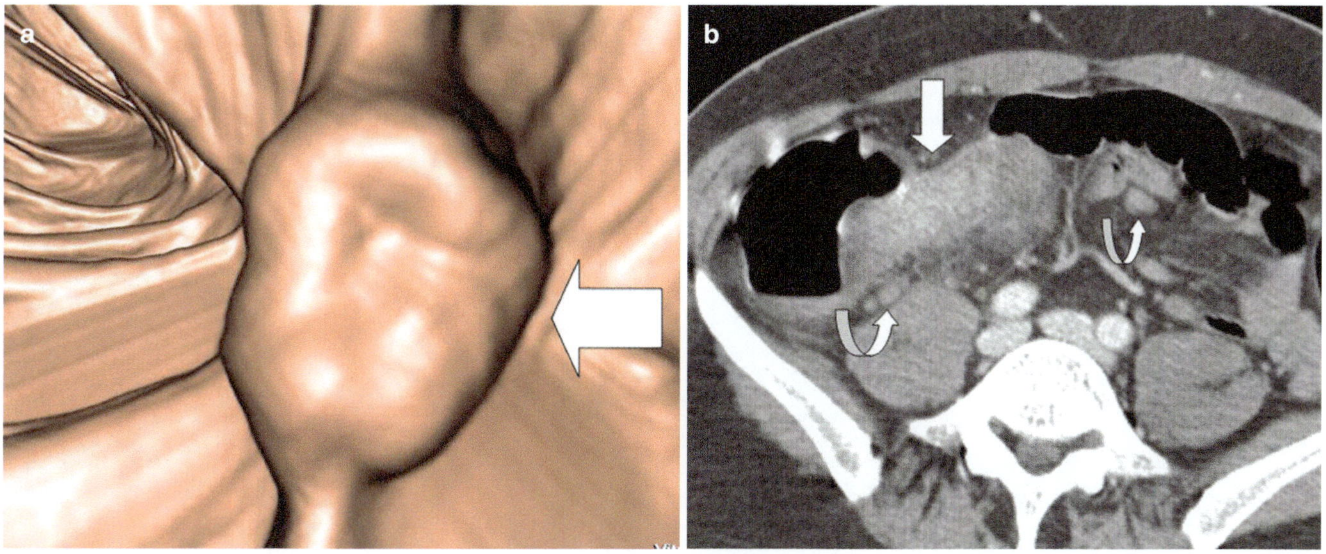

Fig. 8 Shigella. (**a**) Endoluminal view of a bulging and symmetrical ileocecal valve (normal appearance). (**b**) Axial view showing an infiltration of the terminal ileum and the ileocecal valve (*large arrow*) with many small lymph nodes (*curved arrows*) (Courtesy of Dr. F. Iafrate)

Cathartics Abuse

The ileocecal valve will be gapped and flatten in the cathartic colon due to prolonged use of stimulant/irritant cathartics. In this case, the right colon is similar to burned-out chronic ulcerative colitis with absent or diminished haustral marking, but no rigidity: the right colon remains remarkably distensible [23].

Infectious Diseases

The ileocecal valve always appears enlarged by submucosal infiltration in acute enteritis, although it is highly improbable that a virtual colonoscopy will ever be asked for a patient presenting with infections such as typhoid fever, amebiasis, anisakiasis, actinomycosis, tuberculosis, yersinia enterocolitis, or shigellosis (Fig. 8).

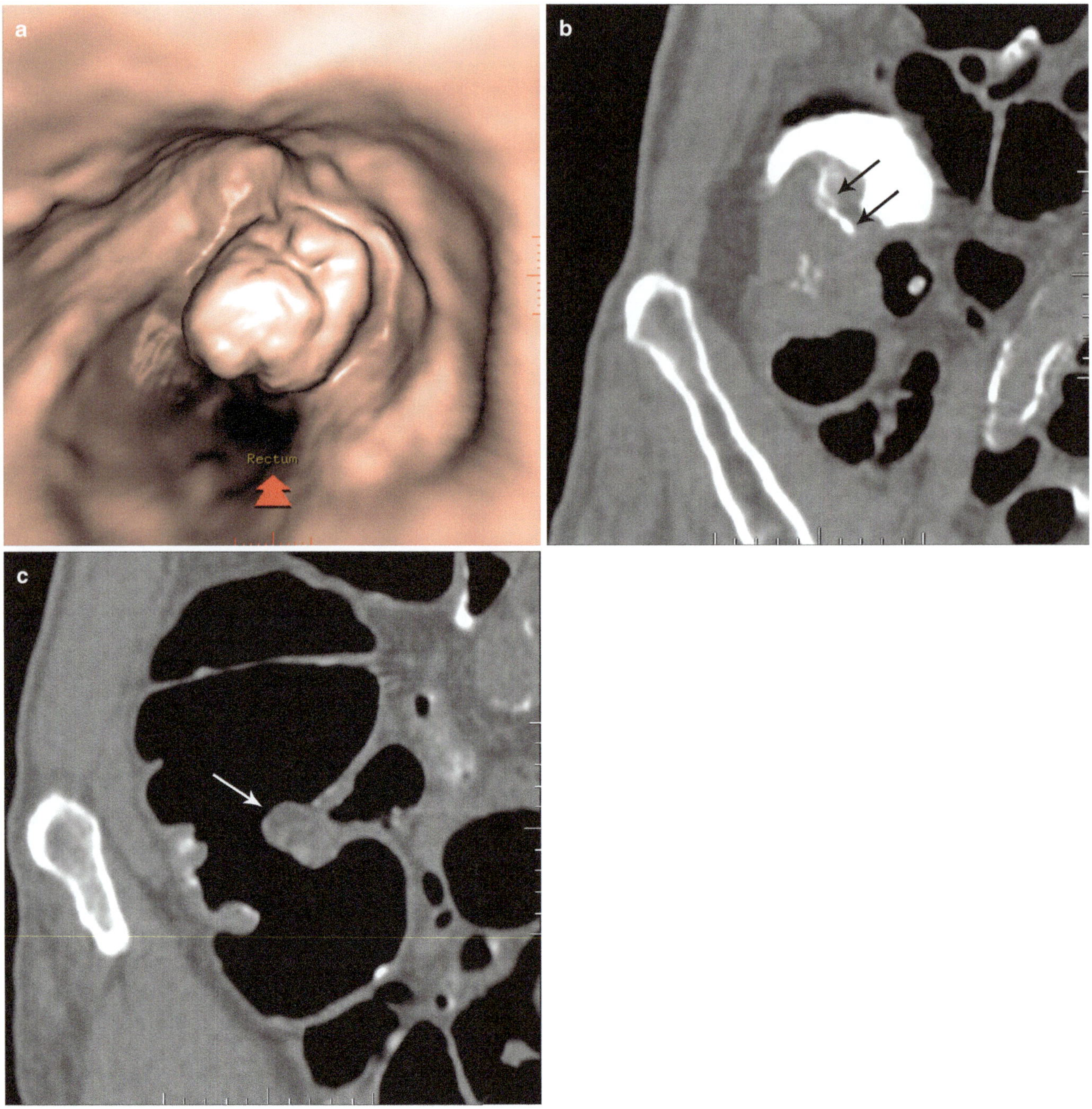

Fig. 9 Intussusception. (**a**) Endoluminal view of a bulging ileocecal valve, supine position. (**b**) Coronal view in supine position: there is an intussusception of the ileocecal valve into the proximal right colon, the lumen of the terminal ileum is opacified by Gastrografin (*arrow*). (**c**) Oblique view in prone acquisition: the intussusception has disappeared, and the lipomatous ileocecal valve appears normal (*arrow*)

Miscellaneous

Intussusception

Intussusception is defined as the invagination of one segment of bowel (intussusceptiens) into the adjacent one (intussusceptum). In children, intussusception is idiopathic, acute, and usually begins in the terminal ileum. In adults, colonic intussusception is most frequently related to colon cancer and often chronic and relapsing [24] (Fig. 9).

References

1. Silva AC, Beaty SD, Hara AK et al (2007) Spectrum of normal and abnormal CT appearances of the ileocecal valve and cecum with endoscopic and surgical correlation. Radiographics 27: 1039–1054
2. Lockart RD, Hamilton GF, Fyfe FW (1959) Large intestine. In: Lockart RD, Hamilton GF, Fyfe FW (eds) Anatomy of the human body. Faber and Faber, London
3. Morson BC, Dawson IMP (1979) Gastrointestinal pathology. Blackwell, Oxford
4. Testut L, Latarjet A (1949) Caecum et appendice. In: Testut L, Latarjet A (eds) Traité d'anatomie humaine, Appareil de la digestion. Doin & Cie, Paris
5. El-Amin LC, Levine MS, Rubesin SE et al (2003) Ileocecal valve: spectrum of normal findings at double-contrast barium enema examination. Radiology 227:52–58
6. Skucas J (2008) Pharmacology. In: Gore RM, Levine MS (eds) Textbook of gastrointestinal radiology, 3rd edn. Saunders WB, Philadelphia
7. Haller JD, Roberts TW (1964) Lipomas of the colon: a clinicopathologic study of 40 cases. Surgery 55:773–781
8. Castro DB, Stearns MW (1972) Lipomas of the large intestine. Dis Colon Rectum 15:441–444
9. Berk RN, Werner LG (1974) The radiology corner: lipoma of the colon. Am J Gastroenterol 61:145–150
10. Yitta S, Tatineny KC, Cipriani NA et al (2006) Characterization of normal ileocecal valve density on CT colonography. J Comput Assist Tomogr 30:58–61
11. Godwin DJ (1975) Carcinoid tumors: an analysis of 2837 cases. Cancer 36:560–569
12. Balthazar EJ (1978) Carcinoid tumors of the alimentary tract. Gastrointest Radiol 3:47–56
13. Fioca R, Capella C, Bufta R et al (1980) Glucagon-like, glicentin-like and pancreatic polypeptide-like immunoreactivities in rectal carcinoids and related colorectal cells. Am J Pathol 100:81–92
14. Berardi SS (1972) Carcinoid tumors of the colon (exclusive of the rectum): review of the literature. Dis Colon Rectum 15:383–391
15. Shulman H, Giustra P (1971) Invasive carcinoids of the colon. Radiology 98:139–143
16. Herrman R, Panahon AM, Barcos MP et al (1980) Gastrointestinal involvement in non-Hodgkin's lymphoma. Cancer 46:215–229
17. Weinsrad D, DeCosse JJ, Sherlock P et al (1982) Primary gastrointestinal lymphoma. Cancer 49:1258–1265
18. Dragosics B, Bauer P, Radaskiewicz T (1985) Primary gastrointestinal non-Hodgkin's lymphoma: a retrospective clinicopathologic study of 150 cases. Cancer 55:1060–1073
19. O'Connell DJ, Thompson AJ (1978) Lymphoma of the colon: the spectrum of radiologic changes. Gastrointest Radiol 2:377–385
20. Wyatt SH, Fishman EK, Jones B (1993) Primary lymphoma of the colon and the rectum: CT and barium correlation. Abdom Imaging 18:376–380
21. Williams SM, Berk RN, Harned RK (1984) Radiologic features of multinodular lymphoma of the colon. AJR Am J Roentgenol 143: 87–91
22. Simpkins KC (1988) Inflammatory bowel disease: ulcerative and Crohn's colitis. In: Simpkins KC (ed) A textbook of radiological diagnosis, vol 4, The alimentary tract: the hollow organs and salivary glands. Lewis HK, London
23. Kim SK, Gerle RD, Rozanski R (1978) Cathartic colitis. AJR Am J Roentgenol 138:825–831
24. Orlando R (1990) Intussusception in adults. In: Welch JP (ed) Bowel obstruction. Saunders WB, Philadelphia

Operated Large Bowel

Stefano Profili and Giovanni Battista Meloni

Contents

S. Profili (✉) • G.B. Meloni
Department of Radiology,
A.S.L Sassari, Sassari, Italy
e-mail: stefanoprofili@gmail.com

Abstract

Surgery of the large bowel includes many different intervention performed in the treatment of a wide spectrum of pathologies. Follow up imaging is needed particularly in patients with neoplastic and flogistic diseases. Contrast CT colonography is an emerging test which allows to obtain during a single examination an accurate assessment of large bowel wall, anastomotic and perianastomotic area, abdominal organs, nodes, and peritoneal cavity. In this chapter the most frequent normal and pathologic Contrast CT colonography pattern are showed.

Introduction

Surgery of the large bowel may be resective or conservative and with or without anastomosis as listed in Table 1.

Indications for colon resection include colon cancer, inflammatory bowel disease, diverticular disease, and gastrointestinal bleeding.

Extent of resection is either based on standard criteria (site, vascular feeding, nodes, etc.) in cases of malignancy suitable for a curative procedure or tailored on the patient in cases of inflammatory disease (longitudinal and axial extension, complications). After surgical removal of the diseased colon, an intestinal anastomosis should be performed: different surgical modalities are showed in Table 2. In describing anastomosis type (e.g. ileo-colonic end-to-side), the first term refers to the proximal segment.

Anastomosis may be done handsewn or more frequently using stapling devices (stapler). In the latter case, a linear (stump closure) or circular (anastomosis) staple line may be demonstrated at CT colonography (computed tomography colonography) examination. Sometimes combined technique using either handsewn suture or staples is employed (mechanical anastomosis and handsewn stump closure or vice versa)

Some demolitive operations include a cutaneous colostomy:

Abdominoperineal resection (Miles operation) is performed when a low rectal anastomosis is not feasible because of dis-

E. Neri et al. (eds.), *CT Colonography Atlas*, Medical Radiology,
DOI 10.1007/978-3-642-11149-5_13,

Table 1 Surgical procedures

Demolitive surgical procedures	Conservative surgical procedures
With anastomosis:	
Ileo-colonic resection	Faecal diversion
Ascending colectomy	Colostomies
Right hemicolectomy	Colon bypass
Transverse colectomy	Polypectomy
Descending colectomy	
Left hemicolectomy	
Sigmoid colectomy	
Low anterior resection	
Subtotal colectomy	
Proctocolectomy	
Colon resection	
Without anastomosis:	
Abdominoperineal resection (Miles operation)	
Hartmann procedure	
Appendectomy	

Table 2 Anastomosis

End-to-end	*End-to-side*
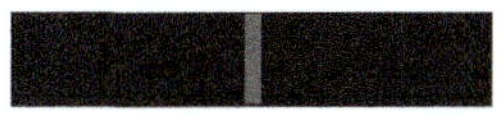	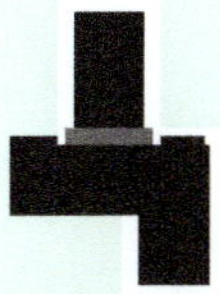
Side-to-end	*Side-to-side*
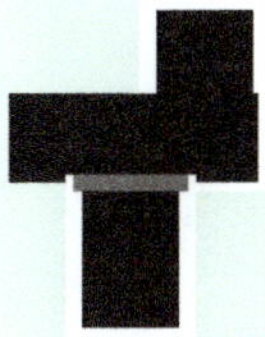	

ease extension and/or location; Hartmann procedure is a two-stage resection: a temporary colostomy is undertaken to allow healing, and an intestinal anastomosis is performed later.

A colostomy or diverting loop ileostomy should be considered if there is any suspicion regarding the technical perfection of the anastomosis and after some difficult resections (e.g. ultra-low anterior resection) to reduce the risk for anastomotic complications.

In the evaluation of flogistic or malignant pathologies, many different complementary tests are routinely employed in the follow-up period to obtain all informations required (laboratory exams, chest x-ray, CT, US, fibre-optic colonoscopy, etc.). CT colonography performed with i.v. contrast media allows to obtain during a single examination an accurate assessment of large bowel wall, anastomotic and perianastomotic area, abdominal organs, nodes, and peritoneal cavity (1.2.3.4.5.6). Total body assessment can also be obtained when needed, extending the examination to the thorax and head.

Case 1. Ileocecal Resection and Ileocolic Side-to-Side Anastomosis

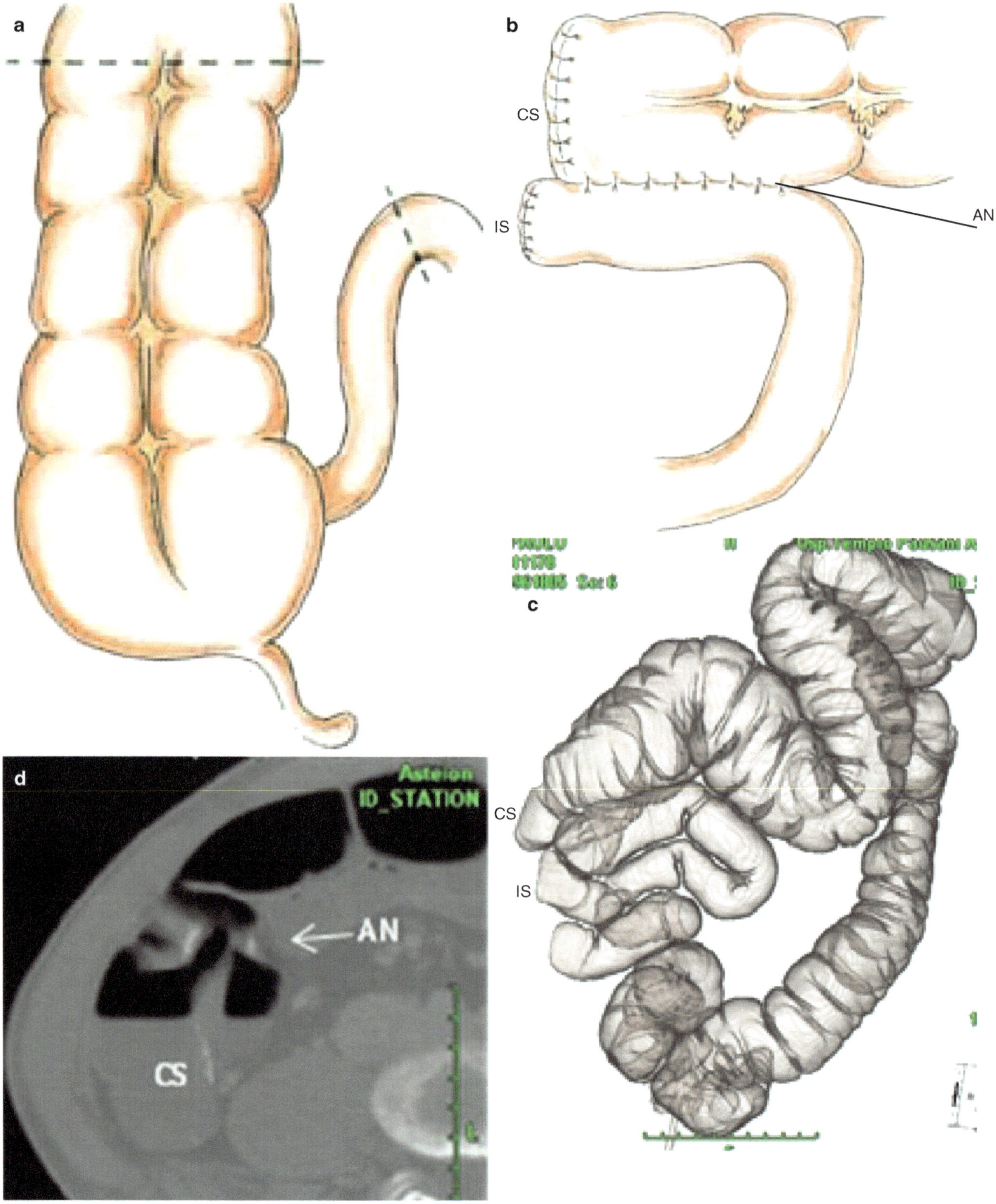

Fig. 1 (**a**) Ileocecal resection: anatomo-surgical pattern, (**b**) ileocolonic side-to-side antiperistaltic anastomosis: anatomo-surgical pattern, (**c**) CT colonography volume-rendering pattern, (**d–f**) CT colonography MPR reformatted images show linear (stump closure) and circular (anastomosis) staple-line sutures, (**g**) CT colonography MIP image oblique view (*cs* colonic stump, *is* ileal stump, *an* anastomosis)

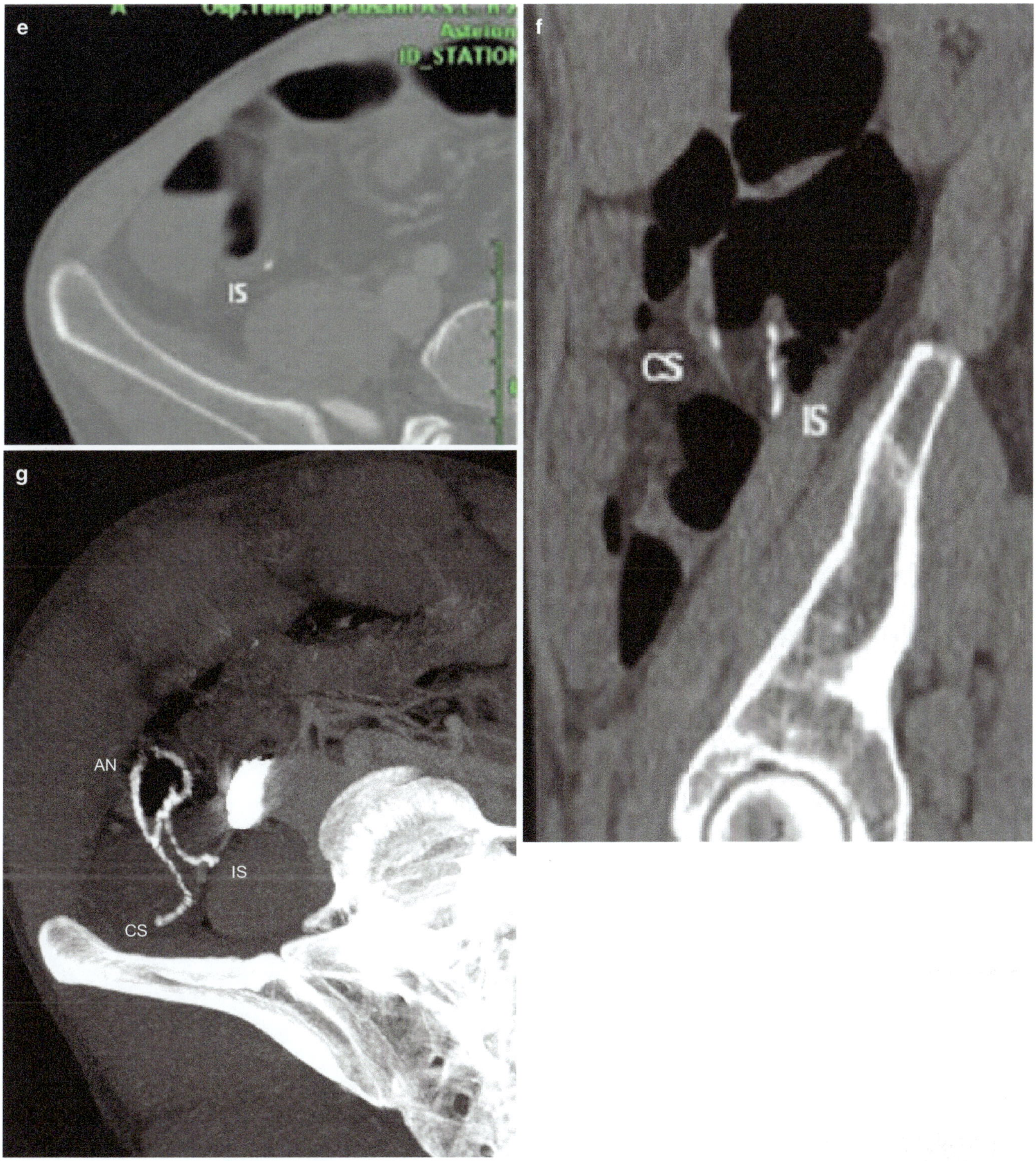

Fig. 1 (continued)

Case 2. Ileocecal Resection and Ileocolic End-to-Side Anastomosis; Crohn Recurrence

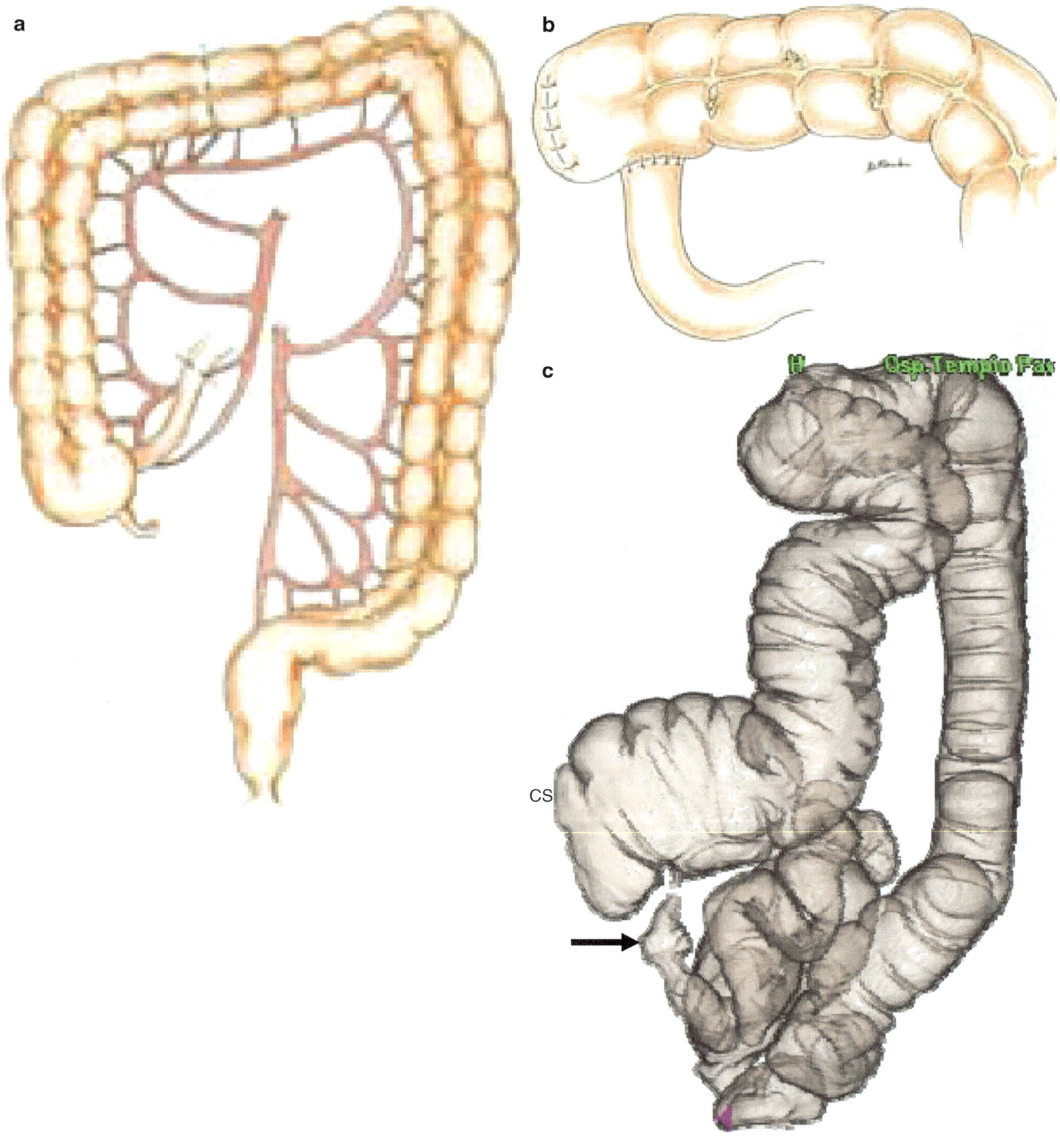

Fig. 2 (**a**, **b**) Ileocecal resection and ileocolic end-to-side anastomosis: anatomo-surgical pattern, (**c**) CT colonography three-dimensional volume-rendering reconstruction shows stricture of the ileal loop (*arrow*) due to Crohn recurrence, (**d**, **e**) CT colonography axial views, (**f**) MPR coronal view

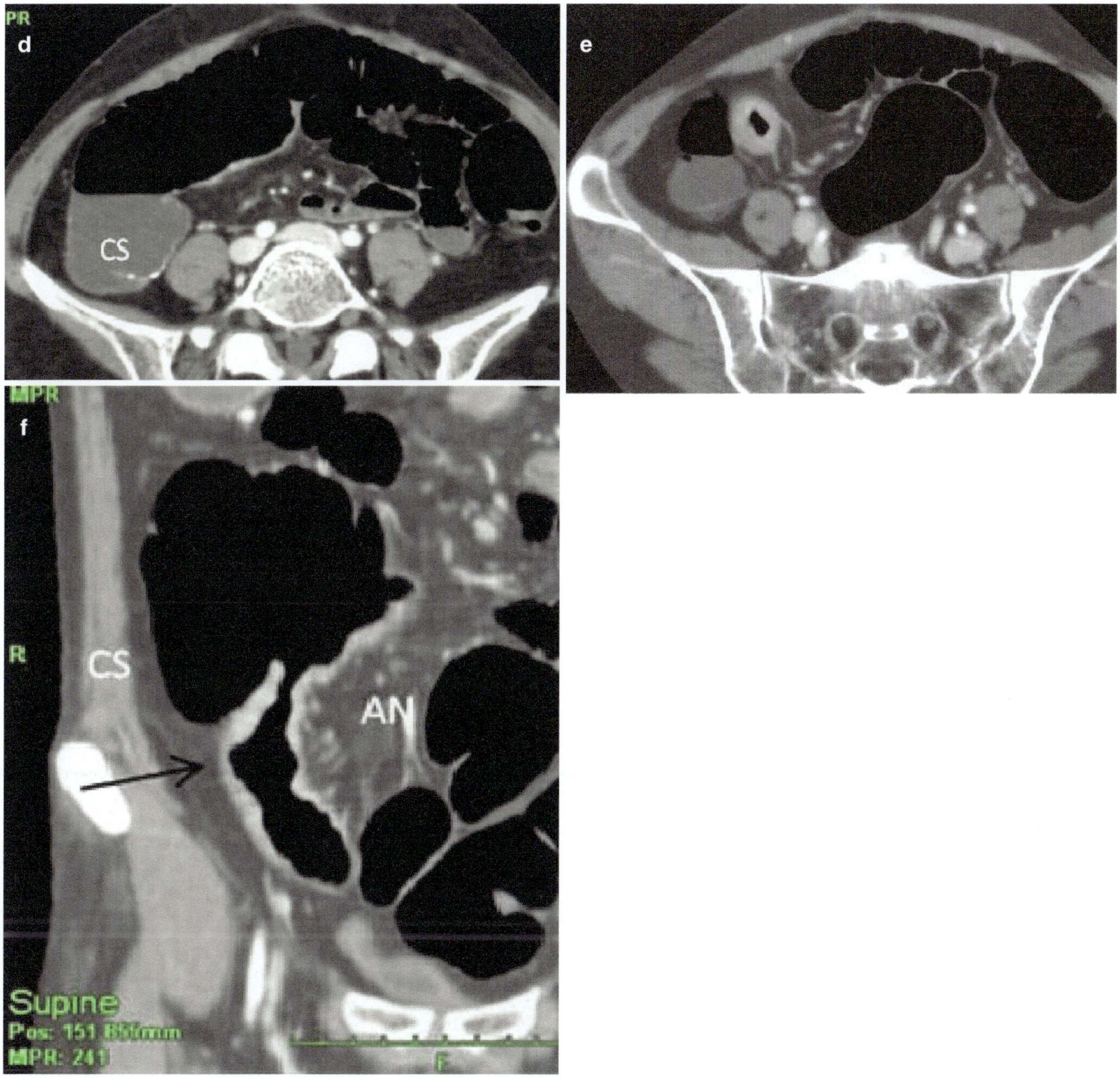

Fig. 2 (continued)

Case 3. Right Hemicolectomy and Ileo-Colonic End-to-Side Anastomosis; Peritoneal Recurrence

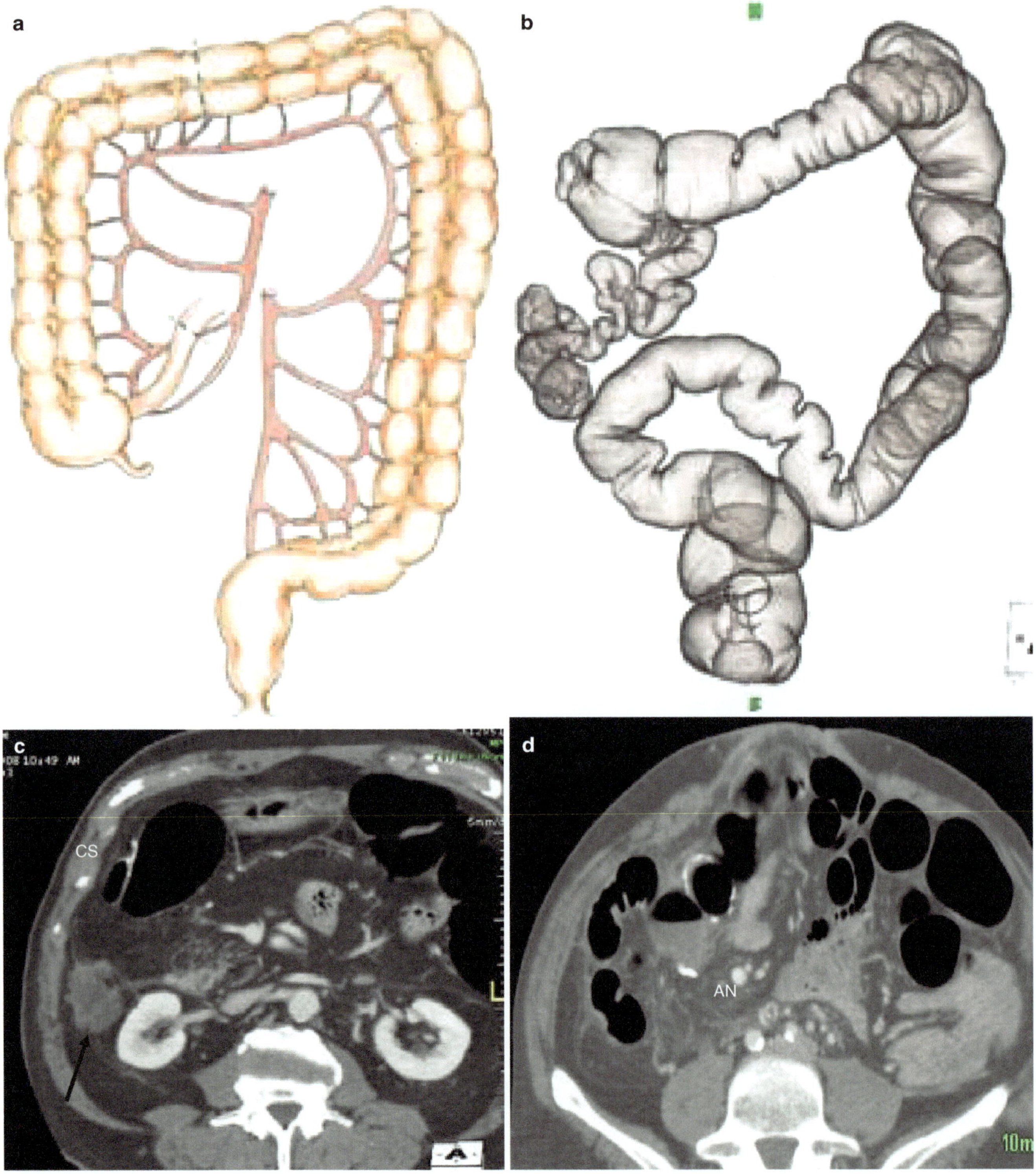

Fig. 3 (**a**) Right hemicolectomy: anatomo-surgical pattern; (**b**) CT colonography volume-rendering view: ileo-colonic end-to-side anastomosis; (**c–e**) CT colonography oblique MPR reconstructed images show peritoneal spread (*black arrow*) and colonic stump (CS); (**c**) anastomosis without complications (**d**, **e**)

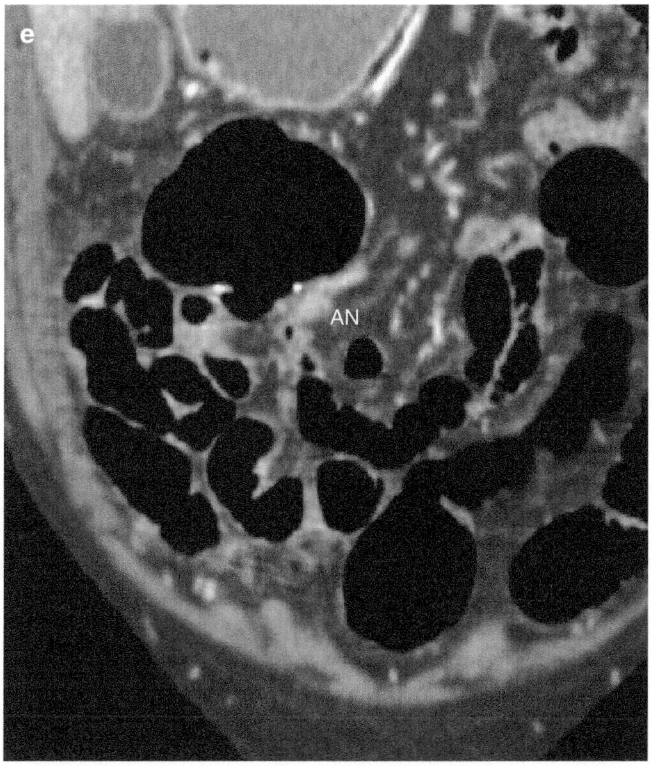

Fig. 3 (continued)

Case 4. Left Hemicolectomy and Colo-Colonic Side-to-Side Anastomosis; Metastatic Nodes

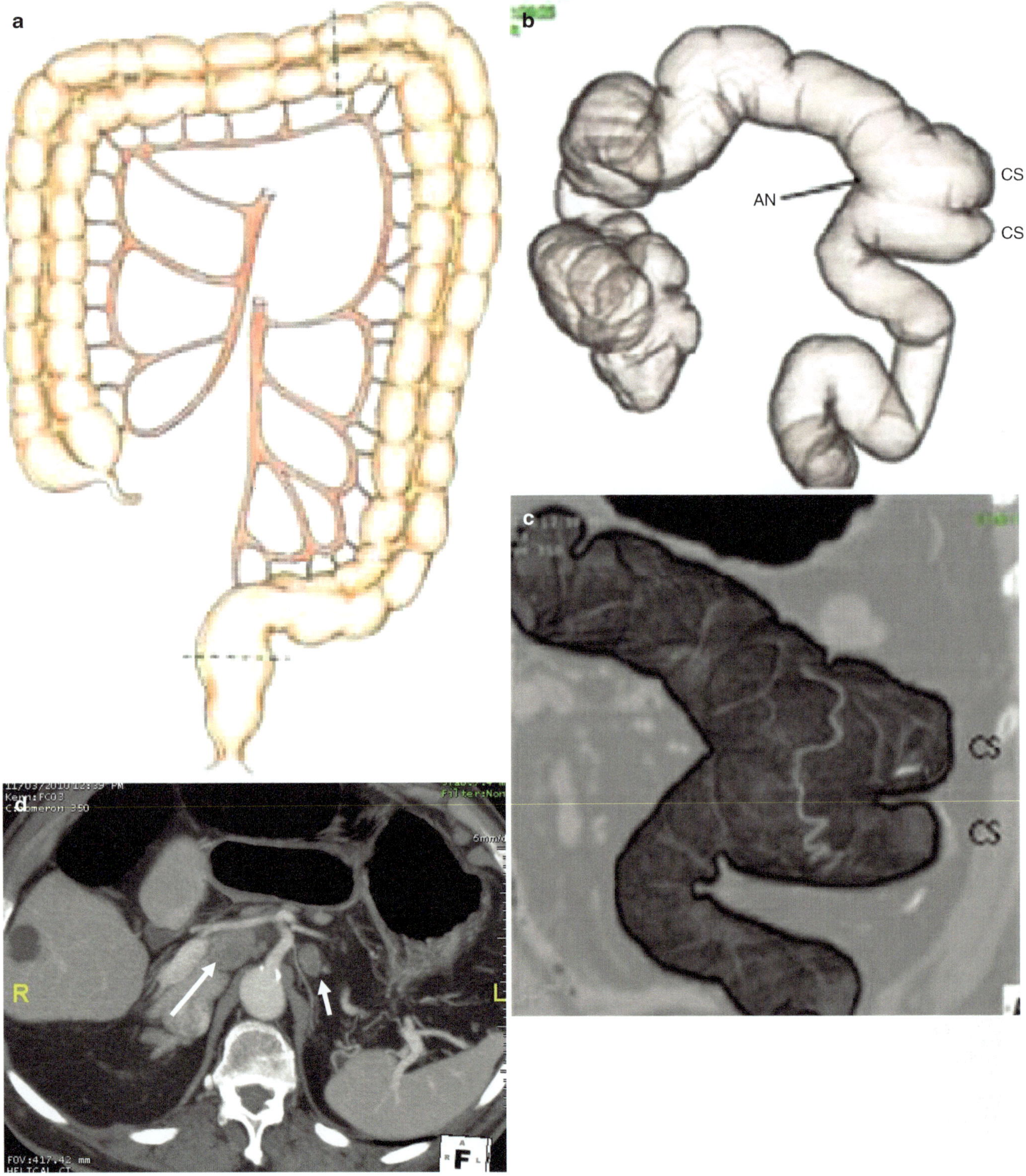

Fig. 4 (**a**) Left hemicolectomy: anatomo-surgical pattern; (**b**, **c**) CT colonography volume-rendering images: colo-colonic side-to-side anastomosis (AN), colonic stump (CS); (**d**) CT colonography axial image: extracolonic recurrence due to metastatic nodes (*arrows*)

Case 5. Anterior Resection of Rectosigmoid: Colorectal End-to-End Anastomosis

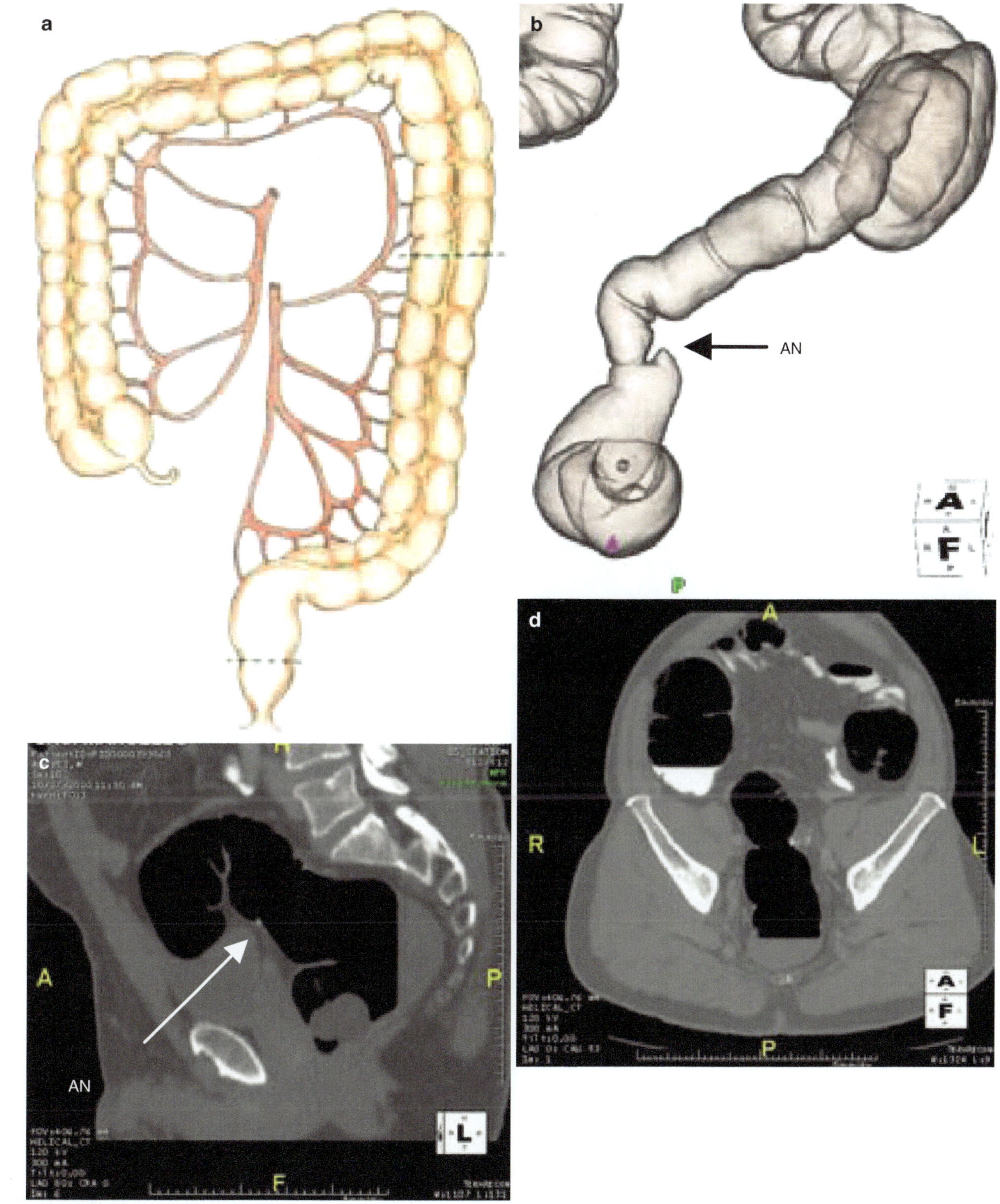

Fig. 5 (**a**) Anterior resection of rectosigmoid: anatomo-surgical pattern; (**b**) CT colonography volume-rendering image: colorectal end-to-end anastomosis (AN); (**c**–**f**) CT colonography MPR, MIP, and virtual endoscopy reconstructed images: normal appearance of anastomotic circular staple line; (**g**) CT colonography axial view: liver metastasis (*arrow*)

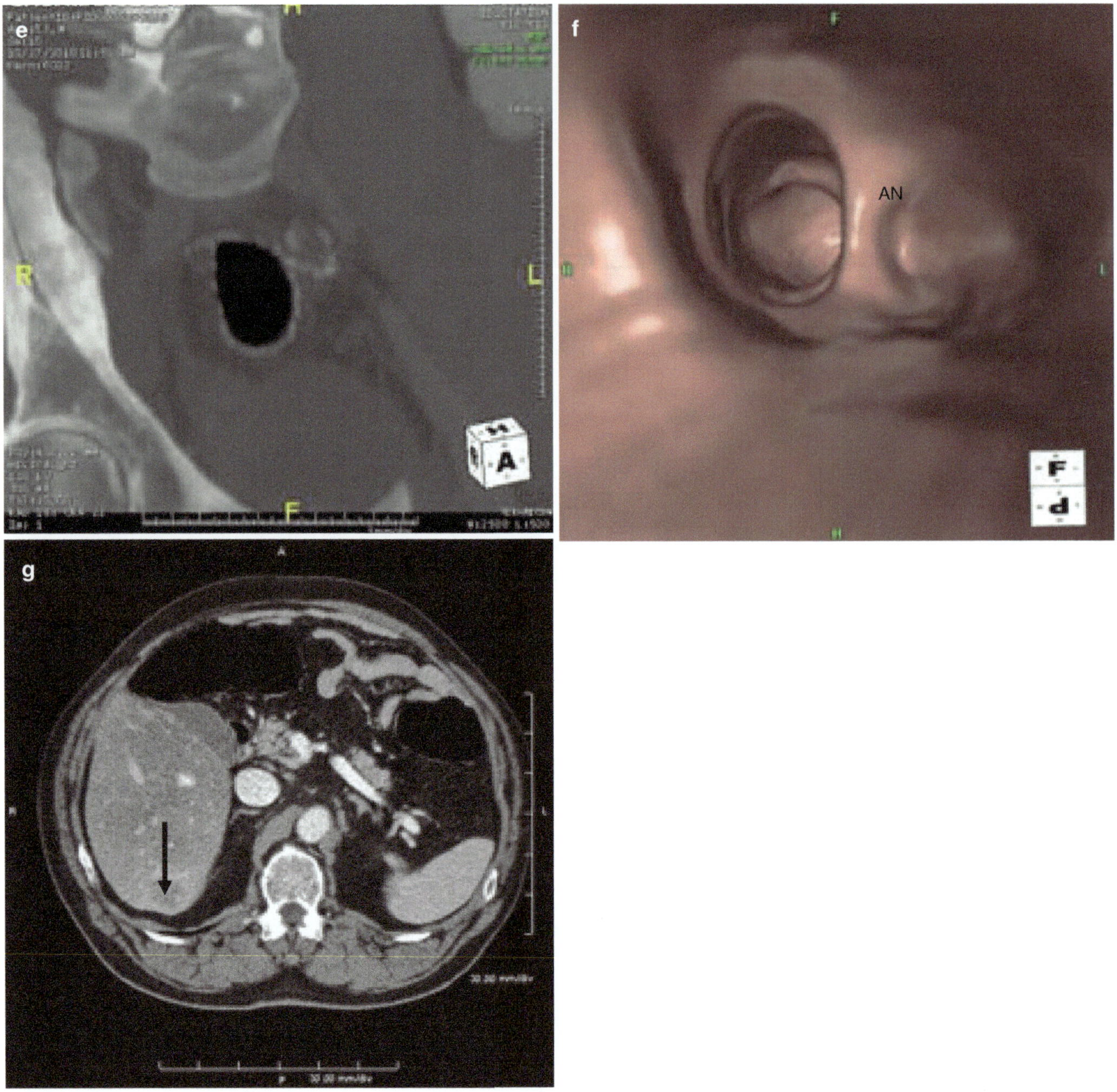

Fig. 5 (continued)

Case 6. Anterior Resection of Rectosigmoid: Colo-Colonic Side-to-End Anastomosis; Inflammatory and Synchronous Adenomatous Polyps

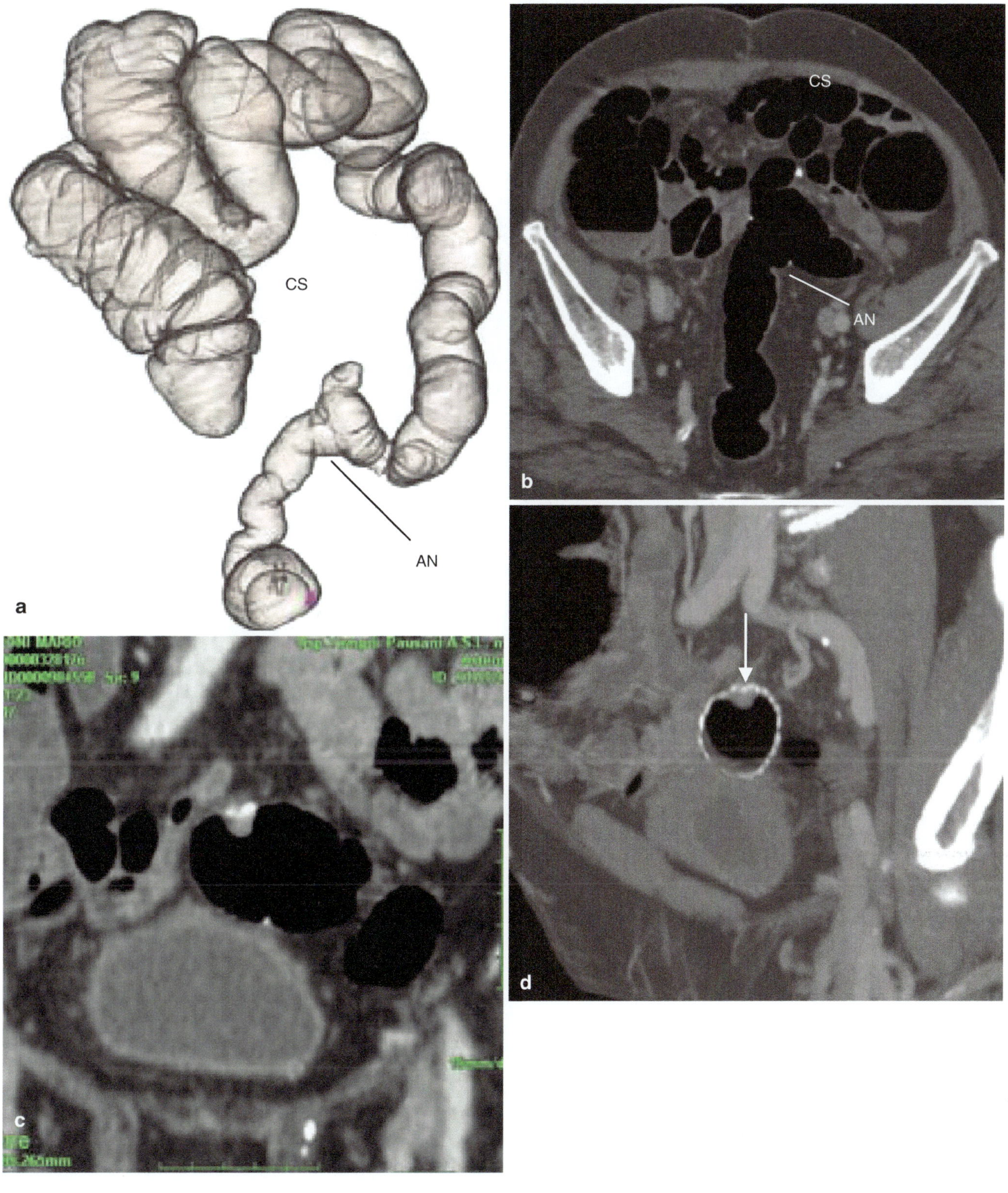

Fig. 6 (**a**) CT colonography volume rendering: anterior resection of rectosigmoid and colo-colonic side-to-end anastomosis (AN), colonic stump (CS); (**b**) MPR oblique pattern; (**c**, **d**) CT colonography MPR and MIP reformatted images show an inflammatory polyp on the side-to-end colorectal anastomosis line (*arrow*); (**e**, **f**) MPR and virtual colonoscopy images: synchronous adenomatous polyp (*arrow*) located in descending colon

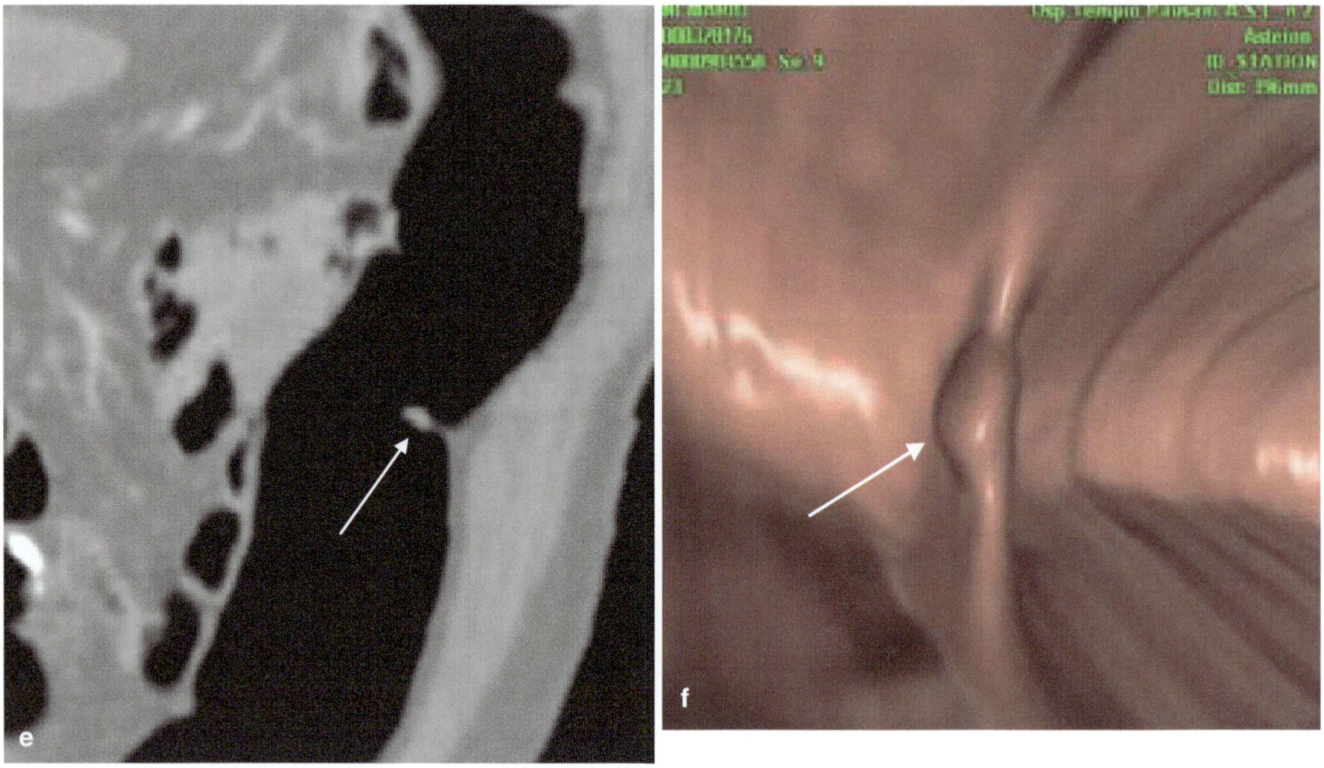

Fig. 6 (continued)

Case 7. Metachronous Colonic Cancer

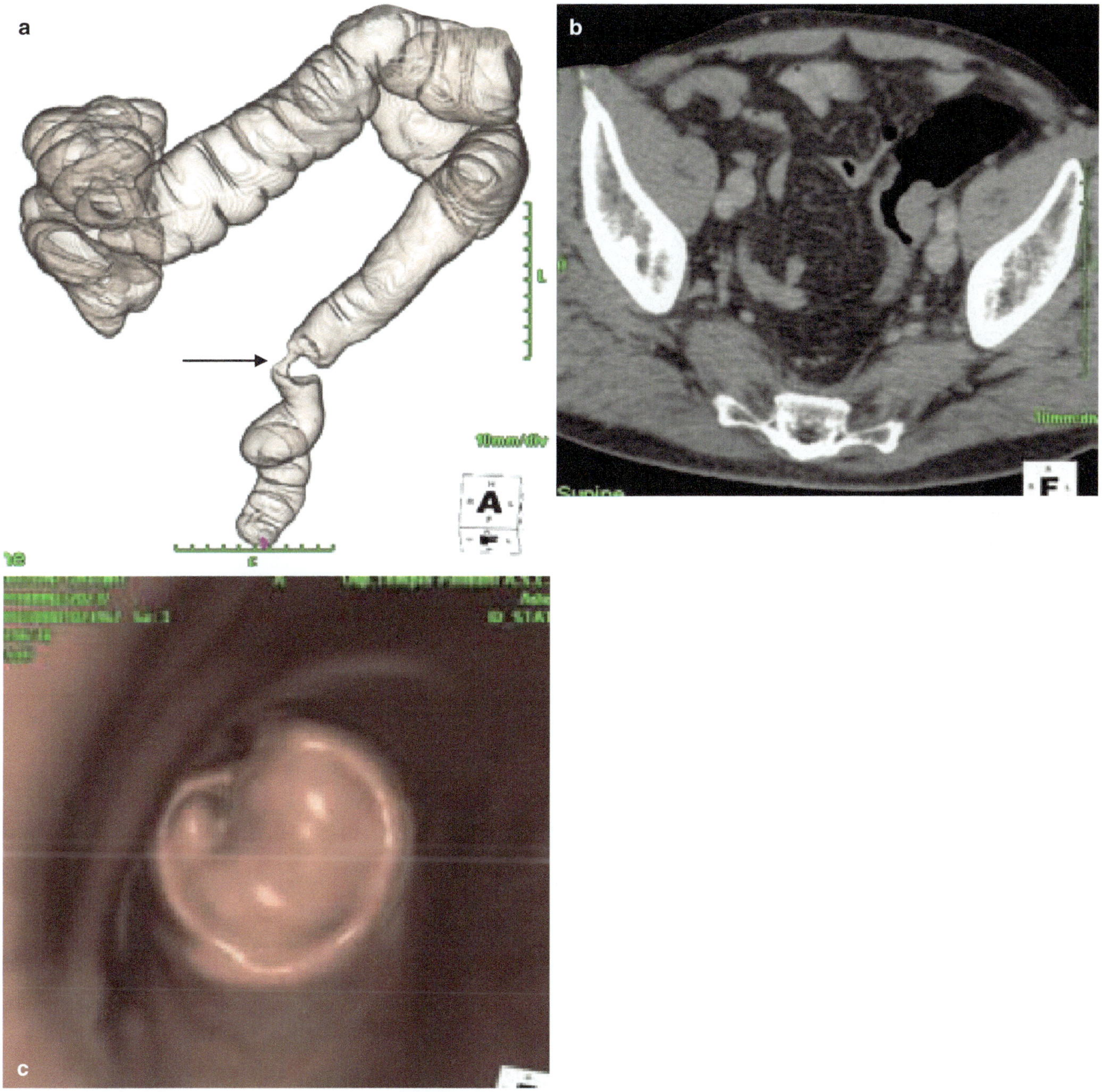

Fig. 7 Anterior resection of rectosigmoid and colorectal ultra-low end-to-end anastomosis: metachronous colonic cancer (*arrow*) in the descending colon; (**a**) CT colonography volume rendering; (**b**) axial view; (**c**) virtual endoscopy

Case 8. Anastomotic Recurrence

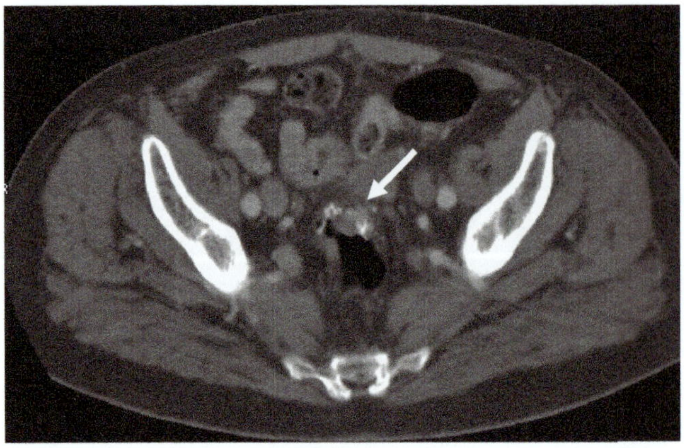

Fig. 8 Anterior resection of rectosigmoid and colorectal end-to-end anastomosis, (**a**) CT colonography axial images show intramural enhancing mass due to anastomotic recurrence (*arrow*)

Case 9. Hartmann Procedure

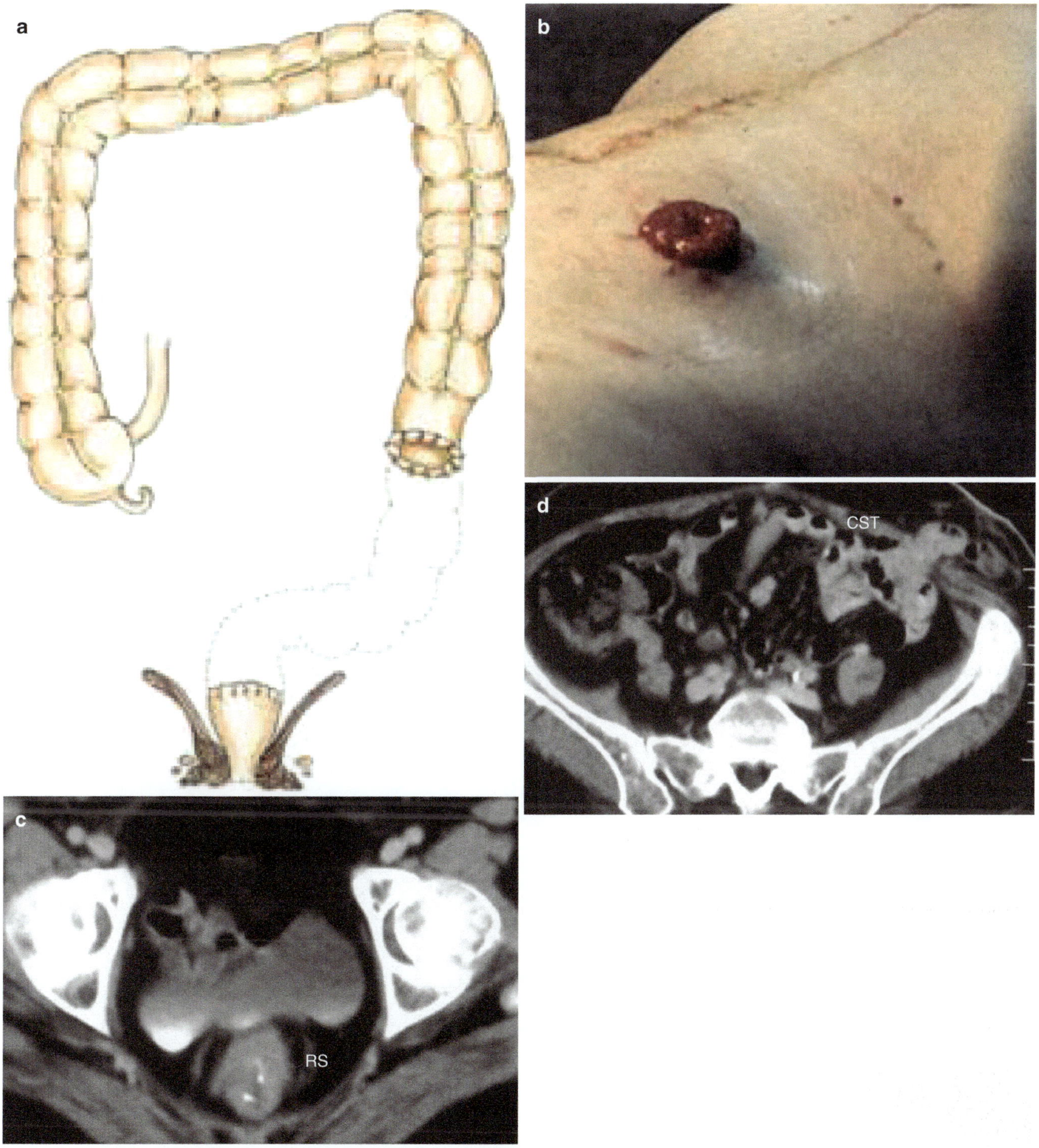

Fig. 9 (**a**) Hartmann procedure: anatomo-surgical pattern. (**b**) Colostomy. (**c**) CT colonography axial images: colostomy can be created by opening the abdominal wall and suturing the distal colon to the skin. (**d**) Rectum is left as a blind pouch (*cst* colononostomy, *rs* rectal stump)

Case 10. Abdominoperineal Resection (Miles); Normal Findings

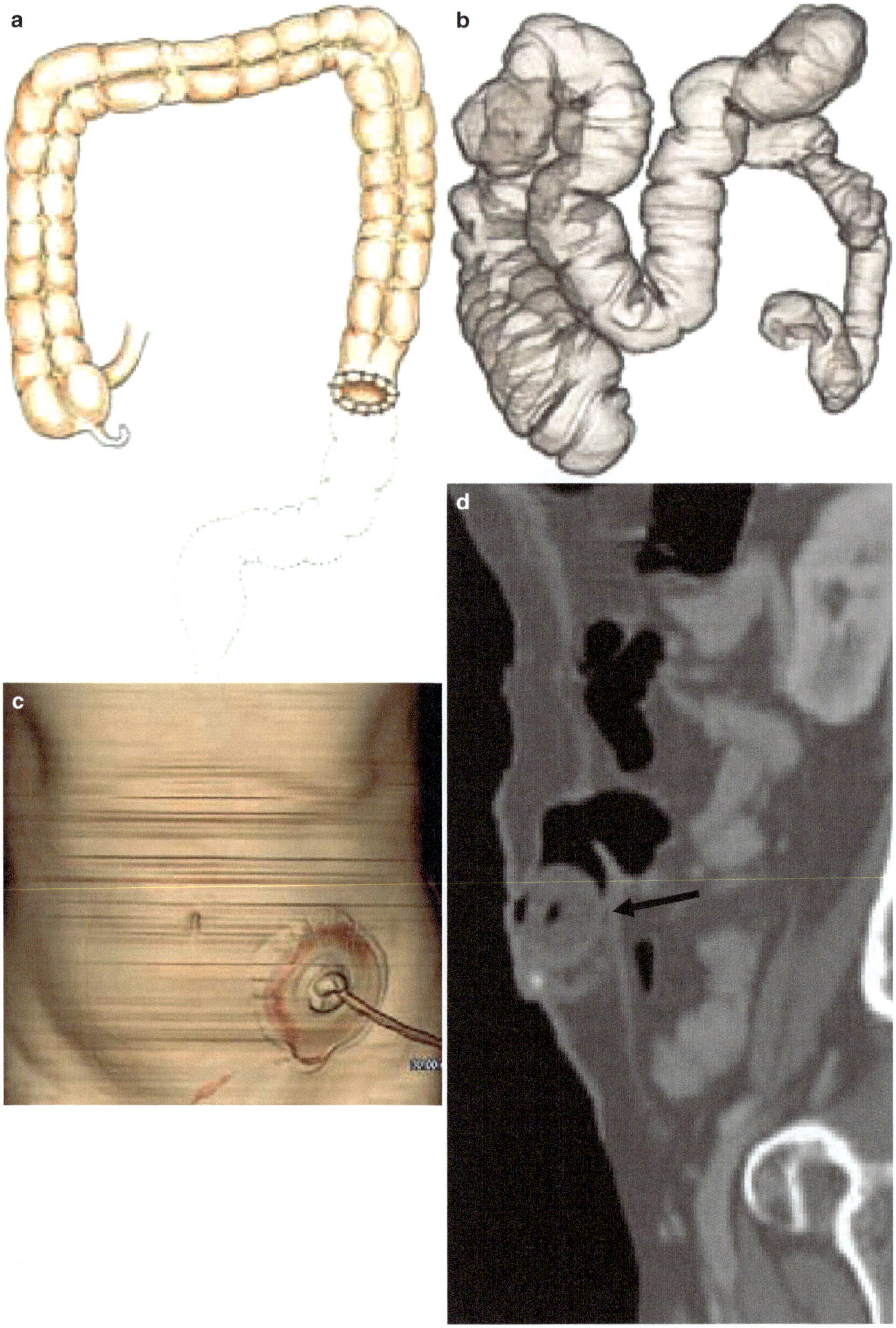

Fig. 10 (**a**) Abdominoperineal resection (Miles procedure): anatomo-surgical pattern. (**b**) CT colonography volume-rendering image. (**c**, **d**) Foley catheter is inserted into colostomy for colon distension. (**e**, **f**) In females CT colonography axial and sagittal images usually show posterior displacement of uterus (*arrow*): differential diagnosis with presacral recurrence is mandatory but sometimes quite difficult (see Fig. 11**c**)

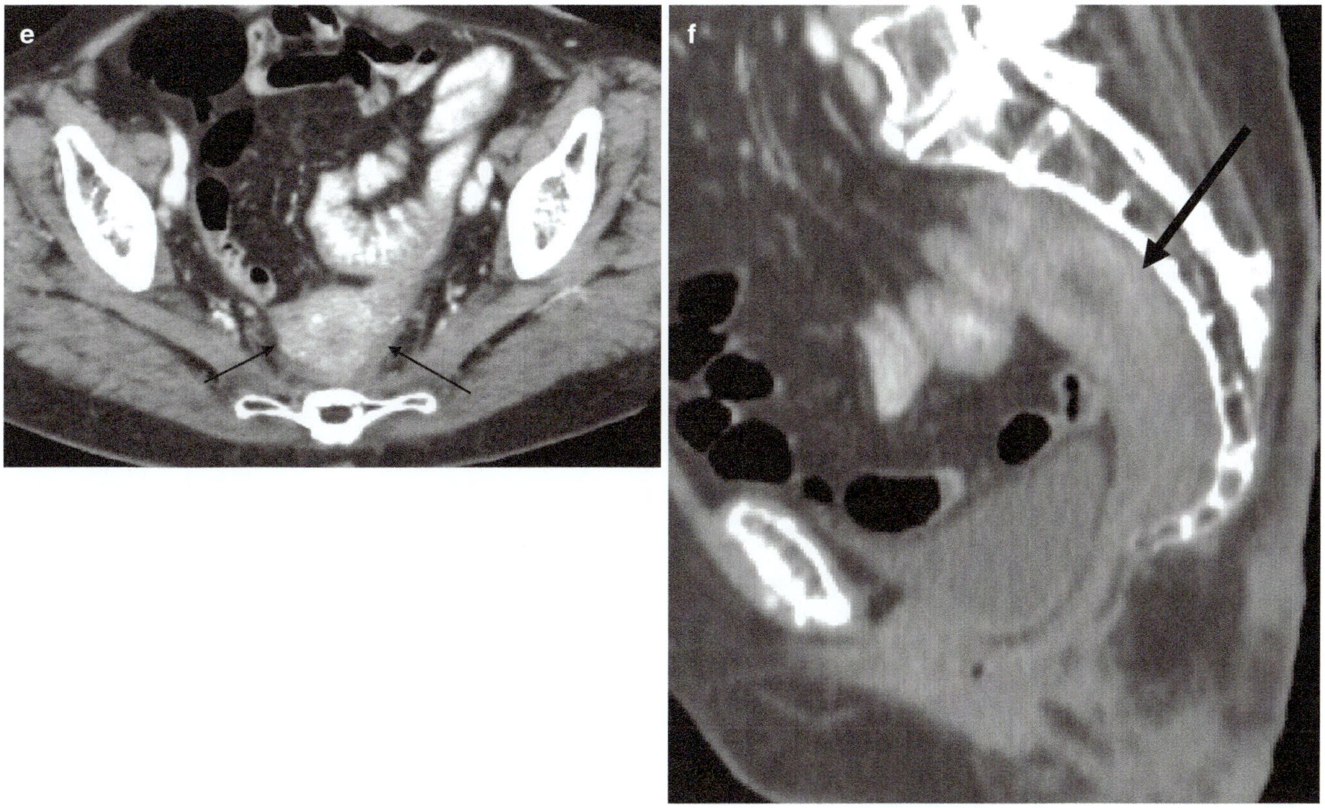

Fig. 10 (continued)

Case 11. Abdominoperineal Resection (Miles); Metachronous Cancer and Presacral Recurrence

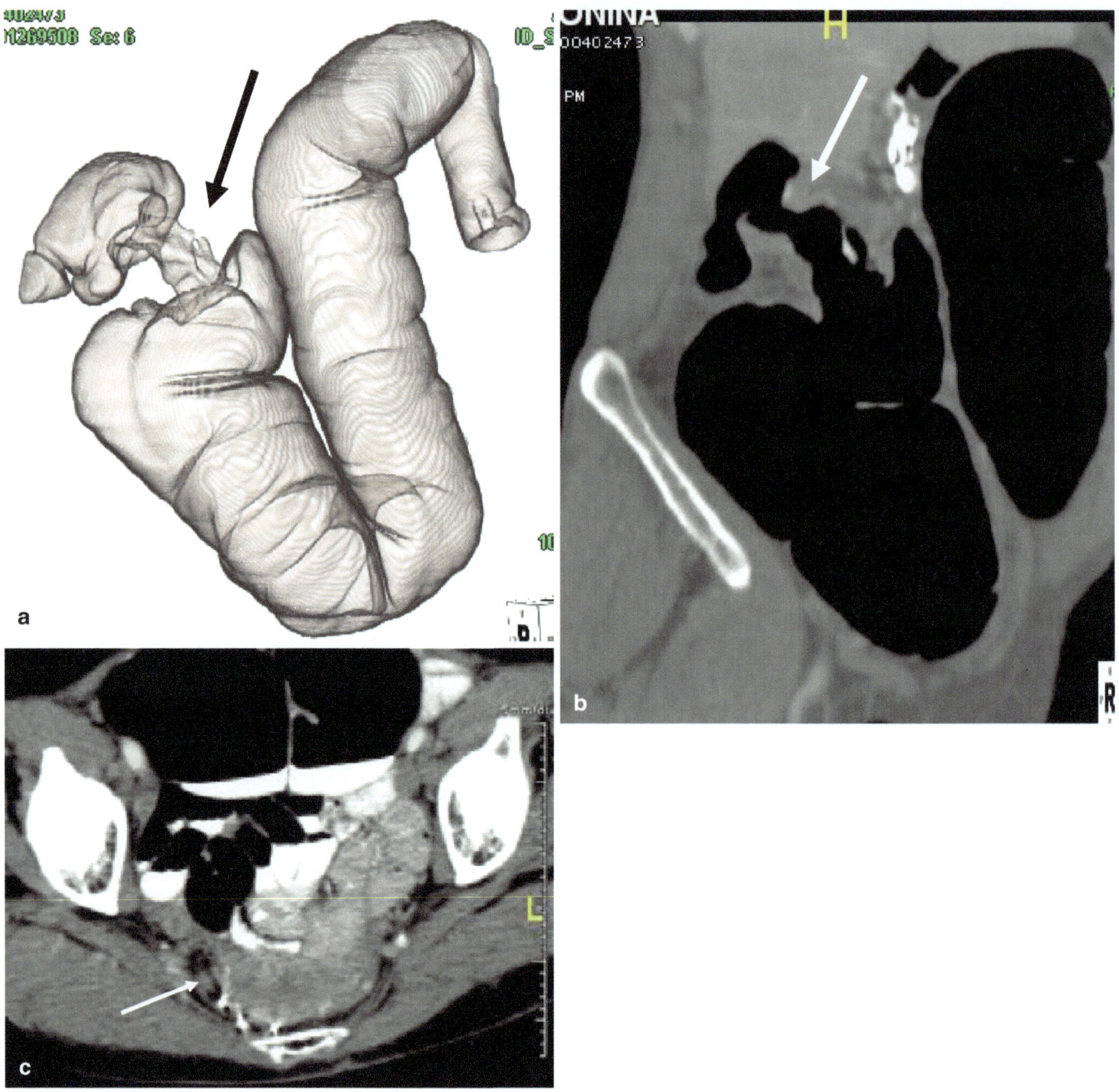

Fig. 11 Abdominoperineal resection (Miles procedure): recurrences. (**a**, **b**) Metachronous cancer (*arrow*) in transverse colon. (**c**) Presacral recurrence (*arrow*)

References

1. Fletcher JG, Johnson CD, Krueger WR, Ahlquist DA, Nelson H, Ilstrup D, Harmsen WS, Corcoran KE (2002) Contrast-enhanced CT colonography in recurrent colorectal carcinoma: feasibility of simultaneous evaluation for metastatic disease, local recurrence, and metachronous neoplasia in colorectal carcinoma. AJR Am J Roentgenol 178:283–290
2. Laghi A, Iannaccone R, Bria E et al (2003) Contrast-enhanced computed tomographic colonography in the follow-up of colorectal cancer patients: a feasibility study. Eur Radiol 13(4):883–889
3. Yau-Tong Y, Chung-Rong CC, Jeng-Yi W et al (2006) Evaluation of contrast-enhanced computed tomographic colonography in detection of local recurrent colorectal cancer. World J Gastroenterol 12(1):123–126
4. Leonardou P, Striggaris K, Pappas P, Filippou D, Bramis I, Tsavaris N, Gouliamos A, Vlachos L (2006) Screening of patients after colectomy: virtual colonography. Abdom Imaging 31(5):521–528
5. Choi YJ, Park SH, Lee SS et al (2007) CT colonography for follow-up after surgery for colorectal cancer. AJR Am J Roentgenol 189(2):283–289
6. Neri E et al (2010) Post-surgical follow-up of colorectal cancer: role of contrast-enhanced CT colonography. Abdom Imaging 35:669–675

GPSR Compliance

The European Union's (EU) General Product Safety Regulation (GPSR) is a set of rules that requires consumer products to be safe and our obligations to ensure this.

If you have any concerns about our products, you can contact us on ProductSafety@springernature.com

In case Publisher is established outside the EU, the EU authorized representative is:

Springer Nature Customer Service Center GmbH
Europaplatz 3
69115 Heidelberg, Germany

Batch number: 10683428

Printed by Printforce, the Netherlands